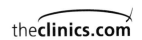

CLINICS IN GERIATRIC MEDICINE

Heart Failure in the Elderly

GUEST EDITOR
Wilbert S. Aronow, MD

February 2007 • Volume 23 • Number 1

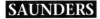

An Imprint of Elsevier, Inc.
PHILADELPHIA   LONDON   TORONTO   MONTREAL   SYDNEY   TOKYO

W.B. SAUNDERS COMPANY
A Division of Elsevier Inc.

Elsevier, Inc. • 1600 John F. Kennedy Blvd., Suite 1800 • Philadelphia, PA 19103-2899

http://www.theclinics.com

CLINICS IN GERIATRIC MEDICINE
February 2007
Editor: Joanne Husovski

Volume 23, Number 1
ISSN 0749-0690
ISBN-13: 978-1-4160-4287-7
ISBN-10: 1-4160-4287-3

Clinics in Geriatric Medicine (ISSN 0749-0690) is published quarterly by Elsevier Inc., 360 Park Avenue South, New York, NY 10010-1710. Months of issue are February, May, August, and November. Business and Editorial Offices: 1600 John F. Kennedy Blvd., Suite 1800, Philadelphia, PA 191023-2899. Customer Service Office: 6277 Sea Harbor Drive, Orlando, FL 32887-4800. Periodicals postage paid at New York, NY, and additional mailing offices. Subscription prices are $178.00 per year (US individuals), $297.00 per year (US institutions), $232.00 per year (Canadian individuals), $362.00 per year (Canadian institutions), $232.00 per year (foreign individuals) and $362.00 per year (foreign institutions). Foreign air speed delivery is included in all *Clinics* subscription prices. All prices are subject to change without notice. POSTMASTER: Send address changes to *Clinics in Geriatric Medicine*, Elsevier Periodicals Customer Service, 6277 Sea Harbor Drive, Orlando, FL 32887-4800. **Customer Service: 1-800-654-2452 (US). From outside of the US, call 1-407-345-4000. E-mail: hhspcs@wbsaunder.com.**

Clinics in Geriatric Medicine is covered in *Index Medicus, EMBASE/Excerpta Medica, Current Contents/Clinical Medicine (CC/CM), and the Cumulative Index to Nursing & Allied Health Literature.*

Printed in the United States of America.

GUEST EDITOR

WILBERT S. ARONOW, MD, FACC, Clinical Professor of Medicine, Divisions of Cardiology, Pulmonary/Critical Care, and Geriatrics; Chief, Cardiology Clinic; and Senior Associate Program Director and Research Mentor for Fellowship Programs, Department of Medicine, New York Medical College, Valhalla, New York

CONTRIBUTORS

ALI AHMED, MD, MPH, FACC, FAHA, FESC, Assistant Professor, Division of Gerontology and Geriatric Medicine, Department of Medicine, School of Medicine, and Department of Epidemiology, School of Public Health; and Director, Geriatric Heart Failure Clinic, Section of Geriatrics, and Scientist, Center for Aging, and Center for Heart Failure Research, University of Alabama at Birmingham, Birmingham, Alabama

WILBERT S. ARONOW, MD, FACC, Clinical Professor of Medicine, Divisions of Cardiology, Pulmonary/Critical Care and Geriatrics; Chief, Cardiology Clinic; and Senior Associate Program Director and Research Mentor for the fellowship Programs, Department of Medicine, New York Medical College, Valhalla, New York

PRADEEP ARUMUGHAM, MD, Research Associate, Division of Clinical Pharmacology, Duke University Medical Center, Durham, North Carolina

JAMIE B. CONTI, MD, Associate Professor of Medicine, Division of Cardiovascular Medicine, University of Florida, Gainesville; and Director, Clinical Cardiac Electrophysiology, University of Florida, Gainesville, Florida

KURT R. DANIEL, DO, Fellow, Section of Cardiology, Department of Internal Medicine, Wake Forest University Health Sciences Center, Winston-Salem, North Carolina

JEROME L. FLEG, MD, Medical Officer, Division of Cardiovascular Diseases, National Heart, Lung, and Blood Institute, Bethesda, Maryland

WILLIAM H. FRISHMAN, MD, Professor of Medicine and Pharmacology and Chairman, Department of Medicine, New York Medical College, Valhalla; Director of Medicine, Westchester Medical Center, Valhalla, New York

TODD W.B. GEHR, MD, Professor of Medicine and Chairman, Division of Nephrology, Virginia Commonwealth University Health System, Richmond, Virginia

ILAN GOLDENBERG, MD, Research Associate Professor, Heart Research Follow-up Program, Cardiology Unit, Department of Medicine, University of Rochester Medical Center, Rochester, New York

DALANE W. KITZMAN, MD, Professor of Medicine, Sections of Cardiology and Geriatrics, Department of Internal Medicine, Wake Forest University Health Sciences, Winston-Salem, North Carolina

JORDANA KRON, MD, Fellow, Division of Cardiovascular Medicine, University of Florida, Gainesville, Florida

STEVEN L. LANSMAN, MD, PhD, Professor of Surgery, New York Medical College; and Chief of Cardiothoracic Surgery, Westchester Medical Center, Valhalla, New York

RAMIN MALEKAN, MD, Assistant Professor, Section of Cardiothoracic Surgery, New York Medical College, Westchester Medical Center, Valhalla, New York

JOHN ARTHUR MCCLUNG, MD, FACC, FAHA, Professor of Clinical Medicine and Associate Professor of Clinical Public Health, New York Medical College, Valhalla; Director, Cardiovascular Fellowship Training Program, Westchester Medical Center/New York Medical College; and Member, Bioethics Institute, New York Medical College, Valhalla, New York

ARTHUR J. MOSS, MD, Professor of Medicine (Cardiology), Director, Heart Research Follow-up Program, Cardiology Unit, Department of Medicine, University of Rochester Medical Center, Rochester, New York

SRIHARI S. NAIDU, MD, Associate Professor of Medicine, Health Sciences Center, State University of New York at Stonybrook; and Director, Cardiac Catheterization Laboratory, Winthrop University Hospital, Mineola, New York

NAVIN C. NANDA, MD, FSGC, FACC, FAHA, Professor of Medicine, Division of Cardiovascular Disease, and Director, Heart Station/Echocardiography Laboratories, University of Alabama at Birmingham, Birmingham, Alabama

CHRISTOPHER M. O'CONNOR, MD, Professor of Medicine, Chief, Division of Clinical Pharmacology, Duke University Medical Center, Durham; Director, Duke Heart Failure Program, Duke Heart Center, Durham, North Carolina

MICHAEL W. RICH, MD, Associate Professor of Medicine, Cardiovascular Division, Washington University School of Medicine, St. Louis, Missouri

DOMENIC A. SICA, MD, Professor of Medicine and Pharmacology; and Chairman, Section of Clinical Pharmacology and Hypertension, Division of Nephrology, Virginia Commonwealth University Health System, Richmond, Virginia

VINCENT L. SORRELL, MD, FACC, FASE, Allan C. Hudson and Helen Lovaas Chair of Cardiac Imaging and Associate Professor of Clinical Medicine and Radiology, Division of Medicine, Section of Cardiology, University of Arizona and the Sarver Heart Center, Tucson, Arizona

RICHARD M. STEINGART, MD, Professor of Medicine, Weill Medical College of Cornell University, New York; Chief, Cardiology Service, Memorial Sloan Kettering Cancer Center, New York; and President, Society of Geriatric Cardiology, New York, New York

SABU THOMAS, MD, Fellow in Cardiology, Division of Cardiology, University of Minnesota, Minneapolis, Minnesota

S. CHIU WONG, MD, Associate Professor of Medicine, Weill Medical College of Cornell University, New York; Director Cardiac Catheterization Laboratory, New York Presbyterian Hospital, New York, New York

CONTENTS

Echocardiography offers comprehensive, noninvasive, and relatively inexpensive tools for diagnosing cardiac pathology in the elderly. With an organized approach using two-dimensional echocardiography and Doppler echocardiography, clinicians can determine the systolic and diastolic left ventricular performance; estimate the cardiac output, pulmonary artery, and ventricular filling pressures; and identify surgically correctable valve disease. Meanwhile, real-time three-dimensional echocardiography provides unprecedented volume data to quantify the left ventricular status. Tissue Doppler-derived myocardial velocity and strain imaging data provide extremely fine details about the regional variations in myocardial synchrony and predict responders to cardiac resynchronization therapy. Thus, echocardiographic tools provide the basis for determining when to attempt to rectify the left ventricular dysfunction with strategically placed, biventricular pacemaker leads.

This article summarizes the four stages of heart failure (HF) as defined by the American College of Cardiology and the American Heart Association and discusses the treatments for elderly patients with HF and abnormal left ventricular systolic function. The article explains the important role of diuretics, the first-line drugs in the treatment of older patients with HF and volume overload. Other treatments described include angiotensin-converting enzyme inhibitors, angiotensin-receptor blockers, β-blockers, aldosterone antagonists, isosorbide dinitrate plus hydralazine, digoxin, and calcium channel blockers. The article explains the role each of these plays and reports on studies that have examined and compared various treatments.

Most elderly patients, particularly women, who have heart failure have a normal ejection fraction. Patients who have this syndrome have severe symptoms of exercise intolerance, frequent hospitalizations, and increased mortality. The pathophysiology and treatment are not well defined. Control of systemic hypertension may be a key to prevention and treatment. Several large trials of specific agents are currently underway.

FORTHCOMING ISSUES

PREVIOUS ISSUES

CLINICS IN
GERIATRIC
MEDICINE

ELSEVIER
SAUNDERS

Clin Geriatr Med 23 (2007) xiii–xiv

Preface

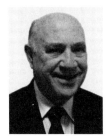

Wilbert S. Aronow, MD
Guest Editor

Heart failure (HF) is the most common cause of hospitalization in the United States. HF affects approximately 5 million people in the United States, and more than 500,000 new cases of HF are reported each year. Approximately 300,000 people die of HF each year. HF is predominantly a disease of the elderly with prevalence rates ranging from 1% in people younger than 50 years to 10% in people aged 80 years and older. Approximately 80% of patients hospitalized with HF are older than 65 years. Aging of the population is contributing to an epidemic of HF.

The prevalence of HF with a normal left ventricular ejection fraction (LVEF) also increases with age and is higher in older women than in older men. Although approximately half of patients older than 60 years of age who have HF have a normal LVEF, there are few randomized controlled trials investigating the use of drugs in the treatment of HF with a normal LVEF. The most important target for basic science and clinical investigation in the years ahead in HF in the elderly is the prevention and treatment of HF with a normal LVEF.

This issue comprises 14 articles on HF in the elderly. The epidemiology, pathophysiology, prognosis, clinical manifestations, diagnostic assessment, etiology, and role of echocardiography in the diagnostic assessment and etiology of HF are discussed. The treatment of HF in the elderly with an abnormal and with a normal LVEF, after acute myocardial infarction, and the use of diuretics, inotropic drugs, neurohormonal antagonists, antiarrhythmic drugs, angioplasty, surgical therapy, cardiac resynchronization therapy, exercise therapy, and use of implantable cardioverter-defibrillators

0749-0690/07/$ - see front matter © 2006 Elsevier Inc. All rights reserved.
doi:10.1016/j.cger.2006.08.012 *geriatric.theclinics.com*

are also discussed. Finally, a very important article on end-of-life care in treating HF in the elderly is discussed.

All of the authors who have contributed to this issue are nationally and internationally recognized experts in cardiovascular disease in the elderly who are dedicated to improving care for older people who have cardiovascular disease. Their many years of personal experience enable them to summarize and synthesize their respective topics with unique insights that are highly beneficial to the reader. My sincere appreciation is extended to each of them for their excellent contributions to the articles in this issue.

Wilbert S. Aronow, MD
Department of Medicine
New York Medical College
Macy Pavilion, Room 138
Valhalla, NY 10595, USA

E-mail address: wsaronow@aol.com

CLINICS IN
GERIATRIC
MEDICINE

ELSEVIER
SAUNDERS

Clin Geriatr Med 23 (2007) 1–10

Epidemiology, Pathophysiology, and Prognosis of Heart Failure in the Elderly

Sabu Thomas, MD, Michael W. Rich, MD*

*Washington University School of Medicine, 660 South Euclid Avenue,
Campus Box 8086, St. Louis, MO 63110, USA*

Although the heart failure (HF) syndrome has been recognized for more than 2000 years, it has been only within the last 25 years that HF has emerged as a major public health concern [1]. A principal reason for this relatively recent development is that HF is primarily a disorder of the elderly, and only in the last half-century has life expectancy increased sufficiently to allow more HF cases to emerge. In the United States, mean life expectancy at birth increased from 49 years in 1900 to 77 years in 2000 [2]. Over the next 25 years, the number of people over age 65 will double from 35 million to more than 70 million, with the largest relative growth occurring in those over age 85 [2]. Furthermore, as treatments and survival rates for other cardiovascular diseases improve, particularly hypertension and ischemic heart disease, more patients will be living and dying with HF.

What accounts for the pronounced association between HF and older age? In effect, HF can be thought of as the quintessential disorder of cardiovascular aging, representing the convergence of age-related changes in cardiovascular structure and function, aging changes in other organ systems, and the progressive increase in cardiovascular diseases in the elderly [3]. Indeed, the median age for patients who have HF in the United States is 75 years (ie, half of all HF cases occur in the 6% of the population 75 years of age or older). Therefore, it is not surprising that the incidence and prevalence of HF will increase proportionately as the population ages.

Heart failure is already the most costly cardiovascular disorder in the United States, and it is the leading cause of hospital admission among Medicare beneficiaries. The estimated total direct and indirect cost for HF in the

---

* Corresponding author.
E-mail address: mrich@im.wustl.edu (M.W. Rich).

0749-0690/07/$ - see front matter © 2006 Elsevier Inc. All rights reserved.
doi:10.1016/j.cger.2006.08.001

United States for 2006 is $29.6 billion. In 2001, $4.0 billion was paid to Medicare beneficiaries for HF hospitalizations, an average of $5912 per discharge [4,5]. In light of the significant societal burden imposed by the emerging HF epidemic, it is essential that health care providers and researchers in the field have an understanding of the epidemiology, pathophysiology, and prognosis of this syndrome, particularly within the geriatric population.

Pathophysiology

HF results from any structural or functional cardiac disorder that impairs the ability of the ventricles to fill with or eject blood, giving rise to a clinical syndrome that represents the end-stage or final common pathway of numerous cardiac diseases. Coronary artery disease is the leading cause of HF in the United States, followed by hypertension, nonischemic cardiomyopathy (especially idiopathic cardiomyopathy), and valvular heart disease [6,7].

In addition to these causes, the effects of aging itself on the cardiovascular system contribute substantially to the development of HF in the elderly (Box 1) [8]. Increased connective tissue deposition in the media and adventitia of the large and medium-sized arteries results in decreased vascular elasticity and increased impedance to left ventricular (LV) ejection [9,10]. These changes lead to a progressive increase in systolic blood pressure with advancing age, which in turn contributes to the development of LV hypertrophy and altered diastolic filling. Increased cardiac interstitial collagen content, compensatory myocyte hypertrophy in response to apoptosis, and impaired calcium flux during diastole further contribute to age-related impairments in LV diastolic relaxation and compliance [11]. These changes lead to an increase in LV end-diastolic pressure and left atrial size and pressure, and they also predispose older individuals to atrial fibrillation.

Although the precise mechanism has yet not been fully elucidated advancing age is associated with a decline in responsiveness to beta-1 and beta-2 adrenergic stimulation, resulting in reductions in maximum heart

---

Box 1. Principal effects of cardiovascular aging

Increased systemic vascular impedance, especially in the larger arteries
Impaired left ventricular diastolic relaxation and compliance
Diminished responsiveness to beta-adrenergic stimulation
Impaired mitochondrial energy production in response to stress
Decline in sinus node function
Impaired endothelial function, especially endothelium-mediated vasodilation

rate and contractility (beta-1 effects) and impaired peripheral vasodilation (beta-2 effect) [12]. Aging is also associated with an impaired capacity of the mitochondria to increase adenosine triphosphate production in response to increased demands imposed by physical activity or illness.

Degenerative changes in the sinus node and atria lead to a progressive decline in sinus node function and increased propensity for atrial arrhythmias, especially atrial fibrillation. Impaired sinus node function further limits the capacity of the aging heart to increase cardiac output in response to stress, and the so-called "sick sinus syndrome" is the leading cause of permanent pacemaker implantation in older adults. Finally, age-associated impairment in endothelium-dependent vasodilation reduces maximum coronary blood flow and predisposes to ischemia, even in the absence of fixed coronary artery stenosis.

The primary clinical implication of these changes is that the capacity of the heart to increase cardiac output in response to increased demands is markedly attenuated with age. This attenuation is perhaps not surprising, because the four physiologic factors that determine cardiac output (ie, heart rate, contractility, preload, and afterload) are all affected adversely by the aging process.

Another implication of cardiovascular aging is that HF in the elderly often is characterized by preserved LV systolic function. Patients who have this syndrome exhibit HF symptoms despite having a normal or near-normal LV ejection fraction (LVEF), as defined by an EF$\geq$45%–50%. This syndrome, often referred to as diastolic HF, occurs in more than 50% of HF patients over age 70 years [13].

Prevalence

More than 5 million Americans have clinical HF, representing an increase of over 150% in the past 20 years, and this figure is expected to double again within the next 25 years because of the aging of the population [5,14]. Similarly, the number of HF cases in Europe is expected to increase substantially over the next two decades [15].

In the United States, the overall population prevalence of HF is about 2.3%, but the proportion increases steeply with age. In the Framingham Heart Study, for example, HF prevalence doubled with each decade after age 50, increasing from 0.8% in people younger than 50 years to 9.1% in people aged 80 to 89 years [6]. Table 1 summarizes prevalence rates of HF as a function of age in various countries [6,16–26]. In Europe, prevalence rates range from 0.4% in people younger than age 65 to 14.1% in those aged 85 years or older [16,17,19].

Gender is also an important factor affecting HF prevalence. The third National Health and Nutrition Examination Survey, conducted from 1988 to 1994, estimated that the number of Americans with HF was 4.7 million, of which 2.3 million were men and 2.4 million were women [27]. Among

Table 1
Prevalence of heart failure in selected countries

Study	Year published	Country	Age	Prevalence (%)
Parameshwar [16]	1992	England	<65	0.4
			>65	2.8
Ho [6]	1993	United States	50–59	0.8
			60–69	2.3
			70–79	4.9
			80–89	9.1
Ambrosio [17]	1994	Italy	65–69	3.6
			75–79	11.1
			>85	14.1
Kupari [18]	1997	Finland	75–86	8.2
Mosterd [19]	1999	Netherlands	55–64	0.7
			65–74	2.7
			75–84	11.7
			55–95 (mean 65)	3.9
Morgan [20]	1999	United Kingdom	70–84 (76)	8.1
Devereaux [21]	2000	United States (SHS-2)	47–81(60)	3.0
Cortina [22]	2001	Spain	>40 (mean 60)	4.9
Nielsen [23]	2001	Denmark	≥50	6.4
Hedberg [24]	2001	Sweden	Mean 75	6.7
Kitzman [25]	2001	United States (CHS)	66–103	8.8
Ceia [26]	2002	Portugal	>25 (68)	4.4

Abbreviations: CHS, Cardiovascular Health Study; SHS, Strong Heart Study.

people less than 70 years of age, HF is predominately a disorder of men, but among those older than age 70, women compose the majority. Higher rates of HF in elderly women can be attributed in part to an increased average life expectancy among women. In addition, women with HF tend to have a somewhat better prognosis than men, in part because they are less likely to have coronary artery disease. Finally, older women have a higher prevalence of diastolic HF than men, owing largely to the fact that hypertension is the most common primary cause of HF in older women [28].

HF prevalence also varies by ethnicity [5]. In the United States there is a higher prevalence of HF in blacks compared with Hispanic or non-Hispanic whites, most likely because of the higher prevalence of hypertension in African Americans [29]. The highest overall prevalence of HF occurs in black women, at 3.5%. This prevalence is followed by that of black men (3.1%), Mexican-American men (2.7%), non-Hispanic Caucasian men (2.5%) and women (1.9%), and finally Mexican-American women (1.6%).

An important aspect of HF in older adults is the striking increase in prevalence of HF with preserved LV systolic function. In patients less than 65 years of age who have HF, approximately 90% have reduced LV ejection fraction because of coronary artery disease or nonischemic dilated cardiomyopathy. In older patients, however, the proportion of HF cases with preserved LV systolic function ranges from 40% to 71%, with a mean of 56%

(Fig. 1) [13]. Moreover, recent data indicate that the proportion of HF cases associated with preserved LV systolic function is increasing as a result of the progressive aging of the population [30]. In the Cardiovascular Health Study (CHS), which enrolled 5888 people 65 years of age or older in four United States communities, among 272 prevalent HF cases 54% were found to have normal LV systolic function, as defined by an LVEF of 55% or greater on echocardiography [25]. In the CHS 67% of older women with HF had normal LV systolic function compared with 41% of older men.

Incidence

It is estimated that approximately 550,000 new cases of HF are diagnosed in the United States each year [5]. Based on 44-year follow-up data from the National Heart, Lung, and Blood Institute's Framingham Heart Study, the incidence of HF approaches 10 per 1000 patient-years after age 65, or approximately 1% per year [6,31]. Data from Olmsted County, Minnesota indicate that the incidence of HF has not declined during the last two decades, although overall survival after the onset of HF has increased [32]. Notably, improvements in survival have been less pronounced in women compared with men, particularly among the elderly, a finding that may reflect the lack of effective therapy for treating diastolic HF, which is more common in women than men.

The incidence of HF is higher in men than in women at all ages. The higher incidence in men is offset by a higher mortality rate in men, however, leading to roughly equal prevalence rates between the sexes.

Among incident HF cases in older adults, approximately 50% have preserved LV systolic function. For example, among 137 patients in Olmsted

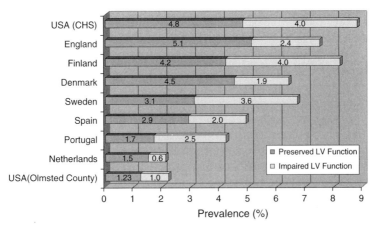

Fig. 1. Prevalence of systolic and diastolic heart failure in the United States and Europe. CHS: Cardiovascular Health Study. (*Adapted from* Hogg K, Swedberg K, McMurray J. Heart failure with preserved left ventricular systolic function. Epidemiology, clinical characteristics and prognosis. J Am Coll Cardiol 2004;43:317–27.)

County, Minnesota presenting with newly diagnosed HF in 1991, 43% had preserved LV systolic function [33]. In the CHS, 57% of 170 patients 65 years of age or older who had incident HF had an LV ejection fraction of 45% or greater [34].

Prognosis and mortality

In the United States, HF is a primary or contributory cause of death in more than 280,000 patients each year [5]. More than 85% of HF deaths occur in patients aged 65 years or older, and approximately 60% occur in patients over age 75. In addition, although the overall mortality rate from HF declined 2% from 1993 to 2003, the actual number of HF deaths increased by 20.5%, reflecting the increasing prevalence of HF and the aging of the population.

Sudden cardiac death and refractory pump failure are the two principal causes of death in patients who have HF, each accounting for about 40% of all deaths, with the remaining 20% of deaths being attributable to other causes. Compared with patients who do not have HF, patients who have HF are 5 to 10 times more likely to die suddenly, primarily as a result of ventricular tachycardia and ventricular fibrillation [35]. Although the prognosis for patients who have established HF has improved over the last two decades [36,37], the overall prognosis remains poor, with median survival rates of less than 5 years among older patients [38]. Moreover, up to one third of older patients die within one year following an initial hospitalization for HF [38]. The overall prognosis of older patients who have HF is worse than for most forms of cancer [39].

In a study of Medicare beneficiaries hospitalized with HF in 1986, the 6-year survival rate was 16% for white men and 19% for black men [38]. Among white and black women, 6-year survival rates were 23% and 25%, respectively. Among patients 67 to 74 years of age, median survival ranged from 2.3 to 3.6 years, depending on gender and race (Figs. 2 and 3). In patients 75 to 84 years of age, median survival ranged from 1.7 to 2.6 years, whereas in patients 85 years of age or older, median survival ranged from just 1.1 to 1.6 years. In all age groups, median survival was longer in women than men, and black men had longer median survival than white men.

In addition to older age, male gender, and white race, other factors associated with worse prognosis in patients who have HF include the presence of coronary artery disease or peripheral arterial disease; more severe symptoms, as defined by higher New York Heart Association functional classification; lower systolic blood pressure; renal insufficiency; hyponatremia; and cognitive impairment. Diastolic HF has a more favorable short-term prognosis than systolic HF, but long-term prognosis is similar [40–42]. Anemia has been associated with worse prognosis in younger patients who have HF, but the importance of anemia in older patients who have HF is unclear.

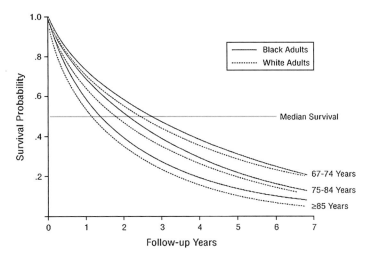

Fig. 2. Survival in men following hospitalization for heart failure in 1986, by age and race. (*From* Croft JB, Giles WH, Pollard RA, et al. Heart failure survival among older adults in the United States: a poor prognosis for an emerging epidemic in the Medicare population. Arch Intern Med 1999;159:505–10; with permission. © Copyright 1999 American Medical Association. All rights reserved.)

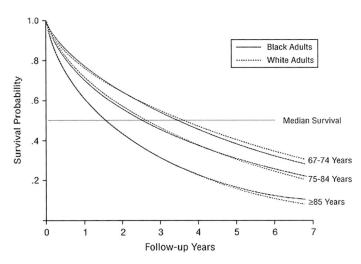

Fig. 3. Survival in women following hospitalization for heart failure in 1986, by age and race. (*From* Croft JB, Giles WH, Pollard RA, et al. Heart failure survival among older adults in the United States: a poor prognosis for an emerging epidemic in the Medicare population. Arch Intern Med 1999;159:505–10; with permission. © Copyright 1999 American Medical Association. All rights reserved.)

Summary

HF is the quintessential disorder of cardiovascular aging, reflecting the convergence of age-related changes in the cardiovascular system and other organ systems and the increasing prevalence of cardiovascular diseases at older age, especially hypertension and coronary artery disease. As a result, the prevalence and incidence of HF increase progressively with advancing age, and HF imposes an enormous burden on society in mortality, morbidity, and associated health care costs. Moreover, as the population ages it is anticipated that the number of older people with HF will increase dramatically over the next several decades. It is essential that substantial resources be devoted to intensive basic, translational, and clinical research designed to develop more effective strategies for the prevention, diagnosis, and treatment of HF in our progressively aging population.

References

[1] Garg R, Packer M, Pitt B, et al. Heart failure in the 1990s: evolution of a major public health problem in cardiovascular medicine. J Am Coll Cardiol 1993;22(Suppl A):3A–5A.
[2] US Census Bureau. Population Division, Population Projections Branch. Available at: http://www.census.gov/ipc/www/usinterimproj. Accessed July 3, 2006.
[3] Rich MW. Heart failure in the 21st century: a cardiogeriatric syndrome. J Gerontol Med Sci 2001;56A:M88–96.
[4] Health Care Financing Review. 2003 Medicare and Medicaid statistical supplement. Available at: http://www.cms.hhs.gov/apps/review/supp/2003. Accessed July 3, 2006.
[5] Thom T, Haase N, Rosamond W, et al. Heart disease and stroke statistics—2006 update. Circulation 2006;113(6):e85–151.
[6] Ho KK, Pinsky JL, Kannel WB, et al. The epidemiology of heart failure: the Framingham Study. J Am Coll Cardiol 1993;22(4, Suppl A):6A–13A.
[7] Gheorghiade M, Bonow RO. Chronic heart failure in the United States: a manifestation of coronary artery disease. Circulation 1998;97:282–9.
[8] Rich MW. Heart failure. Cardiol Clin 1999;17(1):123–35.
[9] Luchi RJ, Taffet GE, Teasdale TA. Congestive heart failure in the elderly. J Am Geriatr Soc 1991;39:810–25.
[10] Lakatta EG, Levy D. Arterial and cardiac aging: major shareholders in cardiovascular disease enterprises: Part I: aging arteries: a "set up" for vascular disease. Circulation 2003;107: 139–46.
[11] Olivetti G, Melissari M, Capasso JM, et al. Cardiomyopathy of the aging human heart. Myocyte loss and reactive cellular hypertrophy. Circ Res 1991;68:1560–8.
[12] Lakatta EG. Diminished beta-adrenergic modulation of cardiovascular function in advanced age. Cardiol Clin 1986;4:185–200.
[13] Hogg K, Swedberg K, McMurray J. Heart failure with preserved left ventricular systolic function. Epidemiology, clinical characteristics and prognosis. J Am Coll Cardiol 2004; 43(3):317–27.
[14] Anderson RN. United States lifetables 1998: national vital statistics reports. 48(18). Hyattsville, MD: National Center for Health Statistics; 2001.
[15] McMurray JJ, Stewart S. Epidemiology, aetiology, and prognosis of heart failure. Heart 2000;83:596–602.
[16] Parameshwar J, Shackell MM, Richardson A, et al. Prevalence of heart failure in three general practices in north west London. Br J Gen Pract 1992;42(360):287–9.

[17] Ambrosio GB, Riva L, Casiglia E, et al. Prevalence of congestive heart failure (CHF) in elderly. Acta Cardiol 1994;49:324–7.

[18] Kupari M, Lindroos M, Iivanainen AM, et al. Congestive heart failure in old age: prevalence, mechanisms and 4-year prognosis in the Helsinki Ageing Study. J Intern Med 1997; 241(5):387–94.

[19] Mosterd A, Hoes AW, de Bruyne MC, et al. Prevalence of heart failure and left ventricular dysfunction in the general population: the Rotterdam Study. Eur Heart J 1999;20: 447–55.

[20] Morgan S, Smith H, Simpson I. Prevalence and clinical characteristics of left ventricular dysfunction among elderly patients in general practice setting: cross-sectional survey. BMJ 1999; 318;368–72.

[21] Devereux RB, Roman MJ, Liu JE. Congestive heart failure despite normal left ventricular systolic function in a population-based sample: the Strong Heart Study. Am J Cardiol 2000;86:1090–6.

[22] Cortina A, Reguero J, Segovia E. Prevalence of heart failure in Asturias (a region in the north of Spain). Am J Cardiol 2001;87:1417–9.

[23] Nielsen OW, Hilden J, Larsen CT, et al. Cross-sectional study estimating prevalence of heart failure and left ventricular systolic dysfunction in community patients at risk. Heart 2001;86: 172–8.

[24] Hedberg P, Lonnberg I, Jonason T, et al. Left ventricular systolic dysfunction in 75-year-old men and women: a population-based study. Eur Heart J 2001;22:676–83.

[25] Kitzman DW, Gardin JM, Gottdiener JS, et al. Importance of heart failure with preserved systolic function in patients ≥ 65 years of age. CHS Research Group. Cardiovascular Health Study. Am J Cardiol 2001;87:413–9.

[26] Ceia F, Fonseca C, Mota T, et al, and the EPICA Investigators. Prevalence of chronic heart failure in Southwestern Europe: the EPICA study. Eur J Heart Fail 2002;4:531–9.

[27] Schocken DD. Epidemiology and risk factors for heart failure in the elderly. Clin Geriatr Med 2000;16(3):407–18.

[28] Levy D, Larson MG, Vasan RS, et al. The progression from hypertension to congestive heart failure. JAMA 1996;275(20):1557–62.

[29] Philbin EF, Weil H, Francis CA, et al. Race-related differences among patients with left ventricular dysfunction: observations from a biracial angiographic cohort. J Card Fail 2000;6: 187–93.

[30] Owan TE, Hodge DO, Herges RM, et al. Trends in prevalence and outcome of heart failure with preserved ejection fraction. N Engl J Med 2006;355:251–9.

[31] Lloyd-Jones DM, Larson MG, Leip EP, et al. Lifetime risk for developing congestive heart failure: the Framingham Heart Study. Circulation 2002;106:3068–72.

[32] Senni M, Tribouilloy CM, Rodeheffer RJ, et al. Congestive heart failure in the community. Arch Intern Med 1999;159:29–34.

[33] Rodeheffer RJ, Jacobsen SJ, Gersh BJ, et al. The incidence and prevalence of congestive heart failure in Rochester, Minnesota. Mayo Clin Proc 1993;68:1143–50.

[34] Aurigemma GP, Gottdiener JS, Shemanski L, et al. Predictive value of systolic and diastolic function for incident congestive heart failure in the elderly: The Cardiovascular Health Study. J Am Coll Cardiol 2001;37(4):1042–8.

[35] Kannel WB, Plehn JF, Cupples LA. Cardiac failure and sudden death in the Framingham Study. Am Heart J 1988;115(4):869–75.

[36] Cleland JGF, Clark A. Has the survival of the heart failure population changed? Lessons from trials. Am J Cardiol 1999;83(Suppl D):112D–9D.

[37] Delahay F, Gevigney G, Delay J. Has the prognosis of congestive heart failure changed over time? Congest Heart Fail 1998;4:27–33.

[38] Croft JB, Giles WH, Pollard RA, et al. Heart failure survival among older adults in the United States: a poor prognosis for an emerging epidemic in the Medicare population. Arch Intern Med 1999;159:505–10.

[39] Stewart S, MacIntyre K, Hole DJ, et al. More "malignant" than cancer? Five-year survival following a first admission for heart failure. Eur J Heart Fail 2001;3(3):315–22.

[40] Gottdiener JS, McClelland RL, Marshall R, et al. Outcome of congestive heart failure in elderly persons: influence of left ventricular systolic function. The Cardiovascular Health Study. Ann Intern Med 2002;137:631–9.

[41] Senni M, Redfield MM. Heart failure with preserved systolic function. A different natural history? J Am Coll Cardiol 2001;38(5):1277–82.

[42] Bhatia RS, Tu JV, Lee DS, et al. Outcome of heart failure with preserved ejection fraction in a population-based study. N Engl J Med 2006;355:260–9.

ELSEVIER
SAUNDERS

CLINICS IN
GERIATRIC
MEDICINE

Clin Geriatr Med 23 (2007) 11–30

Clinical Manifestations, Diagnostic Assessment, and Etiology of Heart Failure in Older Adults

Ali Ahmed, MD, MPH[a,b,*]

[a]*Division of Gerontology and Geriatric Medicine, Department of Medicine,
School of Medicine, and Department of Epidemiology, School of Public Health,
Geriatric Heart Failure Clinic, Center for Aging, and Center for Heart Failure Research,
University of Alabama at Birmingham, 1530 3rd Avenue South,
CH19-219, Birmingham, AL 35294-2041, USA*
[b]*Section of Geriatrics and Geriatric Heart Failure Clinic, Birmingham Veterans Affairs
Medical Center, 700 19th Street South, Birmingham, AL 35233, USA*

Heart failure (HF) is a geriatric syndrome of public health importance. The vast majority of the estimated 5 million HF patients in the United States, half a million who are newly diagnosed with HF every year, and over a million who are hospitalized every year primarily due to HF are 65 years and older. For population 65 years and older, HF is the number one reason for hospitalization. HF is an underlying or contributing cause for about 300,000 deaths annually in the United States; most of these deaths occur in persons 65 years and older. The annual cost of HF is estimated to be $30 billion in 2006. These numbers are projected to double over the next several decades with the projected doubling of the United States population 65 years and older during that period.

Clinical manifestations of heart failure in older adults

Most geriatric HF patients suffer from multiple morbidities and polypharmacy [1]. The management of a 78-year-old woman with HF and left

Dr. Ahmed is supported by the National Institutes of Health through grants from the National Institute on Aging (1-K23-AG19211-04) and the National Heart, Lung, and Blood Institute (1-R01-HL085561-01).
* University of Alabama at Birmingham, 1530 3rd Avenue South, CH19-219, Birmingham AL 35294-2041.
E-mail address: aahmed@uab.edu

doi:10.1016/j.cger.2006.08.002
geriatric.theclinics.com

ventricular ejection fraction (LVEF) greater than 55%, with hypertension, atrial fibrillation, diabetes, arthritis, chronic kidney disease, and depression, and who takes multiple medications, is more difficult than that of a 40-year-old man with LVEF 25%, ischemic heart disease, with no other comorbidity and taking a few medications.

Yet elderly HF patients, many of whom are women and have HF with normal or near normal LVEF, often have been excluded from major randomized clinical trials in HF, which makes the overall management of HF in older adults more challenging [2,3]. That challenge is compounded further by the difficulty in the diagnosis and assessment of HF in older adults [4]. Older adults in general are a heterogeneous group, and as such geriatric HF is characterized by a wide range of phenotypic heterogeneity, as illustrated in the case scenarios presented.

Geriatric heart failure: case scenarios

Case 1

A 79-year-old man with a history of hypertension and an old myocardial infarction presented with a 6-month history of progressive dyspnea on exertion (DOE) and leg swelling. He had no history of dyspnea at rest, orthopnea, paroxysmal nocturnal dyspnea (PND), cough, wheezing, or chest pain. He had no emergency room visits or hospitalizations attributable to dyspnea. His physical examination was remarkable for mild pitting edema around his ankles and lower legs. He had normal jugular venous pressure (JVP), no hepatojugular reflux (HJR), no third heart sound (S3), and no pulmonary râles. His electrocardiogram and chest radiograph were normal. An echocardiogram showed an LVEF of 34%.

Case 2

An 86-year-old woman with a history of HF (LVEF unknown) and hypertension presented with a 4-week history of dyspnea and fatigue on minimal exertion (such as turning over in bed) and orthopnea (she slept in a recliner) but no PND or chest pain. She also complained of weakness, right upper quadrant pain, nausea, loss of appetite, and severe leg swelling. She did not seek emergency room care nor was she hospitalized for her symptoms. Her physical examination was remarkable for a JVP of 15 cm water, a positive HJR, a right-sided S3, no pulmonary rales or wheezing, an enlarged soft tender liver, and severe bilateral lower extremity edema up to midthigh with brown pigmentation and induration of skin and multiple blisters over lower legs. An accentuated second heart sound at the left fourth intercostal space suggested pulmonary hypertension, with an estimated pulmonary artery systolic pressure of 40 to 45 mm Hg. She had a normal electrocardiogram. A chest radiograph revealed marked cardiomegaly and pulmonary congestion. An echocardiogram later showed an LVEF of greater than 55%.

Case 3

An 85-year-old woman with a history of hypertension and atrial fibrillation presented with a 6-month history of progressive dyspnea and fatigue on exertion. She was treated recently in the local emergency department for worsening symptoms, including a two-pillow orthopnea. She had no dyspnea at rest, PND, palpitation, or chest pain. She ran out of her atenolol for several days and was found to have a systolic blood pressure of 202 mm Hg and a pulse of 125 beats per minute. She had a few bibasilar pulmonary rales and lower extremity edema up to mid-leg, but no S3 or elevated JVP. An electrocardiogram was remarkable for atrial fibrillation with a ventricular rate of 102 per minute but no evidence of ischemia. Her cardiac enzymes were normal. A chest radiograph demonstrated cardiomegaly with mild pulmonary edema. An echocardiogram showed an LVEF of 58%.

Case 4

An 84-year-old man with a history of hypertension and diabetes was recently hospitalized with syncope. He was very active physically but noted some mild DOE before hospitalization. He had no dyspnea at rest, orthopnea, PND, or chest pain. He had an enlarged heart by chest radiograph, an LVEF of 25% by echocardiogram, but a normal coronary angiogram. He was discharged on furosemide 80 mg daily, which was later increased to 80 mg twice a day due to his progressive DOE and fatigue. Over the next 2 weeks, he lost more than 20 pounds and his symptoms improved. His blood urea nitrogen to creatinine ratio was 15:1 (normal $\leq$ 10:1) and brain natriuretic peptide (BNP) level was about 400 (normal $<$ 100) pg/ml. He was maintained on furosemide 80 mg twice a day, and several weeks later he started developing fatigue and DOE. Two weeks later he was still symptomatic, and his examination was remarkable for systolic blood pressure of 95 mm Hg and a JVP of 3 cm water.

Case 5

An 82-year-old woman with a history of hypertension and coronary artery disease (CAD) presented with a 1-year history of dyspnea at rest, chest tightness, and dizziness, for which she had three hospitalizations through emergency department visits. During these hospitalizations she underwent comprehensive investigations, including an echocardiogram, a cardiac catheterization, and a magnetic resonance imaging of the brain, none of which revealed any pathology. She had no DOE, orthopnea, PND, or leg swelling. Her physical examination was unremarkable, with no signs of HF. She continued to remain symptomatic, however.

Definition of heart failure

The syndrome of HF is composed of various symptoms that are manifestations of a reduced cardiac output, the hallmark pathology of HF (Table 1).

Table 1
Similar cardiac output and symptoms in systolic and diastolic heart failure despite different
underlying pathology

	EDV (mL)	EF (%)	SV (mL)	HR (bpm)	CO (L/min)	Symptoms
Normal	150	55	75	72	5.4	None
Systolic heart failure	200	25	50	72	3.6	Dyspnea, fatigue, edema
Diastolic heart failure	100	55	50	72	3.6	Dyspnea, fatigue, edema

All data based on left ventricle.
Abbreviations: bpm, beats per minute; CO, cardiac output; EDV, end-diastolic volume; EF, ejection fraction; HR, heart rate; SV, stroke volume.

The cardinal manifestations of HF are dyspnea, fatigue, and edema. Because HF is not a primary disease, it is always associated with one or more underlying causes. HF is also considered the end-stage heart disease. The American College of Cardiology/American Heart Association guidelines for chronic HF define HF as "a complex clinical syndrome that can result from any structural or functional cardiac disorder that impairs the ability of the ventricle to fill with or eject blood" [5]. The Heart Failure Society of America HF guidelines define HF as a "syndrome caused by cardiac dysfunction, generally resulting from myocardial muscle dysfunction or loss and characterized by left ventricular dilation or hypertrophy" [6].

Stages of heart failure

Because HF is a progressive condition, clinical manifestations of HF vary depending on the stages in its natural history. Patients in Stage A and Stage B are asymptomatic and do not have clinical HF. Patients who have Stage A have risk factors for HF, such as hypertension and CAD, but no structural myocardial disorder and no clinical HF. When Stage A patients develop structural myocardial damage, such as left ventricular hypertrophy (LVH) or asymptomatic left ventricular systolic dysfunction, but no clinical HF, they are referred to as Stage B. Most clinical patients who have HF belong to Stage C, with current or past symptoms. Stage D represents end-stage and refractory HF, which may require special therapy, such as temporary circulatory support, cardiac transplant, or palliative care.

Descriptive classification of heart failure

The most clinically relevant descriptive classification of clinical HF is based on LVEF: systolic (low LVEF) HF and diastolic (normal or low-normal LVEF) HF. This classification has prognostic and therapeutic implications. Determination of LVEF is the first crucial step in the assessment of patients diagnosed with HF and is considered a measure of quality of care [7,8]. Other descriptive classifications of HF as described below are less clinically relevant.

Systolic versus diastolic heart failure

Systolic HF is defined by clinical HF with low LVEF. LVEF cutoffs of 35% to 45% have been used variously to define systolic HF [9–15]. Systolic HF typically is characterized by a large thin-walled ventricle that is weak and unable to eject enough blood to produce a normal cardiac output (Table 1). Most randomized clinical trials in HF were restricted to systolic HF [9–15]. It is also the predominant type of HF among younger adults [16].

Epidemiologic data from the past several decades, however, suggest that as many as 50% of all patients who have HF may have diastolic HF [17–22]. Diastolic HF is defined as clinical HF with normal or near-normal LVEF, generally 45% to 55% or greater. Diastolic HF is characterized by a strong thick-walled ventricle that is small and stiff and does not have enough blood to pump to produce a normal cardiac output (Table 1). Although several HF signs, namely elevated JVP and S3, may be more frequent in systolic HF, there is no evidence that the overall clinical manifestations of HF varies by LVEF [5,6,23–25]. *Case 2* presented with classic textbook symptoms and signs of HF and had normal LVEF.

LVEF can be measured using multiple techniques [26]. Transthoracic two-dimensional echocardiography with or without Doppler imaging is usually the preferred technique used to assess LVEF. This technique is widely available, safe, and noninvasive, with little or no patient discomfort, and provides excellent images of not only the heart but also the great vessels and paracardiac structures [27]. Assessment of LVEF is important because it is of crucial therapeutic and prognostic significance [5,6,23,25]. LVEF should not be assessed until after a clinical diagnosis has been made, however.

Most patients who have diastolic HF have significant abnormalities in active and passive relaxation [20,28]. However, it is not essential to determine diastolic abnormalities to make a clinical diagnosis of diastolic HF [21]. Doppler studies of velocity of transmitral blood flow can determine ventricular filling patterns. In diastolic HF, the peak transmitral E velocity (represents Early filling during active ventricular relaxation) is decreased, whereas there is a relative increase in the peak A velocity (because of a compensatory increase in Atrial contraction in late diastole). The E:A ratio thus is decreased in diastolic HF [20,29,30]. However, the E:A ratio is not a reliable marker as it may also be decreased with normal aging [31] and may be normalized with progressive diastolic HF (pseudonormalization) [32,33]. Mitral annular tissue Doppler imaging can distinguish normal from pseudonormal filling patterns, however, and if combined with transmitral flow Doppler imaging and clinical history can determine accurately the severity of diastolic abnormalities [20,32,33]. There is evidence that severity of diastolic dysfunction may be associated with increased mortality [20].

Left-sided versus right-sided heart failure

Left-sided HF occurs when HF predominantly affects the left ventricle. Most early clinical patients who have HF have left-sided HF. Pure left-sided

HF may result in pulmonary congestion, hypoperfusion, or both, and symptoms and signs related to those pathologies, such as dyspnea, cough, wheezing, fatigue, hypotension, tachycardia, confusion, syncope, delirium, oliguria, pulmonary râles, prominent pulmonic component of the second heart sound, and left-sided S3. As HF progresses, left-sided HF eventually leads to right-sided HF.

Right-sided HF occurs when HF predominantly affects the right ventricle. Common symptoms and signs of right-sided HF are often attributable to systemic congestion, resulting in leg swelling, nausea, vomiting, epigastric and upper abdominal pain, elevated JVP, HJR, hepatomegaly, right-sided S3, prominent pulmonic component of the S2, and dependent edema. Dyspnea and fatigue are less common in the early stage of pure right HF, but may be noted in more advanced right HF. Little is known about the parameters of right ventricular function and dysfunction, and the cellular and molecular basis of right-sided HF [34]. Common causes of right HF include pulmonary conditions (cor pulmonale) and left HF.

Most patients who have advanced HF have both left- and right-sided HF, as noted in *Case 2*. Symptoms and signs related to biventricular HF also may be seen in early HF, as in *Cases 1* and *3*, who presented with DOE and leg edema.

Backward versus forward heart failure

The concept of backward failure was first proposed by James Hope in 1832, who suggested that congestion in HF was attributable to backward pressure in the venous and capillary system as a result of the failing heart's inability to pump forward [35]. This notion is supported by the fact that most left HF is associated with some degree of right HF or eventually leads to right HF [36]. It was demonstrated later, however, that edema and congestion in HF are primarily due to salt and fluid retention caused by decreased renal blood flow due to forward failure [37,38]. Diminished renal blood flow contributes to the activation of the renin-angiotensin-aldosterone system and subsequent retention of salt and water in HF [39]. Most patients who have HF have clinical manifestations of both backward and forward HF (*Cases 1–4*). HF may not be clinically distinguished as forward or backward and such distinctions probably have no therapeutic or prognostic implications.

High-output versus low-output heart failure

Most elderly patients who have HF have low-output HF (*Cases 1–4*). High-output HF, characterized by high cardiac output, although rare in older adults, may be associated with hyperdynamic conditions, such as severe anemia, thyrotoxicosis, and arteriovenous fistula, including those used for hemodialysis [40–42]. Although anemia may cause exacerbation of HF symptoms, it rarely causes high-output HF in the absence of other cardiac diseases, or severe anemia (hemoglobin < 5 gm/dL) [5,36]. Thyrotoxicosis alone also rarely causes high-output HF. Clinical features of high- and low-output HF may be indistinguishable. High-output HF patients may have warm extremities. Assessment of all new patients who have HF should include laboratory tests for anemia, kidney function, and thyroid function [5,6,30].

Acute versus chronic heart failure

The concept of acute and chronic HF is generally used in two different contexts: severity (mild to moderate versus severe) and onset (sudden versus gradual) of symptoms. Most patients who have chronic HF undergo acute exacerbations of symptoms from time to time (*Cases 2 and 4*). More than two thirds of all patients hospitalized for acute HF have known chronic HF [43]. Acute worsening of chronic HF may be because of noncompliance with drugs, salt or fluid, acute myocardial ischemia, severe hypertension, or natural disease progression. In many of these patients symptoms are severe and require emergency room visits or hospitalization for acute management. HF is associated with more than 1 million hospitalizations in the United States and is the number one reason for hospitalization for people 65 years of age and older [44,45]. This is despite the fact that elderly patients who have HF often attribute their HF symptoms to aging, and thus delay care even when symptoms are severe (*Case 2*). Clinical manifestations of ambulatory chronic HF and hospitalized acute HF are generally similar but may be more severe in the latter group.

Clinical manifestations of HF may be sudden, such as after a large acute myocardial infarction with or without valve damage, typically leading to systolic HF, and in severe systolic hypertension with flash pulmonary edema, often leading to diastolic HF (*Case 3*) [46,47]. HF may also present acutely with syncope (*Case 4*). Clinical manifestations of HF may be gradual in the presence of chronic myocardial ischemia and less severe hypertension (*Case 1*). Acute exacerbations because of noncompliance may also have a gradual onset (*Case 2*). Both sudden and gradual onset of symptoms may occur in the setting of incident (Stage A or B) or prevalent (Stage C or D) HF.

Symptoms of heart failure in older adults

DOE or exertional fatigue, with or without some degree of lower extremity swelling, is generally the most common early symptom of HF (*Cases 1 and 3*). With progression of disease, especially in the absence of appropriate treatment, DOE or fatigue gradually becomes more severe and appears with decreasing exertion (*Case 2*) and eventually at rest. Older adults often attribute their DOE or fatigue on exertion to aging and respond to their early symptoms by restricting their physical activities, thus delaying clinical manifestations and diagnosis. It is important to take this into consideration while inquiring about DOE from an older adult (Box 1). Clinicians should also routinely screen their geriatric patients who are at high risk for HF (Stage A and Stage B) for symptoms and signs of DOE, exertional fatigue, leg edema, and other common HF symptoms to make an early diagnosis of HF. This screening is important because early initiation of therapy may be

Box 1. Special attributes of symptoms of heart failure in older adults

Dyspnea on exertion (DOE)
If no DOE reported on walking a city block or two, repeat the question with milder forms of activities, such as making bed, walking to the bathroom, taking shower, or changing clothes. Quantify the level or length of activity before dyspnea occurs. DOE may be due to other morbidity, such as lung disease, renal failure, obesity, depression, anemia, and deconditioning. Older adults may not report DOE if they restrict their activity for reasons other than dyspnea, such as pain from severe arthritis, myocardial ischemia, or peripheral arterial disease

Dyspnea at rest
Usually attributable to pulmonary edema, but may also be due to pulmonary embolism and pneumothorax. It is important to quantify the duration. Older adults may restrict their activities in response to DOE and may present with dyspnea at rest. Dyspnea at rest that is not preceded or accompanied by DOE is unlikely to be of organic origin and may represent somatization, and depression should be suspected

Orthopnea
Patients may use multiple pillows, use hospital bed with head-end elevated, or put bricks under head-end of bed to avoid orthopnea. It usually occurs soon after lying down and is relieved promptly by sitting or standing up. Many older adults may sleep in a chair or a recliner to avoid orthopnea and may not report it voluntarily unless specifically asked. Older adults who have COPD rarely also experience orthopnea

Paroxysmal nocturnal dyspnea (PND)
Patients sleeping with multiple pillows or on a recliner may not report PND. PND associated with COPD often can be distinguished by early cough and expectoration, which may or may not be followed by dyspnea. It often is relieved by expectoration of the clogged mucus, with or without sitting up

Cough
May be the early or only symptoms of HF in some older adults

Wheezing
May accompany dyspnea in some older adults who have pulmonary congestion

Swelling
Leg edema is common but not universal. It is also more nonspecific in older than in younger patients. Older adults who have chronic severe edema may develop skin blisters and secondary lymphedema. A mix of pitting and nonpitting edema that may persist despite euvolemia in asymptomatic patients is not uncommon

Fatigue
Fatigue may be attributed to aging and also may be due to depression (typically present at rest without DOE, and often associated with a lack of drive), beta-blocker use (mostly among the very old), and overdiuresis

Weight gain
May be due to depression-associated increased appetite. Depression and late-stage dementia or some medications used to treat them may also cause loss of appetite and weight loss

Syncope
May also be attributable to orthostatic hypotension, in particular postprandial hypotension

Angina
Older adults may have silent angina and may not experience any chest pain

Nocturia
May be due to prostate disorder, diabetes, urinary tract infection, and overactive bladder syndrome

Change in mental status
Common in the very old and frail and often accompanied by dyspnea and fatigue. More common in those who have vascular dementia with extensive cerebrovascular atherosclerosis, or latent Alzheimer disease. Less common in other older adults who are euvolemic, without dyspnea or fatigue

associated with long-term survival benefit [48]. When a patient presents with dyspnea at rest, it is important to determine its duration and if it was preceded by DOE. Dyspnea at rest without DOE almost never is organic in cause and may represent somatization in older adults [36].

Among ambulatory chronic HF patients, ≥65 years (mean age 73 years), who participated in the Digitalis Investigation Group trial, more than 95% had DOE (~75% current and ~20% past), and more than 65% had dyspnea at rest (~25% current and ~50% past) [25]. In another group of ambulatory older adults (mean age 70 years) presenting at the emergency department with dyspnea, approximately 75% had DOE and approximately 25% had dyspnea at rest [49]. In a cohort of hospitalized older adults (mean age 79 years) who had acute HF, approximately 26% had DOE and approximately 90% had dyspnea at rest [50]. The higher prevalence of dyspnea at rest in the latter patient population may be due to the older age of these patients. Reports of DOE have been shown to decline with increasing age and functional impairment [51,52]. Because older adults gradually restrict their activities with increasing DOE, however, it is also possible that by the time they are hospitalized dyspnea at rest becomes the predominant symptom. Dyspnea at rest has high sensitivity (92%) but low specificity (19%) for diagnosis of HF in older adults [4]. When combined with DOE, orthopnea, PND, fatigue, and lower extremity edema, the specificity, positive predictive value, and likelihood ratio positive increased significantly [4].

Orthopnea is a relatively specific symptom for HF in older adults (see Box 1) [4,53]. Orthopnea is particularly helpful if associated with edema (may help distinguish from rare orthopnea due to pulmonary causes). It usually occurs soon after lying down and is also relieved promptly by sitting or standing up. Orthopnea is an infrequent symptom in older adults with HF and may not be reported until fluid overload is severe, as in *Cases 2 and 3* [49,50]. Many older adults may sleep in a chair or a recliner to avoid orthopnea (*Case 3*) and may not report that voluntarily unless specifically asked.

PND is probably a more specific HF symptom [4,53]. Dyspnea in PND occurs 2 to 3 hours after onset of sleep, and causes patients to wake up from sleep with dyspnea, which may be followed by cough or wheezing. Relief starts with sitting up, but complete relief of symptoms may take from 5 to 30 minutes. Patients sleeping with multiple pillows or on a recliner to avoid orthopnea may not experience PND. PND also may be caused by chronic obstructive pulmonary disease (COPD) and usually can be distinguished from HF-associated PND. PND attributable to COPD usually is associated with early onset cough followed by expectoration of mucus. It may or may not be associated with dyspnea and may be relieved with the expectoration of the clogged mucus, even without sitting up (see Box 1) [54]. PND is relatively infrequent in older adults, and none of the cases described above had PND [49,50].

Bilateral lower extremity edema is generally common in older patients who have HF, probably because of age-related decrease in venous tone.

Bilateral leg edema is a relatively nonspecific symptom and also may be caused by chronic venous insufficiency, obesity, prolonged sitting or standing, or medications, such as calcium channel blockers or steroids. Unilateral edema may be caused by cellulitis, past trauma or surgery, deep vein thrombosis, and arthritis. Edema generally begins with the foot and ankle, extending proximally to the leg, but when prolonged and left untreated may also affect the more proximal lower extremity, the perineal area, and the abdomen. Edema associated with HF is always symmetric and pitting. Edema may be marked during evening hours in ambulatory patients and over the sacral area in bed-bound patients. Chronic severe edema may lead to skin changes, including erythema, brown pigmentation, and induration. Older adults are more prone to skin blisters with severe and longstanding edema.

Other less common and atypical symptoms of HF in older adults include fatigue, syncope, angina, nocturia, oliguria, and changes in mental status (see Box 1). Weight gain almost always accompanies symptomatic HF but rarely is reported as a symptom by older HF patients. If educated by their doctors about the importance of daily weight, however, most elderly patients who have HF are likely to monitor and report.

Signs of heart failure in older adults

An elevated JVP is the most specific sign of fluid overload in HF and is the most important physical examination in the initial and subsequent examinations of an elderly patient who has HF [55]. The internal jugular vein (IJV) lies deep in the neck behind the thick sternocleidomastoid muscles and may be difficult to appreciate in chronic HF [54]. In one study of older adults, mean age 70 years, who presented with dyspnea at the emergency department, only 14% had elevated JVP [49]. In two large HF trials, 11% to 13% of patients (mean age 62–64 years) had elevated JVP [56,57]. External jugular veins (EJV) are more superficial and may be more easily visible. An EJV may be distended because of external (compression of platysma muscle) or internal (thrombosis or sclerosis of valves) causes and may not reflect the true JVP [58]. Thus, a distended EJV is unreliable, therefore, and JVP must be estimated. JVP estimation often requires positioning the patients supine (if JVP is low) or sitting (if JVP is high). When estimating a low JVP (*Case 4*), the distance between the top of the venous wave and sternal angle must be subtracted from the distance between right atrium and sternal angle (which is considered constant and represents 5 cm water pressure regardless of body positions). Using EJV and the right technique, JVP can be estimated in 90% to 95% of all elderly HF patients.

HJR reflects the inability of the right ventricles to respond to increased venous return, which is caused by pressure over an abdomen whose veins may already be congested with blood [59]. HJR is considered positive if the JVP increases by 2 to 3 cm and remains elevated for about 10 seconds when sustained pressure is applied to the mid-abdomen area. In one study,

a positive HJR predicted right atrial pressure greater than 9 mm Hg (equivalent to ~12 cm water) with high sensitivity (100%) and specificity (85%)
[60]. A positive HJR in the presence of high JVP confirms fluid overload
[59,60]. A positive HJR in the presence of normal or low JVP indicates
mild residual fluid overload and may be baseline for some patients who
have HF.

Pulmonary rales are not commonly heard in chronic HF, even in the presence of pulmonary congestion (*Case 2*), due to compensatory increase in pulmonary lymphatic drainage, and may also be present in bronchitis or
pneumonia [55]. An S3 is a more specific sign of HF than a fourth heart
sound in older adults. Leg edema, ascites, and pleural effusion are nonspecific
signs and must be coordinated with other symptoms and signs. It is estimated
that 5 liters of extra fluid must accumulate before edema becomes clinically
manifest [36]. Chronic venous insufficiency is common in older adults and
may also cause pitting edema. Chronic lower extremity edema associated
with both HF and chronic venous insufficiency may cause secondary lymphedema and nonpitting edema [61,62]. It is not uncommon to see a mix of pitting and nonpitting edema, and some residual leg edema, in otherwise
euvolemic and asymptomatic elderly patients who have HF.

Diagnostic assessment of heart failure in older adults

Primary care physicians should be familiar with one of the major national
HF guidelines and follow their recommendations regarding appropriate diagnostic assessment for HF [5,6,30]. Initial diagnostic assessment of HF by
primary care physicians may be completed in a 5-step process, which can be
remembered using the mnemonic DEFEAT HF: (1) to establish a clinical
Diagnosis of HF (2) to identify an underlying Etiology for HF, (3) to determine Fluid status, (4) to determine LV Ejection frAction and (5) to provide
evidence based Therapy (Box 2).

Clinical diagnosis of heart failure

HF is a clinical diagnosis and a diagnosis of HF should be established
before an echocardiogram is ordered. This practice is especially important
in patients who have limited (*Case 1*) or atypical (*Case 4*) clinical manifestations of HF. In these patients, a normal LVEF may bias diagnostic assessment. For example, *Case 1* had only DOE and edema, two nonspecific
symptoms, and *Case 4* had a syncopal episode, which is an atypical HF
symptom. If a diagnosis of HF is not already made, a normal LVEF may
increase the risk for a false-negative diagnosis, leading to worsening of
symptoms, possible emergency room visits or hospitalizations, and delays
in diagnosis and therapy. When a classic constellation of symptoms and
signs of HF is present, however, and a clinical diagnosis of HF can be

---

Box 2. DEFEAT HF: A simple 5-step protocol for the diagnostic assessment and management of geriatric heart failure

D—Diagnosis	A thorough history and a careful physical examination should allow a proper clinical **D**iagnosis of HF in most cases
E—Etiology	An underlying **E**tiology for HF must be identified, preferably in collaboration with a cardiologist
F—Fluid	All HF patients should be assessed carefully for **F**luid volume status to achieve euvolemia
EA—Ejection frAction	LV **E**jection fr**A**ction is of prognostic and therapeutic significance and must be determined in all HF patients
T—Therapy	All HF patients should be treated with evidence-based **T**herapy according to the recommendations of a major national HF guideline

---

established without difficulty (*Cases 2 and 3*), a normal LVEF does not question the diagnosis, but instead helps classify HF as diastolic HF.

Functional, physiologic, and psychologic heterogeneity of older adults should be taken into consideration when evaluating clinical manifestations in the diagnostic assessment of HF. DOE is a nonspecific symptom. That was the basis of a presumptive clinical diagnosis of HF for *Case 1*. He was a very active man who refused to restrict his activities because of his DOE, which could not be explained otherwise by another illness. In addition, his DOE was accompanied by new-onset leg edema, and he had several risk factors for HF. All these pointed toward a clinical diagnosis of HF. This diagnosis would be difficult if he were obese, deconditioned, or had COPD. *Case 5* had dyspnea at rest, but no DOE, which is almost always due to nonorganic causes. Further questioning also revealed that about a year ago she lost her husband of many years and moved to a new home close to her children. She was diagnosed with depression and therapy with antidepressants completely resolved her symptoms.

In *Case 4*, a diagnosis of HF was almost missed because of his atypical presentation (syncope) and would probably have been delayed if he had normal LVEF. BNP may be useful when a clinical diagnosis of HF is uncertain, especially when other competing causes of dyspnea, such as COPD or obesity, exist. Too much reliance on BNP should be discouraged, however [63]. As illustrated in *Case 4*, after his furosemide was increased he became euvolemic and asymptomatic. His BNP remained relatively high, however, and he was continued on the same dose of furosemide. Subsequent overdiuresis led to hypovolemia, hypoperfusion, and recurrence of symptoms. After his furosemide dose was decreased he gained about 10 pounds over the next week and his symptoms improved.

Determination of etiology of heart failure

An etiology for HF must be established for all patients who have HF. HF in older adults may be associated with more than one etiologic factor. Primary care physicians should consider referring all new geriatric patients who have HF to cardiologists for evaluation of underlying etiology, especially myocardial ischemia, which can cause continued myocardial damage. Collaboration between generalist and cardiologists may be the preferred model of care for older adults who have HF who also suffer from multiple noncardiac morbidities [5,50,71]. *Case 1* underwent a nuclear stress test that showed myocardial ischemia, which possibly played an etiologic role, along with hypertension, in his HF, and which prompted his referral for cardiology consultation. *Case 4* had a long history of hypertension and diabetes, two known predictors of HF in older adults [72]. He had a normal coronary angiogram. Microvascular dysfunction, however, in the absence of epicardial CAD, also has been shown to cause HF [73,74].

Hypertension and CAD are the two most common causes of HF in all ages, including older adults [72,75]. In the Cardiovascular Health Study, 5888 community-dwelling older adults (65 years of age and older, mean age 73 years) without HF at baseline were followed for a median of 5.5 years and 597 developed new-onset HF. Individuals who had CAD and hypertension had, respectively, 87% and 36% increased risk for incident HF. Because of the high prevalence of hypertension (41% versus 17% for CAD), the population-attributable risk for CAD and hypertension were similar (both 13%). If CAD and hypertension were removed as risk factors, each would prevent HF in about 13% of the population. Relative risk for other risk factors were: diabetes (78%), serum creatinine 1.4 mg/dL or greater (81%), LVH by electrocardiogram (129%), low LVEF (180%), and atrial fibrillation (106%) [72]. Because the prevalence of these conditions was low, however, their population-attributable risks also were low (8% for diabetes and 2% for atrial fibrillation, and others in between).

Presence of these risk factors often may be determined from history and other tests. It is important to identify the presence of these comorbidities, whether they are causally associated with HF or not. The presence of most of these comorbidities is associated with poor outcomes in HF, and thus should be managed according to established guidelines. With the exception of CAD and valvalar heart disease, primary care physicians should be able to identify and manage most of these comorbidities. Because many older adults might have silent ischemia, which may further myocardial damage and disease progression, all patients who have HF, including those who have diastolic HF, should be referred to cardiologists for appropriate assessment and treatment of ischemic heart disease [76].

Determination of fluid volume status

Once a diagnosis of HF has been made, one of the most important assessments is to determine the fluid status. This determination is important because a euvolemic state is essential not only to reduce symptoms and hospitalizations and improve quality of life but also to initiate and maintain life-saving therapy. Careful estimation of JVP, HJR, and pulmonary artery systolic pressure, and assessment of daily weight charts would allow accurate assessment of fluid balance in almost all elderly patients who have HF. Weight gain or loss in the range of 2 to 3 pounds in 2 to 3 days is almost always due to fluid overload or diuresis. If educated and encouraged to do so, most elderly patients who have HF will monitor and report daily weight. Assessment, achievement, and maintenance of euvolemia ensure proper physical functioning, which is particularly important in older adults because they are likely to decondition quickly. Physical activity and exercise reduce deconditioning, improve quality of life, and also may reduce mortality in HF [64–66]. If not properly assessed by clinicians, however, elderly patients who have HF may not report DOE and other exertional symptoms. Instead, they might restrict their activities in response to those symptoms and become deconditioned.

Determination of left ventricular ejection fraction

Once a diagnosis of HF is established, every patient who has HF should have an echocardiographic determination of LVEF. In patients who have systolic HF, there is no need to repeat the procedure unless indicated by major changes in clinical conditions [5]. LVEF should be checked periodically in patients who have diastolic HF because many of these patients eventually develop systolic HF [67,68].

Other diagnostic assessments

Initial evaluation for HF should also include a 12-lead electrocardiogram, a chest radiograph, and a laboratory workup, including serum electrolytes, renal function, liver function, thyroid function, lipid profile, complete cell count, fasting blood glucose, and hemoglobin A1C. All newly diagnosed patients who have HF should be screened for depression using a 15-item Geriatric Depression Scale. Functional status should be ascertained using New York Heart Association (NYHA) functional class. Higher NYHA class is associated with poor outcomes [69,70].

Evidence-based therapy for heart failure

Evidence-based therapy for geriatric HF should be primarily guided by LVEF. Systolic HF patients (low LVEF) should be treated with an ACE inhibitor [5,77]. For patients who cannot tolerate an ACE inhibitor, an angiotensin receptor blocker is a reasonable alternative [5]. Chronic kidney disease is common in HF and should not be considered a contraindication to ACE inhibitor or angiotensin receptor blocker [78,79]. Elderly systolic HF patients should be treated with approved beta-blockers [5]. Metoprolol extended release may be more appropriate in frail elderly systolic HF patients with low blood pressure because it is a selective beta-1 receptor blocker and it has minimal effect on blood pressure [80,81]. Low-dose digoxin should be used for elderly systolic HF patients who are symptomatic despite therapy with an ACE inhibitor and a beta-blocker [11,82]. Aldosterone antagonists should be used in advanced symptomatic HF patients with normal potassium and normal renal function [5]. Evidence-based therapy for diastolic HF (normal or near normal LVEF) is limited. However, recent data suggest that digoxin and candesartan may be beneficial in reducing HF hospitalizations in these patients [83,84]. Diuretics are essential for the management of fluid overload in both systolic and diastolic HF. However, there is little or no data on the long-term safety and should be used with caution in HF patients who are asymptomatic or minimally symptomatic [85].

Summary

Clinical manifestation of HF in older adults may be atypical and diagnostic assessment might be delayed. Assessment of HF in older adults may be made simple by following a simple 5-step process, **DEFEAT** HF: **D**iagnosis, **E**tiology, **F**luid status, **E**jection fra**A**cion, and **T**reatment for HF (see Box 2). A thorough history and a careful physical examination should allow proper clinical diagnosis of HF in most cases. An underlying cause for HF must be identified, preferably in collaboration with a cardiologist. All patients who have HF should be assessed carefully for volume status to achieve euvolemia. LVEF must be determined in all patients with a clinical diagnosis of HF to assess prognosis and guide therapy. All HF patients should be treated with evidence-based therapies according to the recommendations of a major national HF guideline.

Acknowledgments

The author thanks Robert C. Bourge, MD, FACC, Professor and Director, Cardiovascular Diseases, Department of Medicine, School of Mediine, University of Alabama at Birmingham, Birmingham, Alabama for his review of the manuscript and constructive comments.

References

[1] Aronow WS. Epidemiology, pathophysiology, prognosis, an treatment of systolic and diastolic heart failure. Cardiol Rev 2006;14:108–24.

[2] Aronow WS. Drug treatment of systolic and of diastolic heart failure in elderly persons. J Gerontol A Biol Sci Med Sci 2005;60:1597–605.

[3] Ahmed A. American College of Cardiology/American Heart Association chronic heart failure evaluation and management guidelines: Relevance to the geriatric practice. J Am Geriatr Soc 2003;51:123–6.

[4] Ahmed A, Allman RM, Aronow WS, et al. Diagnosis of heart failure in older adults: predictive value of dyspnea at rest. Arch Gerontol Geriatr 2004;38:297–307.

[5] Hunt SA, Abraham WT, Chin MH, et al. ACC/AHA 2005 guideline update for the diagnosis and management of chronic heart failure in the adult: a report of the American College of Cardiology/American Heart Association task force on practice guidelines (writing committee to update the 2001 guidelines for the evaluation and management of heart failure): developed in collaboration with the American College of Chest Physicians and the International Society for Heart and Lung Transplantation: endorsed by the Heart Rhythm SocietyCirculation 2005;112:e154–235.

[6] Adams K, Lindenfeld J, Arnold J, et al. Executive Summary: HFSA 2006 comprehensive heart failure practice guideline. J Card Fail 2006;12:10–38.

[7] Centers for Medicare & Medicaid Services. Overview of specifications of measures displayed on hospital compare as of December 15, 2005. Available at: http://www.cms.hhs.gov/HospitalQualityInits/10_HospitalQualityMeasures.asp#TopOfPage. Accessed June 3, 2006.

[8] Joint Commission on Accreditation of Healthcare Organizations. A comprehensive review of development and testing for national implementation of hospital core measures. Available at: http://www.jointcommission.org/NR/exeres/5A8BFA1C-B844-4A9A-86B2-F16DBE0E20C7.htm. Accessed June 3, 2006.

[9] The SOLVD Investigators. Effect of enalapril on survival in patients with reduced left ventricular ejection fractions and congestive heart failure. N Engl J Med 1991;325: 293–302.

[10] Pfeffer MA, Braunwald E, Moye LA, et al. Effect of captopril on mortality and morbidity in patients with left ventricular dysfunction after myocardial infarction. Results of the survival and ventricular enlargement trial. The SAVE Investigators. N Engl J Med 1992;327:669–77.

[11] The Digitalis Investigation Group. The effect of digoxin on mortality and morbidity in patients with heart failure. N Engl J Med 1997;336:525–33.

[12] Packer M, Bristow MR, Cohn JN, et al. The effect of carvedilol on morbidity and mortality in patients with chronic heart failure. US Carvedilol Heart Failure Study Group. N Engl J Med 1996;334:1349–55.

[13] MERIT-HF Study Group. Effect of metoprolol CR/XL in chronic heart failure: Metoprolol CR/XL Randomised Intervention Trial in Congestive Heart Failure (MERIT-HF). Lancet 1999;353:2001–7.

[14] Pitt B, Zannad F, Remme WJ, et al. The effect of spironolactone on morbidity and mortality in patients with severe heart failure. Randomized Aldactone Evaluation Study Investigators. N Engl J Med 1999;341:709–17.

[15] Pitt B, Poole-Wilson PA, Segal R, et al. Effect of losartan compared with captopril on mortality in patients with symptomatic heart failure: randomised trial–the Losartan Heart Failure Survival Study ELITE II. Lancet 2000;355:1582–7.

[16] Hogg K, Swedberg K, McMurray J. Heart failure with preserved left ventricular systolic function; epidemiology, clinical characteristics, and prognosis. J Am Coll Cardiol 2004;43: 317–27.

[17] Vasan RS, Larson MG, Benjamin EJ, et al. Congestive heart failure in subjects with normal versus reduced left ventricular ejection fraction: prevalence and mortality in a population-based cohort. J Am Coll Cardiol 1999;33:1948–55.

[18] Gottdiener JS, McClelland RL, Marshall R, et al. Outcome of congestive heart failure in elderly persons: influence of left ventricular systolic function. The Cardiovascular Health Study. Ann Intern Med 2002;137:631–9.

[19] Senni M, Redfield MM. Heart failure with preserved systolic function. A different natural history? J Am Coll Cardiol 2001;38:1277–82.

[20] Redfield MM, Jacobsen SJ, Burnett JC Jr, et al. Burden of systolic and diastolic ventricular dysfunction in the community: appreciating the scope of the heart failure epidemic. JAMA 2003;289:194–202.

[21] Zile MR, Gaasch WH, Carroll JD, et al. Heart failure with a normal ejection fraction: is measurement of diastolic function necessary to make the diagnosis of diastolic heart failure? Circulation 2001;104:779–82.

[22] Kitzman DW, Little WC, Brubaker PH, et al. Pathophysiological characterization of isolated diastolic heart failure in comparison to systolic heart failure. JAMA 2002;288: 2144–50.

[23] Ahmed A, Roseman JM, Duxbury AS, et al. Correlates and outcomes of preserved left ventricular systolic function among older adults hospitalized with heart failure. Am Heart J 2002;144:365–72.

[24] Ahmed A, Nanda NC, Weaver MT, et al. Clinical correlates of isolated left ventricular diastolic dysfunction among hospitalized older heart failure patients. Am J Geriatr Cardiol 2003;12:82–9.

[25] Ahmed A. Association of diastolic dysfunction and outcomes in ambulatory older adults with chronic heart failure. J Gerontol A Biol Sci Med Sci 2005;60:1339–44.

[26] Radford MJ, Arnold JM, Bennett SJ, et al. ACC/AHA key data elements and definitions for measuring the clinical management and outcomes of patients with chronic heart failure: a report of the American College of Cardiology/American Heart Association task force on clinical data standards (writing committee to develop heart failure clinical data standards): developed in collaboration with the American College of Chest Physicians and the International Society for Heart and Lung Transplantation: endorsed by the Heart Failure Society of America. Circulation 2005;112:1888–916.

[27] Cheitlin MD, Armstrong WF, Aurigemma GP, et al. ACC/AHA/ASE 2003 guideline update for the clinical application of echocardiography: summary article: a report of the American College of Cardiology/American Heart Association task force on practice guidelines (ACC/AHA/ASE committee to update the 1997 guidelines for the clinical application of echocardiography). Circulation 2003;108:1146–62.

[28] Zile MR, Baicu CF, Gaasch WH. Diastolic heart failure–abnormalities in active relaxation and passive stiffness of the left ventricle. N Engl J Med 2004;350:1953–9.

[29] Thomas JD, Choong CY, Flachskampf FA, et al. Analysis of the early transmitral Doppler velocity curve: effect of primary physiologic changes and compensatory preload adjustment. J Am Coll Cardiol 1990;16:644–55.

[30] Swedberg K, Cleland J, Dargie H, et al. Guidelines for the diagnosis and treatment of chronic heart failure: executive summary (update 2005): The task force for the diagnosis and treatment of chronic heart failure of the european society of cardiology. Eur Heart J 2005;26: 1115–40.

[31] Fleg JL, Shapiro EP, O'Connor F, et al. Left ventricular diastolic filling performance in older male athletes. JAMA 1995;273:1371–5.

[32] Nagueh SF, Middleton KJ, Kopelen HA, et al. Doppler tissue imaging: a noninvasive technique for evaluation of left ventricular relaxation and estimation of filling pressures. J Am Coll Cardiol 1997;30:1527–33.

[33] Sohn DW, Chai IH, Lee DJ, et al. Assessment of mitral annulus velocity by Doppler tissue imaging in the evaluation of left ventricular diastolic function. J Am Coll Cardiol 1997;30: 474–80.

[34] The National Heart Lung, and Blood Institute. Working group on cellular and molecular mechanisms of right heart failure: Executive summary. October 6–7, 2005. Available at: www.nhlbi.nih.gov/meetings/workshops/right-heart.htm. Accessed June 3, 2006.

[35] Cosentino AM. The congested state in renal failure: A historical and diagnostic perspective. Semin Dial 1999;12:307–10.

[36] Braunwald E, Colluci WS, Grossman W. Clinical aspects of heart failure: high-output heart failure; pulmonary edema. In: Braunwald E, editor. Heart disease: a text book of cardiovascular medicine. Volume 1. 5th edition. Philadelphia: W.B. Saunders Company; 1997. p. 445–70.

[37] Warren JV, Stead EA Jr. Fluid dynamics in chronic congestive heart failure. Arch Intern Med 1944;73:138–47.

[38] Merrill AJ. Edema and decreased renal blood flow in patients with chronic congestive heart failure: evidence of "forward failure" as the primary cause of edema. J Clin Invest 1946;25: 389–400.

[39] Francis GS, Goldsmith SR, Levine TB, et al. The neurohumoral axis in congestive heart failure. Ann Intern Med 1984;101:370–7.

[40] Ingram CW, Satler LF, Rackley CE. Progressive heart failure secondary to a high output state. Chest 1987;92:1117–8.

[41] Froeschl M, Haddad H, Commons AS, et al. Thyrotoxicosis-an uncommon cause of heart failure. Cardiovasc Pathol 2005;14:24–7.

[42] Ahearn DJ, Maher JF. Heart failure as a complication of hemodialysis arteriovenous fistula. Ann Intern Med 1972;77:201–4.

[43] Gheorghiade M, Zannad F, Sopko G, et al. Acute heart failure syndromes: current state and framework for future research. Circulation 2005;112:3958–68.

[44] Haldeman GA, Croft JB, Giles WH, et al. Hospitalization of patients with heart failure: National Hospital Discharge Survey, 1985 to 1995. Am Heart J 1999;137:352–60.

[45] Thom T, Haase N, Rosamond W, et al. Heart disease and stroke statistics–2006 update: a report from the American Heart Association statistics committee and stroke statistics subcommittee. Circulation 2006;113:e85–151.

[46] Nieminen MS, Bohm M, Cowie MR, et al. Executive summary of the guidelines on the diagnosis and treatment of acute heart failure: the task force on acute heart failure of the European Society of Cardiology. Eur Heart J 2005;26:384–416.

[47] Kramer K, Kirkman P, Kitzman D, et al. Flash pulmonary edema: association with hypertension and reoccurrence despite coronary revascularization. Am Heart J 2000;140: 451–5.

[48] Jong P, Yusuf S, Ahn SA, et al. Effect of enalapril on 12-year survival and life expectancy in patients with left ventricular systolic dysfunction: a follow-up study. Lancet 2003;361: 1843–8.

[49] Mueller C, Scholer A, Laule-Kilian K, et al. Use of B-type natriuretic peptide in the evaluation and management of acute dyspnea. N Engl J Med 2004;350:647–54.

[50] Ahmed A, Allman RM, Kiefe CI, et al. Association of consultation between generalists and cardiologists with quality and outcomes of heart failure care. Am Heart J 2003;145: 1086–93.

[51] Ahmed A, Allman RM, DeLong JF, et al. Age-related underutilization of angiotensin-converting enzyme inhibitors in older hospitalized heart failure patients. South Med J 2002;95: 703–10.

[52] Ahmed A, Weaver MT, Allman RM, et al. Quality of care of nursing home residents hospitalized with heart failure. J Am Geriatr Soc 2002;50:1831–6.

[53] Wang CS, FitzGerald JM, Schulzer M, et al. Does this dyspneic patient in the emergency department have congestive heart failure? JAMA 2005;294:1944–56.

[54] Perloff JK, Braunwald E. Physical examination of the heart and circulation. In: Braunwald E, editor. Heart disease: a text book of cardiovascular medicine. Volume 1. 5th edition. Philadelphia: W.B. Saunders Company; 1997. p. 15–52.

[55] Butman SM, Ewy GA, Standen JR, et al. Bedside cardiovascular examination in patients with severe chronic heart failure: importance of rest or inducible jugular venous distension. J Am Coll Cardiol 1993;22:968–74.

[56] Drazner MH, Rame JE, Stevenson LW, et al. Prognostic importance of elevated jugular venous pressure and a third heart sound in patients with heart failure. N Engl J Med 2001;345: 574–81.

[57] Curtis JP, Selter JG, Wang Y, et al. The obesity paradox: body mass index and outcomes in patients with heart failure. Arch Intern Med 2005;165:55–61.

[58] Chatterjee K. Physical examination in heart failure. In: Hosenpud JD, Greenberg B, editors. Congestive heart failure: pathophysiology, diagnosis, and comprehensive approach to management. Volume 1. 2nd edition. Philadelphia, PA: Lippincott Williams and Wilkins; 2000. p. 615–29.

[59] Ducas J, Magder S, McGregor M. Validity of the hepatojugular reflux as a clinical test for congestive heart failure. Am J Cardiol 1983;52:1299–303.

[60] Sochowski RA, Dubbin JD, Naqvi SZ. Clinical and hemodynamic assessment of the hepatojugular reflux. Am J Cardiol 1990;66:1002–6.

[61] Young JR. The swollen leg. Am Fam Physician 1977;15:163–73.

[62] Donaldson MC. Chronic Venous Insufficiency. Curr Treat Options Cardiovasc Med 2000;2: 265–72.

[63] Aronow WS. Brain natriuretic peptide in heart failure. J Am Geriatr Soc 2006;54:368–9 [author reply: 369].

[64] Coats AJ, Adamopoulos S, Radaelli A, et al. Controlled trial of physical training in chronic heart failure. Exercise performance, hemodynamics, ventilation, and autonomic function. Circulation 1992;85:2119–31.

[65] Ko JK, McKelvie RS. The role of exercise training for patients with heart failure. Eura Medicophys 2005;41:35–47.

[66] Tenenbaum A, Freimark D, Ahron E, et al. Long-term versus intermediate-term supervised exercise training in advanced heart failure: effects on exercise tolerance and mortality. Int J Cardiol 2006; in press.

[67] Cahill JM, Ryan E, Travers B, et al. Progression of preserved systolic function heart failure to systolic dysfunction–a natural history study. Int J Cardiol 2006;106:95–102.

[68] Yu CM, Lin H, Yang H, et al. Progression of systolic abnormalities in patients with "isolated" diastolic heart failure and diastolic dysfunction. Circulation 2002;105: 1195–201.

[69] Scrutinio D, Lagioia R, Ricci A, et al. Prediction of mortality in mild to moderately symptomatic patients with left ventricular dysfunction. The role of the New York Heart Association classification, cardiopulmonary exercise testing, two-dimensional echocardiography and Holter monitoring. Eur Heart J 1994;15:1089–95.

[70] Ahmed A, Aronow WS, Fleg JL. Higher New York Heart Association classes and increased mortality and hospitalization in patients with heart failure and preserved left ventricular function. Am Heart J 2006;151:444–50.

[71] Ahmed A. Heart failure training: care for older adults with chronic heart failure. J Am Coll Cardiol 2005;45:2096–7.

[72] Gottdiener JS, Arnold AM, Aurigemma GP, et al. Predictors of congestive heart failure in the elderly: the Cardiovascular Health Study. J Am Coll Cardiol 2000;35:1628–37.

[73] Rajappan K, Rimoldi OE, Dutka DP, et al. Mechanisms of coronary microcirculatory dysfunction in patients with aortic stenosis and angiographically normal coronary arteries. Circulation 2002;105:470–6.

[74] Cecchi F, Olivotto I, Gistri R, et al. Coronary microvascular dysfunction and prognosis in hypertrophic cardiomyopathy. N Engl J Med 2003;349:1027–35.

[75] Kannel WB. Vital epidemiologic clues in heart failure. J Clin Epidemiol 2000;53:229–35.

[76] Ahmed A, Zile MR, Rich MW, et al. Hospitalizations due to unstable angina pectoris in diastolic and systolic heart failure. Am J Card 2007; in press.

[77] Ahmed A, Maisiak R, Allman RM, et al. Heart failure mortality among older Medicare beneficiaries: association with left ventricular function evaluation and angiotensin-converting enzyme inhibitor use. South Med J 2003;96:124–9.

[78] Ahmed A. Use of angiotensin-converting enzyme inhibitors in patients with heart failure and renal insufficiency: how concerned should we be by the rise in serum creatinine? J Am Geriatr Soc 2002;50:1297–300.

[79] Ahmed A, Kiefe CI, Allman RM, et al. Survival benefits of angiotensin-converting enzyme inhibitors in older heart failure patients with perceived contraindications. J Am Geriatr Soc 2002;50:1659–66.

[80] Ahmed A, Dell'Italia LJ. Use of beta-blockers in older adults with chronic heart failure. Am J Med Sci 2004;328:100–11.

[81] Ahmed A. Myocardial beta-1 adrenoceptor down-regulation in aging and heart failure: implications for beta-blocker use in older adults with heart failure. Eur J Heart Fail 2003;5: 709–15.

[82] Ahmed A, Rich MW, Love TE, et al. Digoxin and reduction in mortality and hospitalization in heart failure: a comprehensive post hoc analysis of the DIG trial. Eur Heart J 2006;27: 178–86.

[83] Yusuf S, Pfeffer MA, Swedberg K, et al. Effects of candesartan in patients with chronic heart failure and preserved left-ventricular ejection fraction: the CHARM-Preserved Trial. Lancet 2003;362:777–81.

[84] Ahmed A, Rich MW, Fleg JL, et al. Effects of digoxin on morbidity and mortality in diastolic heart failure: the ancillary digitalis investigation group trial. Circulation 2006;114:397–403.

[85] Ahmed A, Husain A, Love TE, et al. Heart failure, chronic diuretic use, and increase in mortality and hospitalization: an observational study using propensity score methods. Eur Heart J 2006;27:1431–9.

ELSEVIER
SAUNDERS

CLINICS IN
GERIATRIC
MEDICINE

Clin Geriatr Med 23 (2007) 31–59

Role of Echocardiography in the Diagnostic Assessment and Etiology of Heart Failure in the Elderly—Opacify, Quantify, and Rectify

Vincent L. Sorrell, MD[a], Navin C. Nanda, MD[b],*

[a]Division of Medicine, Section of Cardiology, University of Arizona,
Sarver Heart Center, 1501 N. Campbell Avenue, Tucson, AZ 85724-5037, USA
[b]Division of Cardiovascular Disease and Director, Heart Station/Echocardiography
Laboratories, University of Alabama at Birmingham,
Heart Station SW/S 102 Birmingham, AL 35249, USA

Heart failure (HF) is the number-one cause of cardiovascular hospitalization in older adults in the United States. This disease is common, disabling, and especially deadly in the elderly population. Hypertension and coronary artery disease are the leading causes of HF. A precise diagnosis of the cardiac pathology is paramount for adequate treatment, and echocardiography offers an evaluation that is comprehensive, noninvasive, and relatively inexpensive. With an organized approach using two-dimensional echocardiography (2DE) and Doppler echocardiography, clinicians can determine the systolic and diastolic left ventricular (LV) performance; estimate the cardiac output, pulmonary artery, and ventricular filling pressures; and identify surgically correctable valve disease. Intravenous contrast should be used to opacify the LV cavity and enhance the endocardial border in patients with suboptimal acoustic windows. Real-time three-dimensional echocardiography (3DE) provides unprecedented volume data to quantify the LV status. Imaging data about myocardial velocity and strain, derived from tissue Doppler echocardiography (TDE), provide extremely fine details about the regional variations in myocardial synchrony and predict responders to cardiac resynchronization therapy (CRT). Thus, echocardiographic tools provide the basis for determining when to attempt

---

* Corresponding author.
  E-mail address: authornanda@uab.edu (N.C. Nanda).

to rectify the LV dysfunction with strategically placed, biventricular pacemaker leads.

More than 10% of those aged 80 to 89 years have HF, making congestive HF extremely common in the elderly [1]. Although HF remains a clinical diagnosis, echocardiography assists in determining the etiology, systolic and diastolic function, and hemodynamic state. The cardiovascular systems of elderly people have important differences from those of the general population and those differences need to be taken into consideration. For example, the rate of myocardial contraction and relaxation in the elderly is prolonged. This abnormality in relaxation may account for the higher prevalence of normal LV systolic function seen in elderly patients with HF, where more than 50% of patients older than 80 years have normal or near-normal systolic function [2].

The clinical findings in systolic and diastolic HF are indistinguishable, making the history and physical examination inadequate for estimating LV function. Although HF patients with a diastolic blood pressure ≥ 105 mm Hg and no jugular venous distention have been shown to have a normal LV systolic ejection fraction (EF) with a positive predictive value of 100%, this combination of findings is uncommon [3]. Most other historical variables (eg, age, symptom duration, hypertension, ischemia) and clinical variables (eg, S3 gallop, edema, cardiomegaly, pulmonary or peripheral edema) are not significantly different in HF patients with normal or abnormal LV EF [4]. Echocardiography should be performed in all patients with new-onset or worsening HF symptoms and provides critical information to assist in the subsequent management of the patient. This article is considerably different from the authors' previous report on this subject [5]. First, the authors have organized this into anatomic (gray scale) and hemodynamic (Doppler) echocardiographic data with expanded references; second, the authors have introduced a number of important new diagnostic echocardiographic techniques and expanded the figures; and third, the authors have provided a greater emphasis on outcome and prognostic data.

Anatomic findings (one-, two-, and three-dimensional echocardiography)

Echocardiography is ideal for assessing LV function, and this has become the most common reason for performing the study. Echocardiography can accurately resolve the endocardial borders throughout the cardiac cycle in multiple well-defined anatomic planes. With M-mode, the fractional shortening ([LV diastolic diameter – LV systolic diameter]/LV diastolic diameter) can be used as a rapid method for estimating LV systolic performance. With 2DE, inspection of the initial parasternal long-axis view will often correctly identify patients with either normal or severely reduced LV EF (Fig. 1). Additional views are required for accuracy.

Using validated geometric equations, 2DE can determine the LV EF, stroke volume and cardiac output. By calculating the LV end-diastolic

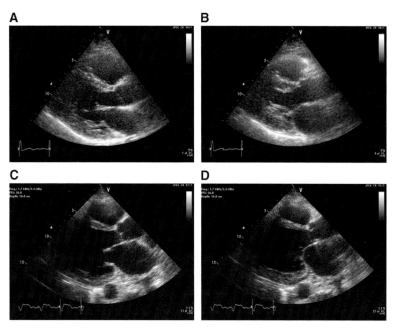

Fig. 1. Parasternal long-axis 2DE view in diastole (*A*) and systole (*B*) in an elderly female with class-III heart failure symptoms. The normal LV EF is immediately evident and raises the likelihood of diastolic dysfunction or transient systolic dysfunction from ischemia or arrhythmias. In contrast, the parasternal long-axis 2DE view ((*C*) Diastole (*D*) Systole) in another elderly patient with class-II symptoms immediately displays a dilated cardiomyopathy with reduced LV EF.

volume (EDV) and end-systolic volume (ESV), the stroke volume (SV) is readily derived (SV = EDV – ESV). In the absence of significant valvular regurgitation, cardiac output is estimated as the product of the SV and heart rate. Furthermore, the EF can then be calculated (EF = SV/EDV).

For determining LV volumes, 2DE offers considerable advantages over M-mode methods and should be used for quantitative assessment. Even in the presence of wall-motion abnormalities, 2DE provides excellent correlation with angiographic techniques [6]. Current ultrasound systems include software that can calculate volumes based on hand-traced regions of interest (Fig. 2). Images with good technical quality are necessary and recently have been improved by the development of second harmonic imaging [7]. When LV border delineation remains suboptimal, intracardiac contrast agents should be employed. These agents cross the pulmonary circuit following intravenous injection and opacify the LV cavity for several cardiac cycles (Fig. 3) [8]. Additionally, newer software allows the LV chamber to be automatically traced on line using real-time, automated border detection, thus providing beat-to-beat estimates of EDV, ESV, and LV EF [9].

3DE has been approved by the US Food and Drug Administration and is commercially available. Modern three-dimensional (3D) techniques have

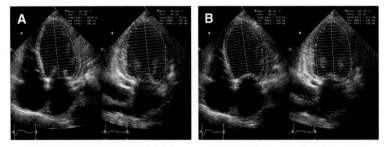

Fig. 2. Apical four-chamber (*left*) and two-chamber (*right*) views in diastole (*A*) and systole (*B*) with the manual endocardial borders traced allowing the computer to determine the LV volumes using the modified Simpson's method-of-discs rule. The two views are averaged to create diastolic (LVd) and systolic (LVs) volumes and the LV EF = (LVd – LVs)/LVd = (231 cc – 198 cc)/231 cc = 14%.

evolved from the necessity to integrate multiple two dimensional (2D) imaging planes to generate a 3D reconstruction, to the intelligent acquisition of near–real-time volume data (Fig. 4). This has catapulted 3DE into the clinical arena. 3DE is able to produce LV EF values similar to other imaging reference standards and offers incremental benefit over 2D techniques with improved accuracy and reproducibility [10]. 3DE has also been investigated as a tool to quantify LV dyssynchrony in patients being considered for CRT (Fig. 5).

In addition to providing a quantitative assessment of EF, many echocardiography laboratories, including those the authors use, visually estimate this important parameter. In experienced hands, visual estimates are associated with a standard error of ≤11%, which compares favorably with quantitative echocardiographic methods (10%) and radionuclide angiographic methods (7%) [11]. Despite experience, visual estimates are only accurate when the LV function is either normal or severely reduced. When the LV

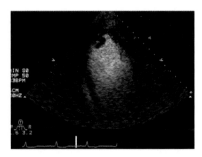

Fig. 3. Apical four-chamber view after the injection of a 1-cc bolus of activated perflutren. The cavity is enhanced and brighter than the relatively darker myocardium. A thrombus is also seen as a filling defect in the LV apex.

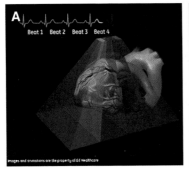 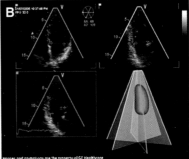

Fig. 4. With a matrix array probe, sets of three-dimensional volume data are acquired within a few cardiac cycles (A). Four individual 15° sectors of volume data are stacked together and stored as a single image, allowing optimal assessment of cardiac volumes. With triplane imaging (B), the apical two-, three-, and four-chamber views can be simultaneously displayed to allow volume assessment via the modified Simpson's method. (Courtesy of GE Healthcare, Chalfont St. Giles, United Kingdom.)

function is intermediate or indeterminate, 2D or 3D quantitative techniques should be employed.

Determining the etiology of HF is paramount to developing an adequate treatment regimen. In addition to numerous myocardial diseases, the clinical findings of HF may be due to such diverse causes as unsuspected valvar stenosis or regurgitation, chronic pulmonary disease, or pericardial constraint. One-dimensional (M-mode) echocardiography and 2DE provide excellent spatial resolution to evaluate the anatomy of the myocardium and cardiac valves. Each of the four major World Health Organization classifications of cardiomyopathies can be reasonably categorized with echocardiography [12].

Dilated cardiomyopathy (DCM), a primary myocardial disease, is usually idiopathic and creates a spherically enlarged LV with normal or thin-walled muscle and reduced LV EF. While late-stage DCM is easy to

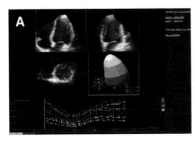 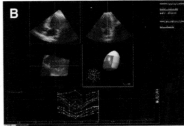

Fig. 5. Sets of three-dimensional volume data enable the creation of a volume-rendered image and regional time/volume curves. In a normal left ventricle, these 17-segment curves reach end-systole at nearly the same time (A), but in a patient with LV dyssynchrony, these curves are chaotic (B). (Courtesy of Philips Medical Systems, New York, NY; with permission.)

recognize, DCM is often difficult to detect in its early stages. Early anatomic echocardiography features that may precede a detectable drop in LV systolic function include a decrease in the descent of the cardiac base, an increase in sphericity, and a rise in ESV index, which appears to be sensitive to changes in global contractility [13–15].

A hypertrophic cardiomyopathy is a primary cardiomyopathy that results in a markedly thickened LV myocardial wall with normal LV contractility until very late in the disease process. This late presentation is not uncommon in the elderly population. A restrictive cardiomyopathy is an unusual classification in that it requires one to combine Doppler information with the usual 2D cardiac appearance of normal or small LV cavity and markedly dilated left and right atria. DCM and hypertrophic cardiomyopathy both have a notoriously grave outcome.

Arrhythmogenic right ventricular cardiomyopathy (dysplasia) is difficult to detect in the early concealed phase, but once fully developed, results in a dilated, dysfunctional right ventricle with a normal left ventricle (Fig. 6). This is a diagnosis of exclusion and should not be considered if significant pulmonary hypertension exists. Other characteristic features of this rare cardiomyopathy include focal aneurysms or thinning at the "triangle of dysplasia," which includes the right ventricular (RV) inflow, the RV outflow and the RV apex [16].

Although echocardiography is rarely able to establish the exact cause of myocardial pathology, some diseases have characteristic echocardiographic features that raise their likelihood. Regional wall-motion abnormalities typically occur in patients with underlying coronary artery disease, but are also present in patients with advanced DCM. However, an area of normal myocardial thickening with abrupt transition to an area of thin, hyperechoic, scarred myocardium is more characteristic of an ischemic cardiomyopathy. For serial comparisons of regional wall-motion assessment and greater consistency among all imaging modalities, a 17-segment myocardial model should be used [17].

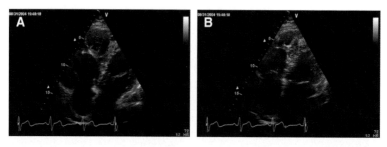

Fig. 6. Apical four-chamber view, tilted rightward for maximal visualization of the right ventricular (RV) cavity, in an elderly male with known arryhthmogenic RV dysplasia. The left ventricle is mildly dilated and dysfunctional (common in late stages), but the RV cavity is markedly dilated, has a prominent moderator band and trabeculae in the absence of pulmonary hypertension, and a focal wall-motion abnormality in the RV apex. (*A*) Diastole. (*B*) Systole.

A sparkled appearance within the myocardium is said to be highly predictive of amyloidosis, but the authors believe that any cause of LV hypertrophy may have this appearance with modern ultrasound transducers. When dramatic and accompanied by other echocardiographic features of amyloidosis, such as a pericardial effusion and myocardial, valvar, and atrial septal thickening, this diagnosis becomes more likely. Occurring in patients with a travel or immigration history from South and Central American countries, the finding of a segmental cardiomyopathy, without coronary artery disease, raises the possibility of Chagas' disease. The most common abnormality is an apical aneurysm, which, unlike coronary disease, spares the interventricular septum [18]. As this disease progresses, the echocardiographic appearance may mimic DCM.

LV noncompaction is an uncommon cause of a DCM that results from intrauterine arrest of compaction of the loose interwoven meshwork that makes up the fetal myocardial primordium. This disorder should be suspected when unexpectedly heavy LV trabeculation is noted, particularly toward the apex. This disease entity has only recently been identified in elderly populations and the diagnosis is aided with the use of contrast, with or without 3DE (Fig. 7) [19].

Normal-appearing LV size and function associated with an enlarged RV cavity, reduced RV function, and an elevated pulmonary artery pressure raise the suspicion of pulmonary artery thromboemboli or primary lung disease (Fig. 8) [20,21]. If the RV free wall (best seen with subcostal imaging) is not thickened (≥ 5 mm), then chronic elevation of the pulmonary artery pressure is unlikely, further reducing the etiology to a more acute diagnosis.

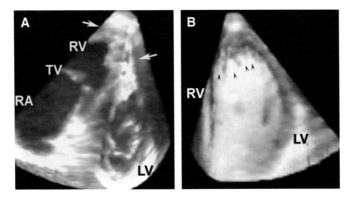

Fig. 7. (*A*) Live 3DE in combined LV and RV noncompaction. White arrows point to massive trabeculations with deep recesses in both the left ventricle and the right ventricle with the diagnosis of isolated noncompaction of the left ventricle (and right ventricle). (*B*) Live 3DE contrast study using activated perflutren microspheres showing filling of intertrabecular recesses with the contrast agent (*black arrows*). RA, right atrium; TV, tricuspid valve. (*From* Bodiwala K, Miller AP, Nanda NC, et al. Live three-dimensional transthoracic echocardiographic assessment of ventricular non-compaction. Echocardiography 2005;22:615.)

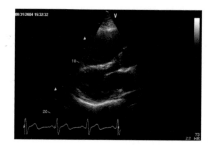

Fig. 8. Parasternal long-axis 2DE view in an elderly male with class-III heart failure symptoms. The diagnosis of cor pulmonale is immediately suggested by the massive RV on this initial 2DE view.

Aortic valve disease is extremely common in the elderly and ranges from calcific degeneration (aortic sclerosis) to severe, critical aortic stenosis. Despite a detailed and careful physical examination, the severity of aortic stenosis is often in doubt, especially in the elderly [22]. 2DE combined with conventional Doppler is well suited to investigate the severity of aortic stenosis. The modified Bernoulli equation converts measured velocities to mean- and peak-pressure gradients and the continuity equation provides an estimate of the aortic valve area. Color flow Doppler can assist in obtaining an accurate estimate of the aortic valve area [23]. When the transthoracic echocardiographic findings are uncertain, transesophageal echocardiography or stress echocardiography can provide additional insight into the severity of the valve lesion [24,25]. Also, real-time 3DE enables direct visualization and measurement of the stenotic aortic valve opening. Real-time 3DE may be more accurate than 2DE with Doppler [26].

Mitral valve disease may also result in the clinical presentation of HF. Mitral regurgitation (MR) is nearly universal when the LV EF is reduced and the left ventricle is enlarged. With mitral annular dilatation, coaptation of the valve is compromised and secondary, central MR occurs. The 2D appearance of the valve is often normal and the degree of MR is rarely severe until late in the disease progression. When LV dysfunction is secondary to mitral regurgitation, the 2D appearance of the mitral valve is universally abnormal. In this situation, the degree of MR is often severe, and the direction of the regurgitant jet is commonly eccentric (directed away from a prolapsing or flail leaflet, or toward a restricted or scarred leaflet). Quantifying the degree of MR is vitally important when considering surgery and real-time 3DE supplements 2DE and color Doppler in the assessment of MR severity [27–29]. If possible, severe MR should be repaired early to minimize progression of LV systolic dysfunction. In rare cases, this repair provides a surgical cure for HF [30].

The right ventricle is notoriously difficult to completely analyze due to its complex, non-geometric shape and a high degree of normal variability in shape and regional motion. Using the apical four-chamber view, simple endocardial tracing in diastole and systole provides a reliable, albeit not highly accurate, estimate of systolic function, expressed as a percentage of fractional area change (FAC) (Fig. 9). Although not specifically investigated in elderly individuals, a FAC >32% (35% is easier to remember) has been found in normal controls [16]. A useful and easily obtained measurement of RV function is the tricuspid annular plane systolic excursion (descent of the base). In one report, an excursion of 14 mm added significant prognostic information to other clinical and echocardiographic findings in dilated cardiomyopathy [31].

The most significant recent advance in systolic HF treatment has been achieved with the placement of strategically positioned biventricular pacemaker leads to create an improved pattern of myocardial contraction. This is CRT. Numerous trials have shown improved outcomes. The effect of CRT in elderly patients has also been shown to be beneficial. In 170 consecutive patients with clinical and echocardiographic improvements after CRT at 6 months, survival at 2 years was similar in patients older than 70 years compared with those patients younger than 70 years [32].

The echocardiography community has known for years that the placement of a RV pacemaker is associated with an abnormal, paradoxical distal septal motion due to pre-activation at the site of the RV apical lead. In the setting of a left bundle branch block (LBBB) pattern ECG, the native septum has a variable degree of paradoxical motion that can be witnessed with 2DE or 3DE. The more abnormal the LBBB pattern, the more abnormal is the 2DE motion. It is intuitive that this dyssynchronous pattern of contraction could be improved by placing a pacemaker lead in the lateral wall and causing pre-activation of this relatively delayed myocardial segment. In essence, this is what CRT does. Although echocardiographic findings can often predict responders of CRT, echocardiography is not a perfect tool. However, it can reliably predict nonresponders by recognizing lateral wall scars. These nonresponders will improve contraction with pacing and

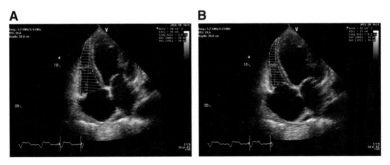

Fig. 9. Apical four-chamber view tilted rightward allows the assessment of the RV function using the FAC method of tracing the endocardial borders in diastole (*A*) and systole (*B*). FAC = (RV diastole – RV systole)/RV diastole = (38-16)/38 = 57%.

therefore should not undergo attempted CRT. Furthermore, echocardiography is the basis for CRT since, in theory, a patient with an EF of 36% would not benefit from CRT but a patient with an EF of 34% would. This is further justification of the need for quantification of LV EF.

To more precisely identify regions of myocardial dyssynchrony, numerous techniques are available, but none have proven superior over the others. Certainly, one of the simplest, most reproducible methods is 3DE (see Fig. 5). This method is criticized for having a low temporal resolution. Others have carefully analyzed the subtle gray-scale relationships of 2DE, known as speckle tracking, as a means to improve upon this temporal resolution issue and have shown early success [33].

Finally, dobutamine infusion has a role in elderly patients with LV systolic dysfunction. If the global dysfunction improves with a low dose, then the left ventricle is viable and worthy of continued investigation for an ischemic etiology. If it does not improve, then there is no reason to pursue this line of investigation. If improvement occurs at low dose and is sustained at higher, target doses, then a nonischemic etiology should be considered. If the low-dose improvement worsens again at higher doses, then ischemia is suggested and revascularization should be advised.

Many patients with HF have a normal LV EF. Although this is often presumed to be due to diastolic dysfunction, it may not be that simple and some of these patients have subtle, undetectable changes in systolic function and are at the early stages of progressive LV systolic dysfunction. The natural history of structural and functional changes of the left ventricle in this patient population is poorly reported. In 38 patients (mean age: 72) with HF and preserved systolic function (LV EF $\geq$45%), repeat echocardiography in 3 months confirmed that 21% had either global (n = 6) or regional (n = 3) LV dysfunction with LV EF <45% [34]. None of these patients had a change in their clinical status, further emphasizing that subclinical LV systolic dysfunction is common.

Hemodynamic data (conventional and tissue Doppler)

Pulsed- or continuous-wave wave Doppler echocardiography quickly and accurately estimates cardiac output. By placing the sample volume within the LV outflow tract (LV OT), the Doppler envelope can be obtained and traced to provide the time velocity integral (TVI). This "stroke distance" is then multiplied by the LV OT area (LV OT diameter^2 $\times$ 0.785) to obtain the stroke volume. Stroke volume multiplied by heart rate provides cardiac output [35]. Using continuous-wave Doppler, the cardiac output is determined by multiplying the TVI by the diameter of the sino-tubular junction (in the absence of aortic stenosis). The validity of the cardiac output has been shown even in the presence of a low-output state or significant tricuspid regurgitation [36]. A global index of myocardial performance that combines both systolic and diastolic parameters has been described for both the

right and left ventricles, but the clinical utility of this index in older congestive HF patients has not yet been well validated [37,38].

Although diastolic dysfunction has been defined clinically as HF in the
presence of a normal ejection fraction, an echocardiographic assessment
of diastolic function is important in confirming the diagnosis [39]. Importantly, any process that impairs the systolic function of the myocardium affects diastolic function as well. No noninvasive technique can directly
measure diastolic function, but Doppler echocardiography uses diastolic filling parameters to infer diastolic function parameters. The various physiologic factors that affect mitral inflow velocities have been studied in
experimental settings, allowing the individual contributions of each to be
considered [40]. These experiments have shown that (1) elevated left atrial
pressure causes an increased acceleration rate, shortened isovolumic relaxation time (IVRT), and increased peak velocities; (2) slowing relaxation
causes a delay in filling, and lower peak velocities and acceleration; (3) increasing ventricular stiffness blunts the E-wave velocity; and (4) reducing
systolic function causes a similar effect as increasing stiffness.

Transmitral flow incorporates early filling (E wave), passive filling (dia-
stasis), and atrial contraction (A wave). The initial systolic forward flow
(S_1 wave) in pulmonary veins occurs because of atrial relaxation (x-descent)
and a second systolic flow (S_2) is the result of the descent of the base of the
left ventricle during contraction. A late forward flow enters the left atrium
during ventricular diastole (D wave) and is roughly timed with the mitral
E wave. In most cases, a careful assessment of the transmitral, tissue Doppler and pulmonary venous flow patterns, combined with Valsalva maneuver,
can provide an accurate estimate of diastolic performance and allow catego-
rization into clinical grades I to IV (Box 1).

Simple pattern recognition allows the identification of three common abnormal pulsed-wave Doppler patterns of mitral valve inflow: a LV "relaxation abnormality" pattern (mild; grade I); a "pseudonormal" pattern
(moderate; grade II); and a "restrictive physiology" pattern (severe; grade
III (reversible) or grade IV (fixed)) [41].

Two predominant mitral inflow patterns exist: (1) impaired LV relaxation
(grade I); and (2) restrictive LV filling (grade III or IV) (Fig. 10). Grade-I
diastolic dysfunction includes a reduced E wave and increased A wave,
with resultant reversal of the normal E/A ratio. An increase in the left atrial
pressure is a reliable marker for grade I. However, such a pattern is also
noted in patients with normal aging (or reduced left atrial pressure). Therefore, this pattern in isolation should be interpreted with caution. Other
echocardiographic findings that support a grade-I pattern include prolongation of the IVRT (>90 ms) and deceleration time of the E wave (>240 ms).
The pulmonary vein diastolic (PV-D) wave parallels the mitral E wave and is
decreased with an associated increase in the pulmonary vein systolic (PV-S)
wave (ratio of systolic pulmonary vein inflow velocity (S) to diastolic pulmonary vein inflow velocity (D) ([S/D ratio] >1.1).

Box 1. Echocardiographic classification of LV diastolic function

Normal diastolic function
- DT 200 ± 40 ms
- E/A ratio 1.0–2.0 (Valsalva change <0.5)
- IVRT 80 ± 10 ms
- PV S/D ratio 1.0 ± 0.1
- TDE e'/a' ratio >1.0
- E/e' ratio <8
- Vp >50 cm/s
- No structural heart disease

Grade I diastolic dysfunction (impaired relaxation pattern)
- DT >240 ms
- E/A ratio <1.0 (very elderly <0.6)
- IVRT >90 ms
- PV S/D ratio >1.1
- TDE e'/a' ratio <1.0
- E/e' >8 (occasionally >15; increased LAP)

Grade II diastolic dysfunction (pseudonormalized pattern)
- DT 200 ± 40ms
- E/A ratio 1–1.5; (Valsalva change >0.5)
- IVRT <90 ms
- PV S/D ratio <1.0
- AR >35 cm/s
- TDE e'/a' ratio <1.0
- E/e' ratio >8 (often >15)
- Evidence of structural heart disease

Grades III and IV diastolic dysfunction (restrictive filling pattern)
- DT <160 ms
- E/A ratio > 1.5–2.0 (Valsalva change <0.5 = grade 4)
- IVRT <70 ms
- PV S/D ratio <0.6
- AR >35 cm/s
- TDE e' very low (usually <3–4cm/s)
- TDE e'/a' variable
- E/e' ratio >15 (rarely 8–15)
- Evidence of structural heart disease

Abbreviations: A, late atrial mitral valve inflow velocity; a', late TDE velocity; AR, atrial reversal pulmonary vein velocity; D, diastolic pulmonary vein inflow velocity; DT, deceleration time; E, early mitral valve inflow velocity; e', early TDE velocity; E/e', ratio of mitral E to TDE e' velocities; PV, pulmonary vein; S, systolic pulmonary vein inflow velocity.

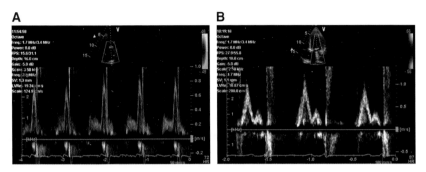

Fig. 10. Mitral inflow pulsed-wave spectral Doppler envelope in an elderly heart failure patient with grade-I diastolic dysfunction (*A*) and grade-III diastolic dysfunction (*B*). Although both patients had identical symptoms and LV EF, patient represented in *A* has a better prognosis than the patient in *B*.

Despite the limitations of echocardiography for evaluating lesser degrees of diastolic dysfunction, the presence of a "restrictive" mitral inflow filling pattern (grade III) is fairly specific for the combination of reduced ventricular compliance and elevated left atrial filling pressure. The reduction in ventricular compliance may be due to a primary abnormality of diastolic performance or secondary-to-marked systolic dysfunction. Additional Doppler alterations associated with severe diastolic dysfunction include reduced deceleration time (<160 ms), reduced IVRT (<70 ms), reduced S/D ratio (usually <0.6), and an increased atrial reversal velocity (>35 cm/s). When this restrictive filling pattern is persistent despite aggressive medical therapy or fixed and unaltered during Valsalva maneuver (E/A ratio change <0.5), then this pattern is advanced to grade IV (Fig. 11) [42].

With normal aging, grade-I patterns are common and the filling pressure of the left ventricle is usually normal due to the brief presystolic rise in pressure

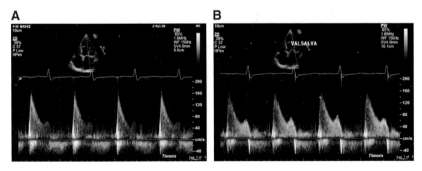

Fig. 11. Grade-III or -IV mitral inflow (restrictive filling pattern) is displayed by the high-velocity E wave, high E/A ratio, and short deceleration time (*A*). However, Valsalva maneuver is required to confirm that this is grade IV (E/A ratio change during Valsalva <0.5) and the prognosis is significantly worse than grade III (*B*).

induced by atrial contraction being compensated by the normal pressure pre-
vailing during the remainder of diastole. Age-associated nomograms have
been developed to identify acceptable values for different age groups [43].
For individuals over 60 years old, the following "extreme values" (two standard errors above the normal mean value) may be used as a reference guide:

- E/A ratio <0.60
- Deceleration time >260 ms
- Atrial reversal pulmonary vein velocity >43 cm/s
- IVRT >101 ms

These "extreme values" are unlikely be exceeded in normal aging and
may be useful for evaluating the elderly patient with HF.

The most difficult mitral inflow pattern to understand is grade II, the so-
called "pseudonormal" filling pattern. This pattern resembles a normal pattern but is actually in transition between delayed relaxation (grade I) and
restriction (grades III or IV). It should be standard practice to perform
a Valsalva maneuver during echocardiography when a "normal" pattern is
detected in an elderly patient (Fig. 12). If the mitral pattern is due to mildly
elevated filling pressure, this maneuver will briefly lower that pressure and
transiently convert this pattern to one of delayed relaxation (grade I) [44].

TDE is an important adjunct for the clarification of this "pseudonormal"
pattern and is simple to acquire, relative to pulmonary vein flow analysis.
This technique is similar to the use of Doppler ultrasound to assess blood
flow, but with a focus on the lower velocity frequency shifts of myocardial
tissue motion. By providing a quantitative representation of the motion of
the longitudinal axis of myocardial contraction and relaxation, TDE provides a new method of analyzing the extent and timing of diastolic wall motion [45]. It is important to have patients hold their breath during TDE

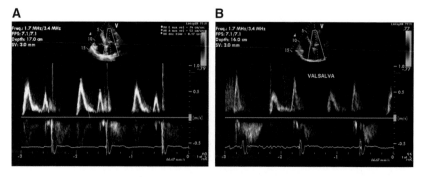

Fig. 12. Grade-II (pseudonormal) mitral inflow Doppler filling pattern may be misinterpreted
as a normal filling pattern (A). The late low-velocity slowing of the E wave is a clue to Grade-II
diastolic dysfunction, but this is dramatically shown with Valsalva, which reverses the E/A ratio
to an obvious grade-I pattern (B).

recordings to minimize artifacts from cardiac translation, since this technique is exquisitely sensitive to small alterations in cardiac motion.

The TDE-derived mitral annular velocity measured at the septal or lateral mitral annulus in the apical four-chamber view reflects changes in the long axis dimension of the left ventricle. The velocity of diastolic movement of the mitral annulus away from the cardiac apex has two peaks roughly corresponding to the E and A waves of Doppler transmitral flow. For clarification, these low velocities are referred to as e' and a' to be distinguished from the higher velocity E and A waves of mitral inflow. The transition from normal to pathologic myocardial velocities is distinct and consistent, and unlike the mitral inflow transition, it does not progress through a "pseudonormal" stage (Fig. 13). Also, the ratio of the E/e' has been repeatedly confirmed as a valid measure of left atrial pressure. The major strength is that ratios <8 and >15 (>12 if using the higher velocity lateral wall e') can confidently separate normal from elevated filling pressures.

Interrogating the pattern of pulmonary vein flow is both feasible and helpful, especially when the tissue Doppler findings are inadequate or unreliable. The pulmonary vein is assessed by using color Doppler guidance to assist in placing a pulsed Doppler sample volume in the right upper

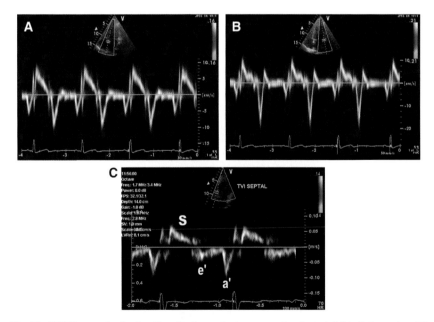

Fig. 13. TDE image obtained at the mitral annulus in a normal patient. (*A*) Medial annulus. (*B*) Lateral annulus. (*C*) TDE display in an elderly patient with class-II heart failure symptoms and a "normal appearing" mitral Doppler filling pattern. With an early TDE (e') velocity much lower than the late TDE velocity (a'), the patient is certain to have grade-II diastolic dysfunction. S, systolic wave.

pulmonary vein, located along the atrial septum (apical four-chamber view). Three distinct waves are seen: the PV-S, PV-D, and atrial reversal waves (Fig. 14). Often, the sample volume must be repositioned more distally to optimize the atrial reversal Doppler velocity envelope.

Also, in healthy older adults, the systolic fraction of pulmonary venous forward flow is greater than 50% due to a decrease in LV compliance resulting in more vigorous atrial contraction and enhanced atrial relaxation [46]. However, during faster heart rates, diastole shortens and the presystolic rise in pressure is one of the mechanisms of exercise intolerance with aging.

Another limitation of current methods for evaluating diastolic filling is that they have been well validated in sinus rhythm only. Many elderly patients have atrial fibrillation with variable cardiac cycle lengths and no organized atrial contraction. More studies are needed to optimize the assessment of diastolic function in patients with atrial fibrillation. However, the peak acceleration rate of the E wave appears to correlate well with the LV filling pressure [47]. Also, it appears that the deceleration time of the mitral valve inflow and the E/e' ratio remains prognostic [48].

The pulmonary artery pressure is readily determined by the peak velocity of tricuspid regurgitation on Doppler echocardiography. Also, Doppler echocardiography detects some degree of pulmonary regurgitation on most echocardiographic exams. This is usually of minimal hemodynamic significance and is often secondary to pulmonary hypertension, but it provides a wonderful opportunity for determining the diastolic pressure of the pulmonary artery. A pulmonary regurgitation end-diastolic velocity of ≥ 110 cm/s (equivalent to 5 mm Hg) predicts an overall worse cardiac prognosis—higher New York Heart Association functional class, higher brain natriuretic peptide, and poorer exercise tolerance—than patients with a pulmonary regurgitation end-diastolic velocity of ≤ 5 mm Hg [49]. This is equivalent to the prognostic capabilities of a tricuspid regurgitation gradient of ≥ 30 mm Hg and may be used in place of the tricuspid regurgitation when this is not present. This pulmonary regurgitation end-diastolic velocity

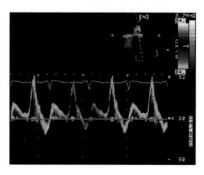

Fig. 14. PV Doppler flow display in an elderly patient with heart failure symptoms. The S/D ratio of <0.6 is consistent with elevated left-atrial pressure.

correlates with the pulmonary artery wedge pressure, regardless of the etiology of HF or severity of tricuspid regurgitation and can be used to assess changes in LV filling pressures resulting from therapy [50].

Color M-mode is another technique that allows determination of LV filling pressure and is predictive of in-hospital HF and short-term survival after a myocardial infarction [51–53]. When the ratio of the mitral inflow peak E-wave velocity to flow propagation velocity (E/Vp), as determined by the color M-mode, is >1.5, then long-term survival after a myocardial infarction is unlikely. A Vp <45 cm/s is itself a predictor of worse outcomes and a Vp <40 cm/s correlates with elevated left atrial pressure (Fig. 15).

Myocardial strain and strain-rate imaging techniques have progressed beyond research tools and entered into the clinical arena. The term "strain" refers to an object's fractional or percentage change from its original, unstressed, dimension (eg, a change in length corrected for the original length) [54]. It reflects deformation of a structure and, when applied to the myocardium, strain directly describes the contraction–relaxation pattern. Strain can be calculated in several dimensions: longitudinal, circumferential, or radial. Strain rate is the rate of this deformation. A variety of methods for measuring strain and strain rates have been developed. Tissue Doppler imaging measures the velocity of myocardial segments, either relative to the echocardiographic transducer or to the surrounding myocardium. Regression analysis and then integration of the raw velocity data produces measures of instantaneous strain. These findings have been well studied to assess for myocardial dyssynchrony and to predict a successful response to CRT (Fig. 16). These parameters have also been used to detect early, preclinical diseases of the myocardium [55].

In summary, through an extensive use of Doppler techniques, one can obtain comprehensive hemodynamic data at bedside [56]. This can be used to provide valuable diagnostic and prognostic information in the elderly patient with known or suspected HF. Doppler echo provides a useful tool for

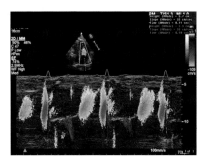

Fig. 15. Color M-mode display of the mitral inflow allows measurement of the velocity of flow propagation (Vp). In this elderly patient with grade-I mitral inflow filling pattern, the slow Vp of 33cm/s confirms that the left atrial pressure is elevated and that the filling pattern is pathologic and not a normal variation for age.

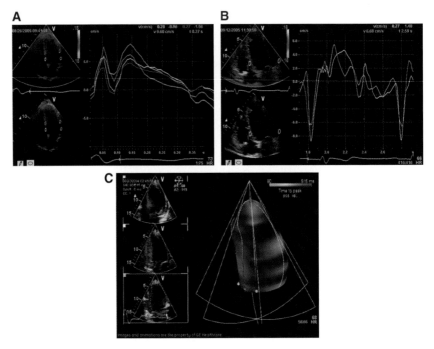

Fig. 16. Parametric color map and quantitative display of the TDE-obtained tissue velocity imaging in a normal elderly patient (*A*). Note the overlapping velocity contours from the basal septal, mid-septal and lateral walls confirming LV synchrony. In an elderly patient with a DCM, the basal septal (*yellow*) and lateral (*blue*) velocity curves do not overlap and are dyssynchronous (*B*). The same display mode can be switched from velocity, to strain and strain-rate imaging displays from the same acquired set of data. With three-dimensional acquisition modes, tissue synchronous imaging can be used to provide a three-dimensional model with thresholds for normal (*green* or *yellow*) or delayed (*red*) time-to-peak velocity graphically displayed (*C*). This elderly heart failure patient has an LBBB ECG, LV EF <30%, and is a candidate for CRT (see text for details).

assessing diastolic function in elderly patients. Because no absolute variables are available to categorize patients into mild, moderate, or severe diastolic dysfunction, all available measurements must be evaluated to minimize interpretive error. Normal aging alters these parameters and the aforementioned extreme values are provided in an effort to minimize false diagnoses.

Prognosis determination

Symptoms or exercise tolerance have no predictable relationship to the LV EF. Some patients are asymptomatic with an LV EF below 20%, while others are moribund with an LV EF above 30%. In general, survival is shorter in patients with lower LV EF [57,58]. The differentiation of normal versus reduced LV systolic function is not only vitally important for subsequent treatment considerations, but it also impacts prognosis. In one study, the single greatest predictor of mortality in elderly patients with HF (and associated coronary artery disease) was the EF [59]. This prospective evaluation revealed that 47% of all elderly patients with congestive HF had normal LV systolic function. Despite having coronary heart disease, 41% of these patients still had normal systolic function. Survival rates in this group were 78% at 1 year, 62% at 2 years, and 44% at 4 years. In contrast, survival rates for patients with reduced LV systolic function were only 53% at 1 year, 29% at 2 years, and 15% at 4 years. In the Vasodilator Heart Failure Trial, patients with congestive HF and normal EFs had an average annual mortality rate of 8%, but those with abnormal EFs had an annual mortality rate of 19% [60]. Thus, echocardiography can assist in determining prognosis (Table 1).

LV EDV index often exceeds 100 mL/m^2 (upper normal is approximately 70 mL/m^2). LV size is another critical predictor of outcome and a LF EDV index >120 mL/m^2 predicts a worse outcome for HF patients [61]. ESV index of 45 mL/m^2 identifies patients with a poor outcome [62].

Death from HF or an appropriate implantable–cardioverter-defribrillator shock was evaluated in 84 patients with chronic HF and a mean LV EF of 29% [63]. Of those 84 patients, 22 (26%) had experienced an event by the time of the 1-year follow-up. Seven of those 22 died. In

Table 1
Studies using echocardiography to predict survival of elderly patients with heart failure

Population	Echocardiographic data	Survival after 1 year	After 2 years
Elderly with HF [57]	Normal LV EF	78%	62%
	Reduced LV EF	53%	29%
Vasodilator Heart Failure Trial [58]	Normal LV EF	92%	
	Reduced LV EF	81%	
HF, ICD, mean EF 29% (n = 84) [61]	Grade ≥III	72%	
	Grade <III	38%	
Chronic HF (n = 173) [65]	Grade I or II DD	94%	
	Grade III DD	81%	
	Grade IV DD	45%	
CM (76% CAD) (n = 144) [66]	Grade III		89%
	Grade IV		63%
DSE (elderly HF) [67]	Grade III (rev w/ Dob)	79%	
	Grade IV (fix w/ Dob)	49%	
98% Male (n = 4000) [68]	IVC >50% collapse	95%	
	IVC <50% collapse	67%	
Class II, III HF [69]	RV EF >35%		93%
	RV EF 25%–35%		77%
	RV EF <25%		59%

Abbreviations: CAD, coronary artery disease; CM, cardiomyopathy; DD, diastolic dysfunction; DSE, dobutamine stress echo; fix w/ Dob, restrictive filling pattern remains unchanged with dobutamine; HF, heart failure; IVC, inferior vena cava; rev w/ Dob, restrictive filling pattern improves with dobutamine.

comparison to the patients who did not have an event, those 22 patients had longer QRS durations (169 versus 146ms), higher mitral E/e' ratios (16.0 versus 12.8), and a more frequent filling pattern (44% versus 9%). Multivariate regression analysis identified a restrictive filling pattern as the only independent predictor of an event (hazard ratio = 3.65) and the event-free survival rate was 38% versus 72% compared with those without a restrictive filling pattern.

Echocardiography and catheterization were performed in elderly patients (mean age: 64) and a multiple regression model of all echocardiographic variables showed that the addition of the E/e' ratio to the clinical history and LV EF provided incremental prognostic information [64]. An E/e' ratio of ≥ 15 identified those with a higher risk of new-onset or recurrent HF.

The presence of restrictive filling pattern has significant prognostic implications. In patients with dilated cardiomyopathy, this pattern is more predictive of the development of severe symptoms than are indices of systolic function. In patients with amyloidosis, restrictive filling is associated with poor 1-year survival [65,66].

The prognostic value of abnormal mitral flow velocity may be enhanced by assessing changes in this parameter during alterations in loading conditions. This was illustrated in a report of 173 patients with chronic HF. The report measured the outcomes at 17 months in four subgroups that were distinguished by differences in changes in mitral valve flow velocity observed during nitroprusside infusion (resulting in a reversible or nonreversible restrictive pattern) and passive leg lifting (resulting in a stable or unstable nonrestrictive pattern) [67]. In this study, the event rate of cardiac death or urgent transplantation worsened progressively from a stable nonrestrictive pattern (6%), to a reversible restrictive pattern (19%), to an unstable nonrestrictive pattern (33%), and finally to an irreversible restrictive pattern (55%).

In 144 patients with HF (76% with coronary artery disease), an initial restrictive pattern that resolved by 6 months of optimal medical therapy had a lower cardiac mortality (11% versus 37%) at 2 years than those without Doppler improvements. This reversible restrictive filling pattern (grade III) has consistently proven superior for survival relative to a fixed restrictive filling pattern (grade IV) [68]. The Valsalva maneuver is a simple, bedside technique to deliver similar prognostic value and should be performed in all elderly HF patients with a restrictive filling pattern. The effect of dobutamine stress on a restrictive pattern also appears to have prognostic value and a restrictive LV filling at rest, which reverts to a nonrestrictive pattern during dobutamine infusion, has a markedly improved survival (79% versus 49%) over a fixed pattern. Persistence of the restrictive pattern was associated with a marked rise in left atrial pressure and a markedly attenuated inotropic response [69]. During stress echocardiography, this mitral inflow pattern should be sought for its incremental prognostic capability.

A dilated inferior vena cava without collapse during inspiration is associated with worse survival in men independent of a history of HF, other comorbidities, ventricular function, and pulmonary artery pressure (Fig. 17).
The inferior vena cava response to "sniffing," with > 50% reduction in diameter being normal, is not only a predictor of elevated right atrial pressure,
but a predictor of survival. In a series of more than 4000 consecutive outpatient echocardiograms (98% men), survival rates were strongly influenced by
the inferior vena cava appearance. In patients with an inspiratory collapse of
their inferior vena cava, the survival rates were 99% after 90 days and 95%
after 1 year, as compared to 89% after 90 days and 67% after 1 year for
those with < 50% collapse [70].

RV systolic dysfunction also may contribute to prognosis in patients with
HF [71]. Echocardiographic measurements of reduced RV function include
a reduction in RV EF fraction, RV enlargement, and tricuspid regurgitation. In patients with class-II or -III HF, the RV EF was an independent
predictor of 1- and 2-year survival and event-free cardiac survival. At 2
years, the event-free survival rates from cardiovascular mortality and urgent
transplantation was 93% for those with an RV EF of 35%; 77% for those

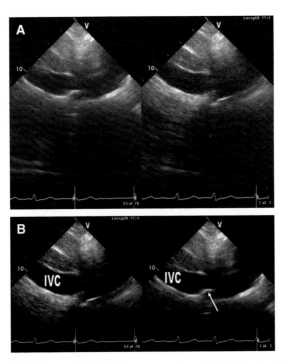

Fig. 17. Subcostal 2DE image of the inferior vena cava in an elderly female with class-III heart
failure (*A*). The inferior vena cava (IVC) is dilated at held expiration (*left*) and does not collapse
with inspiration (*right*). This confirms elevated right atrial pressure and is associated with a poor
prognosis. Note the diaphragm motion during sniffing (*white arrow* in *B*).

with an RV EF ≥ 25 but $<35\%$; and 59% for those with an RV EF $<25\%$. In addition to the RV EF, the severity of tricuspid regurgitation is also associated with prognosis [72].

Discussion

The human and economic burden of HF increases with aging. Only during the past decade have surveys incorporated echocardiography to confirm structural heart disease in people with nonspecific symptoms. Multiple studies have confirmed that the incidence of structural heart disease exceeds the clinical findings [73–77]. In one such cross-sectional observational study of more than 2000 elderly people (60–86 years old), prevalence rates of clinical HF and LV systolic dysfunction (LV EF $\leq 50\%$) were studied [78]. These investigators confirmed that clinical HF increased with advancing age with a 4.4-fold increase from early 1960s to early 1980s. LV systolic dysfunction occurred more commonly than clinical HF, suggesting that symptoms only reveal the tip of the iceberg. Although 21.1% had structural heart disease, only 6.3% had clinical HF. Moreover, of the 5.9% of participants with LV systolic dysfunction, 59% were in the preclinical stage of disease.

In another study, investigators reported a 6% to 10% prevalence of clinical HF in patients over 65 [79]. In this study, HF status was ascertained using clinical scores that have a poor sensitivity and specificity for structural heart disease. Since secondary preventive measures have been shown to be effective for patients with preclinical LV systolic dysfunction, these preclinical disease states must be identified. Targeted screening programs of high-risk people (such as older age groups) should be evaluated for their cost-effectiveness and echocardiography is the ideal tool for this purpose.

Just as systolic dysfunction is frequently preclinical, diastolic dysfunction, even when moderate to severe, may be asymptomatic. In a community-based survey of more than 2000 subjects, 28% had diastolic dysfunction (7.3% moderate to severe), despite only 1% with symptoms [73].

In addition to diastolic dysfunction, transient LV systolic dysfunction, as seen with myocardial ischemia, may also present as congestive HF with normal, resting LV systolic function. A regional wall-motion abnormality, often subtle at rest, may be the only echocardiographic finding. Therefore, in patients with severe HF symptoms, normal wall motion and normal or mildly abnormal diastolic function, myocardial ischemia should be suspected and consideration given for the performance of stress echocardiography. By measuring the degree of LV thickening and the diameter of the LV cavity, the ventricular mass/volume ratio can be obtained and may facilitate the separation of patients likely to have myocardial ischemia, despite similar degrees of diastolic dysfunction and exercise intolerance. Patients with a low ratio (<1.8), indicating less myocardial mass, are more likely to have coronary artery disease with up to 80% having severe coronary artery stenosis [35]. Conversely, in patients with a ventricular mass/volume ratio >1.8, the etiology is more often progressive LV hypertrophy due to hypertension, and these patients are less likely to have coronary artery disease (Fig. 18). This assessment allows therapy to be properly aimed at either LV hypertrophy regression or, more specifically, the improvement of myocardial ischemia.

In addition to the LV EF, the size and shape of the left ventricle, as well as the Doppler findings, may predict the development and severity of congestive HF symptoms. In a substudy of the Studies of Left Ventricular Dysfunction-95, 311 patients with symptomatic LV dysfunction (treatment arm) and 258 patients with asymptomatic LV dysfunction (prevention arm) were evaluated [80]. Compared with patients without symptoms, symptomatic patients had larger LV end-diastolic diameters and LV ESVs, higher sphericity indexes (a measure of the "roundness" of the LV), and a higher E/A ratio. These patients also had a greater incidence of ventricular dysrhythmias. These data suggest that both diastolic properties and the degree of ventricular remodeling affect the clinical status of patients with LV dysfunction, and that echocardiography provides useful information in this assessment.

Few studies have investigated the use and impact of echocardiography in the management of congestive HF. In one such study, the management and clinical outcome of patients with congestive HF were classified according to whether or not an echocardiogram was performed [81]. Although limited by its retrospective design, this study revealed that patients who did not receive an echocardiogram had decreased survival, increased morbidity, and underuse of angiotensin-converting enzyme inhibitor (ACEI) therapy.

With the aid of echocardiography, the elderly patient with HF can be skillfully treated, assessed for treatment response, referred for surgery when indicated, and counseled regarding prognosis. Without knowledge of LV systolic and diastolic function, ACEI, digoxin, and diuretics may

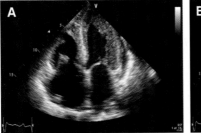 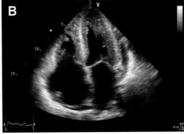

Fig. 18. Apical four-chamber view (A) diastole (B) systole in a 61-year-old female with progressive heart failure symptoms. The LV and RV myocardial walls are thickened, the size of the LV cavity is normal, and the LV mass/volume ratio is > 1.8, lowering the likelihood that the etiology of LV systolic dysfunction is coronary artery disease. This patient had cardiac amyloidosis, which was suggested by the "sparkled" myocardial appearance, thickened valves and atrial septum, small pericardial effusion, and the restrictive 2DE and mitral Doppler inflow.

be used inappropriately in the 40% to 50% of elderly patients who have a normal LV systolic function. Furthermore, the unfortunate patient with unsuspected, surgically correctable, valvular heart disease would go untreated and remain at risk for progressive, irreversible myocardial damage.

Summary

Echocardiography allows the assessment of systolic and diastolic function and identifies many of the common causes of HF. Patients with minimally symptomatic or unsuspected LV systolic dysfunction may be identified and receive the benefits of ACEI therapy. Echocardiography is also useful for assessing the prognosis and can be used serially to evaluate the effectiveness of treatment. Ventricular filling pressures, pulmonary artery pressures, and cardiac output can be sequentially determined.

Box 2. Echocardiographic approach to the elderly patient with heart failure

Step 1. Visually estimate LV systolic function
- If normal (LV EF definitely >55%), proceed to step 2. If intermediate (LV EF 30%–55%), proceed to step 3.
- If indeterminate (unable to assess LV EF), proceed to step 3. If severely reduced (LV EF <30%), proceed to step 4.

Step 2. Evaluate diastolic function
- Use "extreme values" (see text) in the elderly population.
- Consider ischemic heart disease and stress echocardiography.
- Carefully evaluate for valvular heart disease (especially aortic stenosis and mitral regurgitation in elderly). Assess RV function (and pulmonary pressures).

Step 3. Quantify LV systolic function
- Employ volumetric methods (two-dimensional and three-dimensional modified Simpson's rule).
- Obtain three-dimensional volume-rendered echocardiogram.
- Use contrast microbubbles if two consecutive apical wall segments not seen. Proceed to Step 4 and compare results with hemodynamic findings.

Step 4. Hemodynamic and prognostic assessment
- Estimate left atrial pressure (E/e' ratio; Vp; PV S/D ratio; Valsalva response). Determine the right atrial pressure from inferior vena cava (response to "sniff").
- Estimate the pulmonary arterial pressures, RV function.
- Determine LV synchrony and consider CRT candidacy.

The authors believe that all patients with HF should receive careful assessment with 2DE, M-mode echocardiography, and Doppler echocardiography (with strategic use of contrast and 3DE where available) (Box 2). Furthermore, the authors believe the use of echocardiography is especially valuable in the elderly who have the poorest prognosis and are more likely to have HF with a normal LV EF or a reduced LV EF and no clinical symptoms.

References

[1] Kannel WB, Belanger AJ. Epidemiology of heart failure. Am Heart J 1991;121:951–7.

[2] Bonow RO, Udelson JE. Left ventricular diastolic dysfunction as a cause of congestive heart failure: mechanisms and management. Ann Intern Med 1992;117:502–10.

[3] Ihlen H, Amlie JP, Dale J, et al. Determination of cardiac output by Doppler echocardiography. Br Heart J 1984;51:54.

[4] Ghali JK, Kadakia S, Cooper RS, et al. Bedside diagnosis of preserved versus impaired left ventricular systolic function in heart failure. Am J Cardiol 1992;67:1002–6.

[5] Sorrell VL, Nanda NC. Role of echocardiography in the diagnosis and management of heart failure in the elderly. Clin Geriatr Med 2000;16:457–76.

[6] Parisi AF, Moyihan PF, Folland ED, et al. Approaches to determination of left ventricular volumes and ejection fraction by real-time two-dimensional echocardiography. Clin Cardiol 1979;2:257.

[7] Caidahl K, Kazzam E, Lidberg J, et al. New concept in echocardiography: harmonic imaging of tissue without use of a contrast agent. Lancet 1998;352:1264–70.

[8] Senior R. Role of contrast echocardiography for the assessment of left ventricular function. Echocardiogr 1999;16:747–52.

[9] Vandenberg BF, Rath LS, Stuhlmuller P, et al. Estimation of left ventricular cavity area with an on-line, semi-automated echocardiographic edge detection system. Circulation 1992;86: 159–66.

[10] Corsi C, Lang RM, Veronesi F, et al. Volumetric quantification of global and regional left ventricular function from real-time three-dimensional echocardiographic images. Circulation 2005;112:1161.

[11] Marcus ML, Skorton DJ, Schelbert HR, et al, editors. Cardiac imaging—a companion to Braunwald's heart disease. 3rd edition. Philadelphia (PA): W.B. Saunders; 1991. p. 377.

[12] Richardson P, McKenna W, Bristow M, et al. Report of the 1995 World Health Organization/International Society and Federation of Cardiology Task Force on the Definition and Classification of Cardiomyopathies. Circulation 1996;93:841.

[13] Simonson JS, Schiller NB. Descent of the base of the left ventricle: an echocardiographic index of left ventricular function. J Am Soc Echocardiogr 1989;2:25.

[14] Vandenbossche JL, Massie BM, Schiller NB, et al. Relation of left ventricular shape to volume and mass in patients with minimally symptomatic chronic aortic regurgitation. Am Heart J 1988;116:1022.

[15] Gorcsan J III, Denault A, Gasior TA, et al. Rapid estimation of left ventricular contractility from end-systolic relations by echocardiographic automated border detection and femoral arterial pressure. Anesthesiology 1994;81:553.

[16] Yoerger DM, Marcus FL, Sherrill D, et al. Multidisciplinary study of right ventricular dysplasia investigators. Echocardiographic findings in patients meeting task force criteria for arrhythmogenic right ventricular dysplasia: new insights from the multidisciplinary study of right ventricular dysplasia. J Am Coll Cardiol 2005;45:860–5.

[17] Cerqueira MD. Standardized myocardial segmentation and nomenclature for tomographic imaging of the heart. A statement for healthcare professionals from the Cardiac Imaging

Committee of the Council on Clinical Cardiology of the American Heart Association. Circulation 2002;105:539.

[18] Acquatella H, Schiller NB. Echocardiographic recognition of Chagas' disease and endomyocardial fibrosis. J Am Soc Echocardiogr 1988;1:60.

[19] Bodiwala K, Miller AP, Nanda NC, et al. Live three-dimensional transthoracic echocardiographic assessment of ventricular noncompaction. Echocardiogr 2005;22:611–20.

[20] Nanda NC, Gramiak R, Robinson TI, et al. Echocardiographic evaluation of pulmonary hypertension. Circulation 1974;50:575–81.

[21] McConnell MV, Solomon SD, Rayan ME, et al. Regional right ventricular dysfunction detected by echocardiography in acute pulmonary embolism. Am J Cardiol 1996;78:469–73.

[22] Kotler MN, Mintz GS, Parry WR, et al. Bedside diagnosis of organic murmurs in the elderly. Geriatrics 1981;36:107–25.

[23] Fan PH, Kapur KK, Nanda NC. Color-guided Doppler echocardiographic assessment in assessment of aortic valve stenosis. J Am Coll Cardiol 1998;12:441–9.

[24] Naqvi TZ, Siegel RJ. Aortic stenosis: the role of transesophageal echocardiography. Echocardiogr 1999;16:677–88.

[25] Bermejo J, Garcia-Fernandez MA, Antoranz JC, et al. Stress echocardiography in aortic stenosis: insights into valve mechanics and hemodynamics. Echocardiogr 1999;16:689–99.

[26] Vengala S, Nanda NC, Dod H, et al. Usefulness of live three-dimensional transthoracic echocardiography in aortic valve stenosis evaluation. Am J Geriatr Cardiol 2004;13: 279–84.

[27] Bargiggia GS, Tronconi L, Sahn DJ, et al. A new method for quantitation of mitral regurgitation based on color flow Doppler imaging of flow convergence proximal to regurgitant oriface. Circulation 1991;84:1481.

[28] Khanna D, Vengala S, Miller AP, et al. Quantification of mitral regurgitation by live three-dimensional transthoracic echocardiographic measurements of vena contracta area. Echocardiography 2004;21:737–43.

[29] Khanna D, Miller AP, Nanda NC, et al. Transthoracic and transesophageal echocardiographic assessment of mitral regurgitation severity: usefulness of qualitative and semi-quantitative techniques. Echocardiography 2005;22:748–69.

[30] Ling LH, Enriquez-Sarano M, Seward JB, et al. Clinical outcome of mitral regurgitation due to flail leaflet. N Engl J Med 1996;335:1417–23.

[31] Ghio S, Recusani F, Klersy C, et al. Prognostic usefulness of the tricuspid annular plane systolic excursion in patients with congestive heart failure secondary to idiopathic or ischemic dilated cardiomyopathy. Am J Cardiol 2000;85:837.

[32] Bleeker GB, Schalij MJ, Molhoek SG, et al. Comparison of effectiveness of cardiac resynchronization therapy in patients <70 versus >/= 70 years of age. Am J Cardiol 2005; 96:420–2.

[33] Suffoletto MS, Dohi K, Cannesson M, et al. Novel speckle-tracking radial strain from routine black-and-white echocardiographic images to quantify dyssynchrony and predict response to cardiac resynchronization therapy. Circulation 2006;113:960–8.

[34] Cahill JM, Ryan E, Travers B, et al. Progression of preserved systolic function heart failure to systolic dysfunction—a natural history study. Int J Cardiol 2006;106:95–102.

[35] Iriarte M, Murga N, Sagastagoitia D, et al. Congestive heart failure from left ventricular diastolic dysfunction in systemic hypertension. Am J Cardiol 1993;71:308–12.

[36] Gola A, Pozzoli M, Capomolla S, et al. Comparison of Doppler echocardiography with thermodilution for assessing cardiac output in advanced congestive heart failure. Am J Cardiol 1996;78:708.

[37] Tei C, Ling LH, Hodge DO, et al. New index of combined systolic and diastolic myocardial performance: a simple and reproducible measure of cardiac function—a study in normals and dilated cardiomyopathy. J Cardiol 1995;26:357–66.

[38] Tei C, Dujardin KS, Hodge DO, et al. Doppler echocardiographic index for assessment of global right ventricular function. J Am Soc Echocardiogr 1996;9:838–47.

[39] Zile MR, Gaasch WH, Carroll JD, et al. Heart failure with a normal ejection fraction: is measurement of diastolic function necessary to make the diagnosis of diastolic heart failure? Circulation 2001;104:779.

[40] Thomas JD, Weyman AE. Echocardiographic Doppler evaluation of left ventricular diastolic function: physics and physiology. Circulation 1991;84:977.

[41] Nishimura RA, Tajik AJ. Evaluation of diastolic filling of the left ventricle in health and disease: Doppler echocardiography is the clinician's Rosetta Stone. J Am Coll Cardiol 1997;30: 8–18.

[42] Pinamonti B, Zecchin M, Di Lenarda A, et al. Persistence of restrictive left ventricular filling pattern in dilated cardiomyopathy: an ominous prognostic sign. J Am Coll Cardiol 1997;29: 604–12.

[43] Oh JK, Seward JB, Tajik AJ. The echo manual. 2nd Edition. Philadelphia (PA): Lippincott—Raven; 1999. p. 53.

[44] Dumesnil JG, Gaudreault G, Honos GN, et al. Use of Valsalva maneuver to unmask left ventricular diastolic function abnormalities by Doppler echocardiography in patients with coronary artery disease or systemic hypertension. Am J Cardiol 1991;68:515–9.

[45] Marwick TH. Clinical applications of tissue Doppler imaging: a promise fulfilled. Heart 2003;89:1377.

[46] Klein AL, Burstow DJ, Tajik AJ, et al. Effects of age on left ventricular dimensions and filling dynamics in 117 normal persons. Mayo Clin Proc 1994;69:212.

[47] Nagueh SF, Kopellen HA, Quinones MA. Assessment of left ventricular filling pressures by Doppler in the presence of atrial fibrillation. Circulation 1996;94:2138–45.

[48] Hurrell DG, Oh JK, Mahoney DW, et al. Short deceleration time of mitral inflow E velocity: prognostic implication with atrial fibrillation versus sinus rhythm. J Am Soc Echocardiogr 1998;11:450–7.

[49] Ristow B, Ahmed S, Wang L, et al. Pulmonary regurgitation end-diastolic gradient is a Doppler marker of cardiac status: data from the Heart and Soul Study. J Am Soc Echocardiogr 2005;18:885–91.

[50] Drazner MH, Hamilton MA, Fonarow G, et al. Relationship between right and left-sided filling pressures in 1000 patients with advanced heart failure. J Heart Lung Transplant 1999;18:1126.

[51] Sohn DW, Chai IH, Lee DJ, et al. Assessment of mitral annulus velocity by Doppler tissue imaging in the evaluation of left ventricular diastolic function. J Am Coll Cardiol 1997;30: 474–80.

[52] Thomas JD, Greenberg NA, Vandervoort PM, et al. Digital analysis of transmitral color Doppler M-mode data: a potential new approach to the noninvasive assessment of diastolic function. Comput Cardiol 1992;1(1):631–4.

[53] Moller JE, Sondergaard E, Seward JB, et al. Ratio of left ventricular peak E-wave velocity to flow propagation velocity assessed by color M-mode Doppler echocardiography in first myocardial infarction: prognostic and clinical implications. J Am Coll Cardiol 2000;35:363.

[54] Sorrell VL, Reeves WC. Noninvasive right and left heart catheterization: taking the echo lab beyond an image-only laboratory. Echocardiography 2001;18:31–41.

[55] Marwick TH. Measurement of strain and strain rate by echocardiography: ready for prime time? J Am Coll Cardiol 2006;47:1313.

[56] Lee R, Hanekom L, Marwick TH, et al. Prediction of subclinical left ventricular dysfunction with strain rate imaging in patients with asymptomatic severe mitral regurgitation. Am J Cardiol 2004;94:1333.

[57] Wong M, Staszewsky L, Latini R, et al. Severity of left ventricular remodeling defines outcomes and response to therapy in heart failure: Valsartan heart failure trial (Val-HeFT) echocardiographic data. J Am Coll Cardiol 2004;43:2022.

[58] Quinones MA, Greenberg BH, Kopelen HA, et al. Echocardiographic predictors of clinical outcome in patients with left ventricular dysfunction enrolled in the SOLVD registry and trials: significance of left ventricular hypertrophy. J Am Coll Cardiol 2000;35:1237.

[59] Aronow WS, Ahn C, Kronzon I. Prognosis of congestive heart failure in elderly patients with normal versus abnormal left ventricular systolic function associated with coronary artery disease. Am J Cardiol 1990;66:1257–9.

[60] Cohn JN, Johnson G. Veterans Administration Cooperative Study Group. Heart failure with normal ejection fraction. The V-HeFT study. Circulation 1980;81(suppl III): III-48–53.

[61] Grayburn PA, Appleton CP, DeMaria AN, et al. Echocardiographic predictors of morbidity and mortality in patients with advanced heart failure: the Beta-blocker Evaluation of Survival Trial (BEST). J Am Coll Cardiol 2005;45:1064.

[62] White HD, Norris RM, Brown MA, et al. Left ventricular end-systolic volume as the major determinant of survival after recovery from myocardial infarction. Circulation 1987; 76:44.

[63] Bruch C, Gotzmann M, Sindermann J, et al. Prognostic value of a restrictive mitral filling pattern in patients with systolic heart failure and an implantable cardioverter-defibrillator. Am J Cardiol 2006;97:676–80.

[64] Liang HY, Cauduro SA, Pellikka PA, et al. Comparison of usefulness of echocardiographic Doppler variables to left ventricular end-diastolic pressure in predicting future heart failure events. Am J Cardiol 2006;97:866–71.

[65] Klein AL, et al. Prognostic significance of Doppler measures of diastolic function in cardiac amyloidosis: a Doppler echocardiography study. Circulation 1991;83:808.

[66] Vanoverschelde J-LJ, Raphael DA, Robert AR, et al. Left ventricular filling in dilated cardiomyopathy: relation to functional class and hemodynamics. J Am Coll Cardiol 1990;15: 1288.

[67] Pozzoli M, Traversi E, Cioffi G, et al. Loading manipulation improves the prognostic value of Doppler evaluation of mitral valve flow in patients with chronic heart failure. Circulation 1997;95:1222.

[68] Temporelli PL, Corra U, Imparto A, et al. Reversible restrictive left ventricular diastolic filling with optimized oral therapy predicts a more favorable prognosis in patients with chronic heart failure. J Am Coll Cardiol 1998;31:1591.

[69] Duncan AM, Lim E, Gibson DG, et al. Effect of dobutamine stress on left ventricular filling in ischemic dilated cardiomyopathy: pathophysiology and prognostic implications. J Am Coll Cardiol 2005;46:488.

[70] Nath J, Vacek JL, Heidenreich PA. A dilated inferior vena cava is a marker of poor survival. Am Heart J 2006;151:730–5.

[71] De Groote P, Millaire A, Foucher-Hossein C, et al. Right ventricular ejection fraction is an independent predictor of survival in patients with moderate heart failure. J Am Coll Cardiol 1998;32:948.

[72] Hung J, Koelling T, Semigran MJ, et al. Usefulness of echocardiographic determined tricuspid regurgitation in predicting event-free survival in severe heart failure secondary to idiopathic-dilated cardiomyopathy or to ischemic cardiomyopathy. Am J Cardiol 1998; 82:1301.

[73] Redfield MM, Jacobsen SJ, Burnett JC Jr, et al. Burden of systolic and diastolic ventricular dysfunction in the community: appreciating the scope of the heart failure epidemic. JAMA 2003;289:194–202.

[74] Mosterd A, Hoes AW, de Bruyne MC, et al. Prevalence of heart failure and left ventricular dysfunction in the general population: the Rotterdam study. Eur Heart J 1999;20:447–55.

[75] Davies M, Hobbs F, Davis R, et al. Prevalence of left-ventricular systolic dysfunction and heart failure in the Echocardiographic Heart of England Screening Study: a population-based study. Lancet 2001;358:439–44.

[76] McDonagh TA, Morrison CE, Lawrence A, et al. Symptomatic and asymptomatic left-ventricular systolic dysfunction in an urban population. Lancet 1997;350:829–33.

[77] Devereux RB, Roman MJ, Paranicas M, et al. A population-based assessment of left ventricular systolic dysfunction in middle-aged and older adults: the Strong Heart Study. Am Heart J 2001;141:439–46.

[78] Abhayaratna WP, Smith WT, Becker NG, et al. Prevalence of heart failure and systolic ventricular dysfunction in older Australians: the Canberra Heart Study. MJA 2006;184:151–4.

[79] Kannel WB. Epidemiology and prevention of cardiac failure: Framingham Study insights. Eur Heart J 1987;8(Suppl F):23–6.

[80] Koilpillai C, Quinones MA, Greenberg B, et al. Relation of ventricular size and function to heart failure status and ventricular dysrhythmia in patients with severe left ventricular dysfunction. Am J Cardiol 1996;78:606–11.

[81] Senni M, Rodeheffer RJ, Tribouilloy CM, et al. Use of echocardiography in the management of congestive heart failure in the community. J Am Coll Cardiol 1999;33:164–70.

ELSEVIER
SAUNDERS

CLINICS IN
GERIATRIC
MEDICINE

Clin Geriatr Med 23 (2007) 61–81

Treatment of Heart Failure with Abnormal Left Ventricular Systolic Function in the Elderly

Wilbert S. Aronow, MD

Department of Medicine, Divisions of Cardiology,
Geriatrics, and Pulmonary/Critical Care Medicine, Westchester Medical Center,
New York Medical College, Macy Pavilion, Room 138, Valhalla, NY 10595, USA

The American College of Cardiology (ACC)/American Heart Association (AHA) guidelines for the evaluation and management of heart failure (HF) define four stages of HF [1]. Patients with stage-A HF are at high risk of developing HF because of conditions strongly associated with the development of HF [1]. These patients have hypertension, coronary artery disease, diabetes mellitus, a history of cardiotoxic drug therapy, alcohol abuse, a history of rheumatic fever, or a family history of cardiomyopathy. These patients have no evidence of structural heart disease.

Patients with stage-B HF have structural heart disease associated with the development of HF, but have never shown symptoms or signs of HF [1]. These patients have a prior myocardial infarction, left ventricular (LV) hypertrophy or fibrosis, LV dilatation or hypocontractility, or asymptomatic valvular heart disease [1].

Patients with stage-C HF have current or prior symptoms of HF associated with structural heart disease [1]. Patients with stage-D HF have advanced structural heart disease and marked symptoms of HF at rest despite maximal medical therapy. These patients require specialized interventions [1].

Treatment of stage-A heart failure

In patients with stage-A HF, clinicians should treat hypertension [1,2] and lipid disorders [1,3,4]; encourage regular exercise; discourage smoking,

---

E-mail address: WSAronow@aol.com

alcohol consumption, and illicit drug use; control the ventricular rate in patients with supraventricular tachyarrhythmias; and use angiotensin-converting enzyme (ACE) inhibitors in patients with atherosclerotic vascular disease, diabetes mellitus, or hypertension [1]. Diabetics should be treated as if they had coronary artery disease [5]. Educational programs may be needed to increase the use of lipid-lowering drugs [6,7].

Treatment of stage-B heart failure

The ACC/AHA guidelines recommend in patients with stage-B HF treatment with all stage-A measures, treatment with ACE inhibitors and β-blockers, and valve replacement or repair for patients with hemodynamically significant valvular stenosis or regurgitation [1].

General measure for treatment of stage-C heart failure

Underlying and precipitating causes of HF should be identified and treated when possible. Hypertension should be treated with diuretics, ACE inhibitors, and β-blockers. Myocardial ischemia should be treated with nitrates and β-blockers.

Older persons who have HF without contraindications to coronary revascularization, and who have exercise-limiting angina pectoris, angina pectoris occurring frequently at rest, or recurrent episodes of acute pulmonary edema despite optimal medical therapy, should have coronary angiography. Coronary artery bypass graft surgery or percutaneous transluminal coronary angioplasty should be performed in selected patients with myocardial ischemia attributable to viable myocardium subserved by severely stenotic coronary arteries.

If clinically indicated, selected patients should have surgical correction of valvular lesions, surgical excision of a dyskinetic LV aneurysm, surgical correction of a systemic arteriovenous fistula, and surgical resection of the pericardium for constrictive pericarditis. Infective endocarditis should be treated with intravenous antibiotics and with surgical replacement of valvular lesions if clinically indicated. Anemia, infection, bronchospasm, hypoxia, tachyarrhythmias, bradyarrhythmias, obesity, hyperthyroidism, and hypothyroidism should be treated.

Oral warfarin should be given to patients with HF who have prior systemic or pulmonary embolism, atrial fibrillation, or cardiac thrombi detected by two-dimensional echocardiography. The dose of warfarin administered should achieve an International Normalized Ratio of 2.0 to 3.0. A surgical procedure should be performed if anticoagulant therapy fails to prevent pulmonary embolism. Beriberi heart disease should be treated with thiamine. A transvenous pacemaker should be implanted into the right ventricle of a patient with HF and complete atrioventricular block or severe bradycardia.

Patients with HF should have their sodium intake reduced to 1.6 to 2.0 g of sodium (4–5 g of sodium chloride) daily. Spices and herbs instead of sodium chloride should be used to flavor food. Normal fluid intake with sodium restriction is the general recommendation. Fluid intake should be restricted if dilutional hyponatremia develops and the serum sodium concentration falls below 130 mEq/L. Through patient education, patient compliance should be stressed, such as the need for salt restriction, fluid restriction, and daily weights.

Patients with HF should avoid exposure to heavy air pollution. Air conditioning is essential for patients with HF who are in hot, humid environments. Ethyl alcohol intake should be avoided. Medications that precipitate or exacerbate HF, such as nonsteroidal anti-inflammatory (NSAIDs) and antiarrhythmic drugs, other than β-blockers, digoxin, amiodarone, and dofetilide, should be stopped (Box 1) [1]. Regular physical activity, such as walking, should be encouraged in patients with mild-to-moderate HF to improve functional status and to decrease symptoms. Patients with HF who are dyspneic at rest at a low work level may benefit from a formal cardiac rehabilitation program (see Box 1) [1,8]. A multidisciplinary approach to care is useful [9].

Diuretics

Diuretics are the first-line drugs in the treatment of older patients with HF and volume overload (see Box 1). Diuretics decrease venous return, reduce ventricular filling pressures, cause loss of fluid from the body, and decrease symptoms of pulmonary and systemic congestion and edema. Age-related decreases in renal function and in circulating plasma volume may reduce the efficacy of diuretics in elderly patients with HF.

A thiazide diuretic, such as hydrochlorothiazide, may be used to treat elderly patients with mild HF. However, a thiazide diuretic is ineffective if the glomerular filtration rate is less than 30 mL/min. Elderly patients with moderate or severe HF should be treated with a loop diuretic such as furosemide. These patients should not take NSAIDs because these drugs may inhibit the induction of diuresis by furosemide. Elderly patients with severe HF or concomitant renal insufficiency may need the addition of metolazone to the loop diuretic. Severe volume overload should be treated with intravenous diuretics and hospitalization.

Elderly patients with HF treated with diuretics need close monitoring of their serum electrolytes. Hypokalemia and hypomagnesemia, both of which may precipitate ventricular arrhythmias and digitalis toxicity, may develop. Hyponatremia with activation of the renin-angiotensin-aldosterone system may occur.

Elderly patients with HF are especially sensitive to volume depletion. Dehydration and prerenal azotemia may occur if excessive doses of diuretics are given. Therefore, the minimum effective dose of diuretics should be used.

Box 1. Class-I recommendations for treating heart failure with abnormal LV systolic function

- Use all class-I recommendations for treating stage-A and -B heart failure (HF).
- Use diuretics and salt restriction in patients with fluid retention.
- Use angiotensin-converting enzyme inhibitors.
- Use β-blockers (carvedilol, sustained-release metoprolol succinate, or bisoprolol).
- Use angiotensin II receptor blockers (candesartan or valsartan) if intolerant to ACE inhibitors because of cough or angioneurotic edema.
- Avoid or withdraw NSAIDs, most antiarrhythmic drugs, and most calcium channel blockers.
- Recommend exercise training.
- Implant cardioverter-defibrillator in patients with a history of cardiac arrest, ventricular fibrillation, or hemodynamically unstable ventricular tachycardia.
- Implant cardioverter-defibrillator in patients with ischemic heart disease ≥40 days post-myocardial infarction or nonischemic cardiomyopathy, a LV ejection fraction ≤30%, New York Heart Association class-II or -III symptoms on optimal medical therapy, and an expectation of survival of ≥1 year.
- Use cardiac resynchronization therapy in patients with a LV ejection fraction ≤35%, New York Heart Association class-III or -IV symptoms despite optimal therapy, and a QRS duration >120 ms.
- Add an aldosterone antagonist (spironolactone or eplerenone) in selected patients with moderately severe to severe symptoms of HF who can be carefully monitored for renal function and potassium concentration (Serum creatinine should be ≤2.5 mg/dL in men and ≤2.0 mg/dL in women. Serum potassium should be <5.0 mEq/L.).

Adapted from Hunt SA, Abraham WT, Chin MH, et al. ACC/AHA 2005 guideline update for the diagnosis and management of chronic heart failure in the adult—summary article. Circulation 2005;112:1825–52.

The dose of diuretics should be gradually reduced and stopped if possible when fluid retention is not present in patients with HF. Patients on high doses of diuretics have an increased mortality [10]. The use of diuretics in elderly patients with HF is extensively discussed in the article by Sica and colleagues elsewhere in this issue.

ACE inhibitors

ACE inhibitors are balanced vasodilators that decrease both afterload and preload. ACE inhibitors reduce systemic vascular resistance, arterial pressure, LV and right ventricular end-diastolic pressures, cardiac work, and myocardial oxygen consumption; and increase cardiac output. ACE inhibitors decrease circulating levels of angiotensin II, reduce sympathetic nervous system activity, stimulate prostaglandin synthesis, and decrease sodium and water retention by inhibiting angiotensin II stimulation of aldosterone release. ACE inhibitors are very effective in treating HF associated with abnormal LV ejection fraction (Table 1). The ability of ACE inhibitors to block aldosterone production is only partial and limited to approximately the first 6 months of therapy with loss of efficacy afterwards.

ACE inhibitors improve symptoms, quality of life, and exercise tolerance in patients with HF. ACE inhibitors also increase survival in patients with HF and abnormal LV ejection fraction (see Table 1) [11–15] and should be used to treat patients with HF and abnormal LV ejection fraction with a class-I indication (see Box 1) [1]. ACE inhibitors also improve survival and reduce the incidence of HF and coronary events in patients with abnormal LV ejection fraction but without HF [16–19]. ACE inhibitors should be used to treat these patients with a class-I indication [1].

ACE inhibitors should be started in elderly patients with HF in low doses after correction of hyponatremia or volume depletion. Avoid over-diuresis

Table 1
Effect of ACE inhibitors on survival in patients with heart failure and abnormal LV ejection fraction

Study	Results
Cooperative North Scandinavian Enalapril Survival Study [11]	Compared with placebo, enalapril significantly decreased mortality 40% at 6 months, 31% at 1 year, and 27% at end of study.
Veterans Administration Cooperative Vasodilator–Heart Failure Trial II [12]	Compared with hydralazine plus isosorbide dinitrate, enalapril significantly decreased mortality 28% at 2 years.
Studies of Left Ventricular Dysfunction Treatment Trial [13]	At 41-month follow-up, enalapril, compared with placebo, significantly decreased mortality by 16%, death due to progressive HF by 22%, and mortality or hospitalization for worsening HF by 26%.
Acute Infarction Ramipril Efficacy Study [14]	At 15-month follow-up of patients with myocardial infarction and HF, ramipril, compared with placebo, significantly decreased mortality by 36% in patients aged ≥ 65 years.
Overview of 32 randomized trials of ACE inhibitors on mortality and morbidity in patients with HF [15]	Compared with placebo, ACE inhibitors significantly decreased mortality by 23% and mortality or hospitalization for HF by 35%.

Abbreviation: HF, heart failure.

before initiating treatment with ACE inhibitors because volume depletion may cause hypotension or renal insufficiency when ACE inhibitors are started or when the dose of these drugs is increased to full therapeutic levels. After the maintenance dose of ACE inhibitors is reached, it may be necessary to increase the dose of diuretics.

Patients with HF and abnormal LV ejection fraction were randomized to lisinopril 2.5 mg to 5.0 mg daily versus 32.5 mg to 35 mg daily [20]. At 39-month to 58-month follow-up, compared with low-dose lisinopril, high-dose lisinopril caused an 8% insignificant reduction in mortality, a significant 12% reduction in mortality or all-cause hospitalization, and a significant 24% reduction in hospitalization for HF [20]. The discontinuation of study drug was similar for the two treatment groups. These data indicate that patients with HF should be treated with high doses of ACE inhibitors unless low doses are the only doses that can be tolerated.

In the Veterans Administration Cooperative Vasodilator–Heart Failure Trial II, enalapril, compared with isosorbide dinitrate plus hydralazine, significantly reduced 2-year mortality by 28% because of a greater response to enalapril in whites than in African-Americans [12]. This finding led to the study of isosorbide dinitrate versus placebo in African-Americans with HF [21]. A report from the Studies of Left Ventricular Dysfunction databases showed that whites but not African-Americans randomized to enalapril had a significant reduction in the risk of hospitalization for HF [22]. However, a post hoc analysis of the 4054 African-American and white participants in the Studies of Left Ventricular Dysfunction Prevention Trial was performed to investigate whether enalapril had similar efficacy in preventing symptomatic HF in African-Americans versus whites [23]. Despite the increased absolute risk in African-Americans compared with whites for the progression of asymptomatic LV dysfunction, enalapril was equally efficacious in reducing the risk of HF in African-Americans versus whites [23].

Elderly patients at risk for excessive hypotension should have their blood pressure monitored closely for the first 2 weeks of ACE inhibitor therapy and whenever the physician increases the dose of ACE inhibitor or diuretic. Renal function should be monitored in patients administered ACE inhibitors to detect increases in blood urea nitrogen and in serum creatinine, especially in elderly patients with renal artery stenosis. A doubling in serum creatinine should lead the physician to consider renal dysfunction caused by ACE inhibitors, a need to decrease the dose of diuretics, or exacerbation of HF. Potassium supplements and potassium-sparing diuretics should not be given to patients receiving ACE inhibitors because ACE inhibitor therapy may cause hyperkalemia by blocking aldosterone production.

Asymptomatic hypotension with a systolic blood pressure between 80 and 90 mm Hg and a serum creatinine of <2.5 mg/dL are side effects of ACE inhibitors that should not necessarily cause discontinuation of this drug but should cause the physician to reduce the dose of diuretics if the jugular venous pressure is normal and to consider decreasing the dose of ACE inhibitor. Contraindications to the use of ACE inhibitors are symptomatic hypotension, progressive azotemia, angioneurotic edema, hyperkalemia, intolerable cough, and rash.

ACE inhibitors inhibit the metabolic degradation of bradykinin, which promotes vascular synthesis of vasodilating prostaglandins [24]. Aspirin is a cyclooxygenase inhibitor that dose-dependently inhibits synthesis of prostaglandins in vascular tissues [25]. Aspirin in doses of < 100 mg daily provides the desired antiplatelet effect without inhibiting synthesis of prostaglandins.

There are conflicting data about the importance of the negative interaction of aspirin with ACE inhibitors in the treatment of patients with HF. Some hemodynamic studies support the importance of this negative interaction [26,27], whereas other hemodynamic studies do not [28,29]. Retrospective analyses of clinical studies have also shown conflicting data with some studies supporting [30,31] and other studies not supporting [32–34] a negative interaction between aspirin and ACE inhibitors. In a study of elderly patients with HF treated with ACE inhibitors, aspirin did not affect outcomes negatively [34].

Until data from controlled clinical trials are available, a prudent approach to this controversy might be to decrease the dose of aspirin to 80 mg to 100 mg daily or substitute clopidogrel as an antiplatelet drug in patients with HF treated with ACE inhibitors. The dose of ACE inhibitors could also be increased to overcome aspirin-related attenuation.

Angiotensin-receptor blockers

Angiotensin II is a potent vasoconstrictor that may impair LV function and cause the progression of HF through increased impedance of LV emptying, adverse long-term structural effects on the heart and vasculature [35], and activation of other neurohormonal agonists, including norepinephrine, aldosterone, and endothelin [36].

The angiotensin II type-1 receptor blocker losartan significantly reduced the rate of first hospitalization for HF by 32%, compared with placebo, at 3.4-year follow-up of patients with type-2 diabetes mellitus and nephropathy [37]. Losartan also significantly reduced hospitalization for HF by 41% compared with atenolol at 4.7-year follow-up of diabetics with hypertension and electrocardiographic LV hypertrophy [38].

In the Losartan Heart Failure Survival Study (ELITE) II, 3152 patients aged ≥ 60 years with New York Heart Association (NYHA) class-II through -IV HF and a LV ejection fraction of $\leq 40\%$ were randomized in a double-blind trial to receive losartan 50 mg daily or captopril 50 mg three times daily [39]. Median follow-up was 555 days. More patients discontinued captopril because of adverse effects (14.7%) than discontinued losartan (9.7%) for the same reason [39].

Mortality was insignificantly 13% less in patients treated with captopril than in patients treated with losartan, significantly 77% less in patients treated with captopril plus β-blockers than in patients treated with losartan plus β-blockers, and insignificantly 5% less in patients treated with captopril without β-blockers than in patients treated with losartan without β-blockers [39]. Hospital admissions for any cause were insignificantly 4% higher in patients treated with losartan than in patients treated with captopril [39].

The Valsartan Heart Failure Trial randomized 5010 patients with NYHA class-II through -IV HF and an abnormal LV ejection fraction to valsartan 160 mg daily or placebo [40]. Ninety-three percent of the patients were treated with ACE inhibitors, 85% with diuretics, 67% with digoxin, and 35% with β-blockers. At 23-month follow-up, mortality was similar in the two treatment groups [40]. Mortality plus morbidity was significantly reduced 13% in patients treated with valsartan. Valsartan significantly decreased mortality in patients treated with neither an ACE inhibitor nor β-blocker [40].

The Valsartan in Acute Myocardial Infarction trial randomized 14,703 patients after myocardial infarction complicated by LV systolic dysfunction, HF, or both to valsartan 160 mg twice daily, valsartan 80 mg twice daily plus captopril 50 mg three times daily, or captopril 50 mg three times daily [41]. At 25-month median follow-up, all-cause mortality was similar in the three groups. Hypotension and renal dysfunction were more common in patients treated with valsartan, whereas cough, rash, and taste disturbance were more common in patients treated with captopril [41]. Combining valsartan with captopril increased the incidence of adverse effects without improving survival [41].

In the Candesartan in Heart Failure: Assessment of Reduction in Mortality and Morbidity—Alternative Study, 2028 patients with HF, an abnormal LV ejection fraction and intolerance to ACE inhibitors were randomized to candesartan 32 mg once daily or placebo [42]. At 34-month median follow-up, candesartan significantly reduced the incidence of cardiovascular death or hospitalization for HF by 30% [42].

In the Candesartan in Heart Failure: Assessment of Reduction in Mortality and Morbidity—Added Study, 2548 patients with HF and an abnormal LV ejection fraction treated with ACE inhibitors were randomized to candesartan 32 mg daily or to placebo [43]. At 41-month median follow-up, addition of candesartan to the ACE inhibitor significantly reduced cardiovascular death or hospitalization for HF by 15% [43].

On the basis of these data [39–43], the author concurs with the ACC/AHA guidelines [1] that (1) an angiotensin-receptor blocker (ARB) should be used for treating HF if the patient cannot tolerate an ACE inhibitor because of cough or angioneurotic edema with a class-I indication (see Box 1), and (2) an ARB instead of an ACE inhibitor should be used if the patient is already on an ARB with a class-IIa indication (Box 2) [1].

Box 2. Class-IIa recommendations for treating heart failure with abnormal LV systolic function

- Angiotensin II receptor blockers may be used instead of ACE inhibitors if patients are already taking them for other indications.
- Add hydralazine plus a nitrate to patients with persistent symptoms.
- Implant cardioverter-defibrillator in patients with LV ejection fraction of 30%–35% of any origin with NYHA class-II or -III symptoms on optimal medical therapy with a life expectancy of >1 year.
- Digoxin can be used in patients with persistent symptoms to reduce hospitalization for HF.

Adapted from Hunt SA, Abraham WT, Chin MH, et al. ACC/AHA 2005 guideline update for the diagnosis and management of chronic heart failure in the adult—summary article. Circulation 2005;112:1825–52.

β-blockers

Chronic administration of β-blockers after myocardial infarction decreases mortality, sudden cardiac death, and recurrent myocardial infarction, especially in elderly patients [44–46]. These benefits are more marked in patients with a history of HF [47].

β-blockers have been shown to reduce mortality in elderly patients with complex ventricular arrhythmias associated with prior myocardial infarction and abnormal [48] or normal [49] LV ejection fraction. In patients with prior myocardial infarction, abnormal LV ejection fraction, and complex ventricular arrhythmias, β-blockers caused a significant 32% decrease in occurrence of new or worsened HF [48]. The benefit of β-blockers in decreasing coronary events in elderly patients with prior myocardial infarction is also especially increased in patients with diabetes mellitus [50], peripheral arterial disease [51], and abnormal LV ejection fraction [19,52]. β-blockers significantly reduce mortality in elderly patients with HF and abnormal LV ejection fraction (Table 2) [53–57].

β-blockers are effective in antagonizing neurohormonal systems that cause myocyte apoptosis, myocyte necrosis, myocyte hypertrophy, fetal gene program activation, extracellular matrix alterations, and β-receptor uncoupling [58]. β-blockers may prevent or reverse increased systemic vascular resistance and increased afterload caused by excessive sympathetic nervous system activation. β-blockers also reduce levels of atrial natriuretic peptide, brain natriuretic peptide, and tumor necrosis alpha levels [59]. β-blockers are also effective in preventing cardiovascular events because of their

Table 2
Effect of β-blockers on mortality in patients with heart failure

Study	Results
Packer, et al [53] (n = 1,094)	At 6- to 12-month follow-up of patients with NYHA class-II, -III, or -IV HF and abnormal LV ejection fraction, carvedilol, compared with placebo, significantly decreased mortality 65%.
The Cardiac Insufficiency Bisoprolol Study II (CIBIS II) [54] (n = 2,647)	At 1.3-year follow-up of patients with NYHA class-III or -IV HF and abnormal LV ejection fraction, bisoprolol, compared with placebo, significantly decreased mortality 34%.
Metoprolol CR/XL Randomised Intervention Trial in Congestive Heart Failure (MERIT-HF) [55] (n = 3,991)	At 1-year follow-up of patients with NYHA class-II, -III, or -IV HF and abnormal LV ejection fraction, extended-release or controlled-release metoprolol (metoprolol CR/XL), compared with placebo, significantly decreased mortality 34%.
Carvedilol Prospective Randomized Cumulative Survival Trial (COPERNICUS) [56] (n = 2,289)	At 10.4-month follow-up of patients with severe HF and abnormal LV ejection fraction, carvedilol, compared with placebo, significantly reduced mortality 35%.
Randomized trial to determine the effect of nebivolol on mortality and cardiovascular hospital admission in elderly patients with HF (SENIORS) [57] (n = 1,369)	At 32-month follow-up of elderly patients with NYHA class-II or -III HF and LV ejection fraction ≤35%, nebivolol, compared with placebo, significantly reduced mortality or cardiovascular hospital admission by 14%.

Abbreviation: HF, heart failure.

antihypertensive, anti-ischemic, antiarrhythmic, and antiatherogenic effect [60]. The increase in ventricular rate that occurs after exercise can also be prevented with modest doses of β-blockers, especially in elderly patients.

β-blockers reduce all-cause mortality, cardiovascular mortality, sudden death, and death from worsening HF in patients with HF [53–57]. β-blockers significantly reduce mortality in African-Americans [53,55,56] and in whites [53–57] with HF, in women and in men with HF [53–57], in elderly and in younger patients with HF [53–57], in diabetics and in nondiabetics with HF [53–57], and in patients with severe HF and with mild or moderate HF [53–55,57]. β-blockers should be used to treat patients with HF and abnormal LV ejection fraction with a class-I indication (see Table 2) [1] unless there are contraindications to their use. Carvedilol and extended-release or controlled-release metoprolol (metoprolol CR/XL) are the only β-blockers that have been approved by the US Food and Drug Administration for the treatment of HF in the United States. Bisoprolol is also approved for the treatment of HF in Europe.

Patients with prior myocardial infarction and asymptomatic abnormal LV ejection fraction should be treated with ACE inhibitors plus β-blockers [1,19,61,62]. An observational prospective study was performed in 477 patients (196 men and 281 women; mean age: 79 years) with prior myocardial infarction and abnormal LV ejection fraction (mean LV ejection fraction: 31%) [19]. At 34-month follow-up, ACE inhibitors alone significantly reduced new coronary events 17% and new HF 32%, and β-blocker alone significantly reduced new coronary events 25% and new HF 41%, compared with no β-blocker or ACE inhibitor [19]. At 41-month follow-up, ACE inhibitors plus β-blockers significantly reduced new coronary events 37% and new HF 61%, compared with no β-blocker or ACE inhibitor [19]. The significantly longer follow-up time in patients treated with ACE inhibitors plus β-blockers indicates that β-blockers plus ACE inhibitors delayed as well as decreased the occurrence of new coronary events and HF [19].

Patients should be treated with an ACE inhibitor or ARB and be in a relatively stable condition without the need of intravenous inotropic therapy and without signs of marked fluid retention before initiating β-blocker therapy in patients with HF [63]. β-blockers should be initiated in a low dose, such as carvedilol 3.125 mg twice daily or metoprolol CR/XL 12.5 mg daily if there is NYHA class-III or -IV HF, or 25 mg daily if there is NYHA class-II HF. The dose of β-blockers should be doubled at 2- to 3-week intervals with the maintenance dose of β-blockers reached over 3 months (carvedilol 25 mg twice daily or 50 mg twice daily if over 187 pounds or metoprolol CR/XL 200 mg once daily). The patient may experience fatigue during the initiation or up-titration of the dose of β-blockers with this effect dissipating over time. The need to continue β-blockers in this patient must be stressed because of the importance of β-blockers in decreasing mortality.

During titration, the patient should be monitored for HF symptoms, fluid retention, hypotension, and bradycardia [63]. If there is worsening of symptoms, increase the dose of diuretics or ACE inhibitors. Temporarily reduce the dose of β-blockers if necessary. If there is hypotension, decrease the dose of vasodilators and temporarily decrease the dose of β-blockers if necessary. Reduce or discontinue drugs that may decrease heart rate in the presence of bradycardia. Contraindications to the use of β-blockers in patients with HF are bronchial asthma, severe bronchial disease, symptomatic bradycardia, and symptomatic hypotension [63].

Aldosterone antagonists

At 2-year follow-up of 1663 patients (mean age: 65 years) with severe HF and an abnormal LV ejection fraction treated with diuretics, ACE inhibitors, 73% with digoxin, and 10% with β-blockers, spironolactone 25 mg daily significantly reduced mortality by 30% and hospitalization for worsening HF by 35% [64]. At 16-month follow-up of 6632 patients (mean age: 64 years) with acute myocardial infarction complicated by HF and a low LV ejection fraction treated with diuretics, ACE inhibitors, and 75% with β-blockers, eplerenone 50 mg daily significantly reduced mortality by 15% and death from cardiovascular causes or hospitalization for cardiovascular events by 13% [65].

The ACC/AHA guidelines recommend using aldosterone antagonists in selected patients with moderately severe to severe symptoms of HF and an abnormal LV ejection fraction despite treatment with diuretics, ACE inhibitors, and β-blockers if there is preserved renal function and a normal serum potassium with a class-I indication (see Box 1) [1].

Isorbide dinitrate plus hydralazine

Oral nitrates reduce preload and pulmonary congestion in patients with HF. Hydralazine reduces afterload, improving perfusion at the same level of LV filling pressure. In the Veterans Administration Cooperative Vasodilator–Heart Failure Trial I, oral isosorbide dinitrate plus hydralazine, compared with placebo, significantly decreased mortality by 38% at 1 year, 25% at 2 years, and 23% at 3 years in men (mean age: 58 years) with abnormal LV ejection fraction [66].

The African-American Heart Failure Trial randomized 1040 African-Americans with HF and an abnormal LV ejection fraction (only 23% with ischemic heart disease) treated with diuretics, ACE inhibitors, and β-blockers to isosorbide dinitrate plus hydralazine or to placebo [21]. At 10-month follow-up, isosorbide dinitrate plus hydralazine significantly reduced mortality by 43% and rate of first hospitalization for HF by 33% [21].

The ACC/AHA guidelines recommend using isosorbide dinitrate plus hydralazine in patients with persistent symptoms of HF who are being treated with diuretics, ACE inhibitors, and β-blockers with a class-IIa recommendation (see Box 2) [1].

The initial dose of oral isosorbide dinitrate in elderly patients with HF is 10 mg three times daily, with subsequent titration up to a maximum dose of 40 mg three times daily. Nitrates should be given no more than three times daily, with daily nitrate washout intervals of 12 hours to prevent nitrate tolerance from developing. The initial dose of oral hydralazine in elderly patients with HF is 10 mg to 25 mg three times daily, with subsequent titration up to a maximum dose of 100 mg three times daily.

Digoxin

At 37-month follow-up of 6,800 patients (mean age: 64 years) with HF and a LV ejection fraction ≤45% in the Digitalis Investigator Group (DIG) study, mortality was similar in patients treated with digoxin or placebo [67,68]. HF hospitalization was significantly reduced by 28% in patients with an abnormal LV ejection fraction [67,68]. Hospitalization for any cause was significantly reduced 8% in patients with an abnormal LV ejection fraction [68]. Hospitalization for suspected digoxin toxicity in patients treated with digoxin was 0.67% in patients aged 50 to 59 years, 1.91% in patients aged 60 to 69 years, 2.47% in patients aged 70 to 79 years, and 4.42% in patients aged ≥80 years [68].

A post hoc subgroup analysis of data from women with a LV ejection fraction <45% in the DIG study showed by multivariate analysis that digoxin significantly increased the risk of death among women by 23% (absolute increase of 4.2%) [69]. A post hoc subgroup analysis of data from men with a LV ejection fraction <45% in the DIG study showed that digoxin significantly reduced mortality by 6% if the serum digoxin level was 0.5 to 0.8 ng/mL, insignificantly increased mortality by 3% if the serum digoxin level was 0.8 to 1.1 ng/mL, and significantly increased mortality by 12% if the serum digoxin level was ≥1.2 ng/mL [70].

Another post hoc subgroup analysis of data from all 1366 women with HF in the DIG study showed that digoxin significantly increased mortality for women by 80% if the serum digoxin level was ≥1.2 ng/mL and insignificantly increased mortality by 5% if the serum digoxin level was 0.5 to 1.1 ng/mL [71]. If the serum digoxin level was 0.5 to 1.1 ng/mL and the LV ejection fraction was <35%, digoxin significantly reduced HF hospitalization by 37% in women [71].

Digoxin reduces the rapid ventricular rate associated with supraventricular tachyarrhythmias and may be used along with β-blockers to treat elderly patients with HF and supraventricular tachyarrhythmias, such as atrial fibrillation. Digoxin may also be used to treat patients with persistent symptoms of HF and an abnormal LV ejection fraction despite treatment with diuretics, ACE inhibitors, and β-blockers to reduce HF hospitalization with a class-IIa indication (see Box 2) [1]. The maintenance dose of digoxin should be 0.125 mg daily in elderly patients with HF, and the serum digoxin level should be between 0.5 to 0.8 ng/mL.

Digoxin has a narrow therapeutic index, especially in elderly patients. Age-related reduction in renal function increases serum digoxin levels in older persons. The decrease in skeletal muscle mass in elderly patients reduces the volume of distribution of digoxin, increasing serum digoxin levels. Elderly patients are also more likely to be taking drugs that interact with digoxin by interfering with its bioavailability or excretion. For example, spironolactone, triamterene, amiodarone, quinidine, verapamil, propafenone, erythromycin, tetracycline, propantheline, and other drugs increase serum digoxin levels. Therefore, elderly patients receiving these drugs are at increased risk for developing digitalis toxicity. In addition, hypokalemia, hypomagnesemia, myocardial ischemia, hypoxia, acute and chronic lung disease, acidosis, hypercalcemia, and hypothyroidism may cause digitalis toxicity despite normal serum digoxin levels [72].

Other neurohormonal antagonists

Other neurohormonal antagonists have not been shown to be effective in the treatment of HF [73–75]. However, preliminary data with arginine vasopressin antagonists in the treatment of patients with HF are encouraging and warrant further investigation [76,77].

Calcium channel blockers

Calcium channel blockers, such as nifedipine, diltiazem, and verapamil, exacerbate HF in patients with HF and abnormal LV ejection fraction [78]. Diltiazem significantly increased mortality in patients with pulmonary congestion and abnormal LV ejection fraction after myocardial infarction [79]. The Multicenter Diltiazem Postinfarction Trial also showed in patients with a LV ejection fraction <40% that late HF at follow-up significantly increased in patients randomized to diltiazem (21%) compared with patients randomized to placebo (12%) [80].

The vasoselective calcium channel blockers amlodipine [81] and felodipine [82] did not significantly affect survival in patients with HF and abnormal LV ejection fraction. In these studies, incidence of pulmonary edema was significantly higher in patients treated with amlodipine (15%) than in patients treated with placebo (10%) [81] and incidence of peripheral edema was significantly higher in patients treated with amlodipine [81] or felodipine [82] than in those treated with placebo. On the basis of the available data, calcium channel blockers should not be administered to patients with HF and an abnormal LV ejection fraction (see Box 1) [1].

Synchronized pacing and cardioverter-defibrillators

The use of cardiac resynchronization therapy [83–86] in the treatment of elderly patients with HF is discussed in the article by Kron and Conti elsewhere in this issue. The use of implantable cardioverter-defibrillators in the treatment of elderly patients with HF [87] is discussed in an article elsewhere in this issue. The ACC/AHA guidelines recommend using cardiac resynchronization therapy in patients with HF, a LV ejection fraction ≤35%, and class-III or -IV symptoms despite optimal therapy, and a QRS duration >120 ms with a class-I indication (see Boxes 1 and 2) [1].

Inotropic therapy

Inotropic therapy significantly increases mortality in patients with HF and abnormal LV ejection fraction [88–95]. The use of inotropic therapy in the treatment of elderly patients with acute decompensated HF is discussed in the article by O'Connor elsewhere in this issue.

Nesiritide

Intravenous nesiritide (human B-type natriuretic peptide) causes hemodynamic and symptomatic improvement in hospitalized patients with decompensated HF through balanced vasodilatory effects, neurohormonal suppression, and enhanced natriuresis and diuresis [96]. Nesiritide improved hemodynamic function and some self-reported symptoms more effectively than intravenous nitroglycerin or placebo in a randomized, double-blind trial of 489 patients with dyspnea at rest from decompensated HF in the Vasodilation in the Management of Acute CHF (VMAC) study [96].

However, in the VMAC study, intravenous nesiritide, compared with intravenous nitroglycerin, insignificantly increased hospital stay and 30-day and 6-month mortality [96,97]. This trial was also not powered for mortality. A review of US Food and Drug Administration files available via the website also showed that nesiritide (1) significantly increases the risk of worsening renal function in patients with acute decompensated HF [98] and (2) that nesiritide insignificantly increased mortality 1.8 times in patients with acute decompensated HF with an abnormal LV ejection fraction [99]. The European Trial of Nesiritide in Acute Decompensated Heart Failure is randomizing 1900 patients with acute decompensated HF to treatment with nesiritide or placebo. This study should clarify the role of nesiritide in the treatment of patients with acute decompensated HF.

Surgical therapy

Surgical therapy, including surgical ventricular restoration [100], in the treatment of HF is discussed in the article by Malekan elsewhere in this issue. The Surgical Treatment for Ischemic Heart Failure Trial is investigating long-term outcomes in patients with HF and abnormal LV ejection fraction randomized to medical therapy, coronary revascularization, or coronary revascularization plus surgical ventricular restoration.

End-stage heart failure

An implantable LV assist device (LVAD) has benefited patients with end-stage HF as a bridge to cardiac transplantation. However, cardiac transplantation is not a viable option for the vast majority of patients with end-stage HF. One hundred and twenty-nine transplant-ineligible patients (mean age: 67 years) with end-stage HF were randomized to medical therapy or to an LVAD [101]. The 2-year survival was 23% in the LVAD-treated group versus 8% in the medical-therapy–treated group [101]. These data suggest using a LVAD as an alternative therapy in selected patients who are not candidates for cardiac transplantation. Other therapies for elderly patients with end-stage HF include continuous intravenous inotropic infusions for palliation and hospice care [1].

References

[1] Hunt SA, Abraham WT, Chin MH, et al. ACC/AHA 2005 guideline update for the diagnosis and management of chronic heart failure in the adult—summary article. Circulation 2005;112:1825–52.

[2] Aronow WS. What is the appropriate treatment of hypertension in elders? J Gerontol: Med Sci 2002;57A:M483–6.

[3] Aronow WS. Treatment of older persons with hypercholesterolemia with and without cardiovascular disease. J Gerontol Med Sci 2001;56A:M138–45.

[4] Aronow WS, Ahn C. Frequency of congestive heart failure in older persons with prior myocardial infarction and serum low-density lipoprotein cholesterol ≥ 125 mg/dL treated with statins versus no lipid-lowering drug. Am J Cardiol 2002;90:147–9.

[5] Aronow WS, Ahn C. Elderly diabetics with peripheral arterial disease and no coronary artery disease have a higher incidence of new coronary events than elderly nondiabetics with peripheral arterial disease and prior myocardial infarction treated with statins and with no lipid-lowering drug. J Gerontol: Med Sci 2003;58A:M573–5.

[6] Sanal S, Aronow WS. Effect of an educational program on the prevalence of use of antiplatelet drugs, beta blockers, angiotensin-converting enzyme inhibitors, lipid-lowering drugs, and calcium channel blockers prescribed during hospitalization and at hospital discharge in patients with coronary artery disease. J Gerontol: Med Sci 2003;58A:M1046–8.

[7] Ghosh S, Aronow WS. Utilization of lipid-lowering drugs in elderly persons with increased serum low-density lipoprotein cholesterol associated with coronary artery disease, symptomatic peripheral arterial disease, prior stroke, or diabetes mellitus before and after an educational program on dyslipidemia treatment. J Gerontol: Med Sci 2003;58A:M432–5.

[8] Aronow WS. Exercise therapy for older persons with cardiovascular disease. Am J Geriatr Cardiol 2001;10:245–52.

[9] Rich MW, Beckham V, Wittenberg C, et al. A multidisciplinary intervention to prevent the readmission of elderly patients with congestive heart failure. N Engl J Med 1995;333: 1190–5.

[10] Neuberg GW, Miller AB, O'Connor CM, et al. Diuretic resistance predicts mortality in patients with advanced heart failure. Am Heart J 2002;144:31–8.

[11] The CONSENSUS Trial Study Group. Effect of enalapril on mortality in severe congestive heart failure: results of the Cooperative North Scandinavian Enalapril Survival Study (CONSENSUS). N Engl J Med 1987;316:1429–35.

[12] Cohn J, Johnson G, Ziesche S, et al. A comparison of enalapril with hydralazine-isosorbide dinitrate in the treatment of chronic congestive heart failure. N Engl J Med 1991;325: 303–10.

[13] The SOLVD Investigators. Effect of enalapril on survival in patients with reduced left ventricular ejection fractions and congestive heart failure. N Engl J Med 1991;325:293–302.

[14] The Acute Infarction Ramipril Efficacy (AIRE) Study Investigators. Effect of ramipril on mortality and morbidity of survivors of acute myocardial infarction with clinical evidence of heart failure. Lancet 1993;342:821–8.

[15] Garg R, Yusuf S. Overview of randomized trials of angiotensin-converting enzyme inhibitors on mortality and morbidity in patients with heart failure. JAMA 1995;273: 1450–6.

[16] Pfeffer MA, Braunwald E, Moye LA, et al. Effect of captopril on mortality and morbidity in patients with left ventricular dysfunction after myocardial infarction. Results of the Survival and Ventricular Enlargement Trial. N Engl J Med 1992;327:669–77.

[17] The SOLVD Investigators. Effect of enalapril on mortality and the development of heart failure in asymptomatic patients with reduced left ventricular ejection fractions. N Engl J Med 1992;327:685–91.

[18] Kober L, Torp-Pedersen C, Carlsen JE, et al. A clinical trial of the angiotensin-converting-enzyme inhibitor trandolapril in patients with left ventricular dysfunction after myocardial infarction. N Engl J Med 1995;333:1670–6.

[19] Aronow WS, Ahn C, Kronzon I. Effect of beta blockers alone, of angiotensin-converting enzyme inhibitors alone, and of beta blockers plus angiotensin-converting enzyme inhibitors on new coronary events and on congestive heart failure in older persons with healed

myocardial infarcts and asymptomatic left ventricular systolic dysfunction. Am J Cardiol 2001;88:1298–300.

[20] Packer M, Poole-Wilson PA, Armstrong PW, et al. Comparative effects of low and high doses of the angiotensin-converting enzyme inhibitor, lisinopril, on morbidity and mortality in chronic heart failure. Circulation 1999;100:2312–8.

[21] Taylor AL, Ziesche S, Yancy C, et al. Combination of isosorbide dinitrate and hydralazine in blacks with heart failure. N Engl J Med 2004;351:2049–57.

[22] Exner DV, Dries DL, Domanski MJ, et al. Lesser response to angiotensin-converting enzyme inhibitor therapy in black as compared with white patients with left ventricular dysfunction. N Engl J Med 2001;344:1351–7.

[23] Dries DL, Strong MH, Cooper RS, et al. Efficacy of angiotensin-converting enzyme inhibition in reducing progression from asymptomatic left ventricular dysfunction to symptomatic heart failure in black and white patients. J Am Coll Cardiol 2002;40:311–7.

[24] Vanhoutte PM, Auch-schwelk W, Biondi ML, et al. Why are converting enzyme inhibitors vasodilators? Br J Clin Pharmacol 1989;28:95S–104S.

[25] Weksler BB, Pett SB, Alonso D, et al. Differential inhibition by aspirin of vascular and platelet prostaglandin synthesis in atherosclerotic patients. N Engl J Med 1983;308:800–5.

[26] Hall D, Zeitler H, Rudolph W. Counteraction of the vasodilator effects of enalapril by aspirin in severe heart failure. J Am Coll Cardiol 1994;20:1549–55.

[27] Boger RH, Bodeboger SM, Kramme P, et al. Effect of captopril on prostacyclin and nitric oxide formation in healthy human subjects: interaction with low dose acetylsalicylic acid. Br J Clin Pharmacol 1996;42:721–7.

[28] Evans MA, Burnett JC Jr, Redfield MM. Effect of low dose aspirin on cardiorenal function and acute hemodynamic response to enalaprilat in a canine model of severe heart failure. J Am Coll Cardiol 1995;25:1445–50.

[29] Katz SD, Radin M, Graves T, et al. Effect of aspirin and ifetroban on skeletal muscle blood flow in patients with congestive heart failure treated with enalapril. J Am Coll Cardiol 1999; 34:170–6.

[30] Nguyen KN, Aursnes I, Kjekshus J. Interaction between enalapril and aspirin on mortality after acute myocardial infarction: subgroup analysis of the Cooperative New Scandinavian Enalapril Survival Study II (CONSENSUS II). Am J Cardiol 1997;79: 115–9.

[31] Al-Khadra AS, Salem DN, Rand WM, et al. Antiplatelet agents and survival: a cohort analysis from the Studies of Left Ventricular Dysfunction (SOLVD) trial. J Am Coll Cardiol 1998;31:419–25.

[32] Leor J, Reicher-Reiss H, Goldbourt U, et al. Aspirin and mortality in patients treated with angiotensin-converting enzyme inhibitors. A cohort study of 11,575 patients with coronary artery disease. J Am Coll Cardiol 1999;33:1920–5.

[33] Flather MD, Yusuf S, Kober L, et al. Long-term ACE-inhibitor therapy in patients with heart failure or left-ventricular dysfunction: a systematic overview of data from individual patients. Lancet 2000;355:1575–81.

[34] Lapane KL, Hume AL, Barbour MM, et al. Does aspirin attenuate the effect of angiotensin-converting enzyme inhibitors on health outcomes of very old patients with heart failure? J Am Geriatr Soc 2002;50:1198–204.

[35] Dzau VJ. Tissue renin-angiotensin system in myocardial hypertrophy and failure. Arch Intern Med 1993;153:937–42.

[36] Jilma B, Krejcy K, Dirnberger E, et al. Effects of angiotensin-II infusion at pressor and subpressor doses on endothelin-1 plasma levels in healthy men. Life Sci 1997;60:1859–66.

[37] Brenner BM, Cooper ME, de Zeeuw D, et al. Effects of losartan on renal and cardiovascular outcomes in patients with type 2 diabetes and nephropathy. N Engl J Med 2001;345:861–9.

[38] Lindholm LH, Ibsen H, Dahlof B, et al. Cardiovascular morbidity and mortality in patients with diabetes in the Losartan Intervention for Endpoint reduction in hypertension study (LIFE): a randomised trial against atenolol. Lancet 2002;359:1004–10.

[39] Pitt B, Poole-Wilson PA, Segal R, et al. Effect of losartan compared with captopril on mortality in patients with symptomatic heart failure: randomised trial—the Losartan Heart Failure Survival Study ELITE II. Lancet 2000;355:1582–7.

[40] Cohn JN, Tognoni G. A randomized trial of the angiotensin-receptor blocker valsartan in chronic heart failure. N Engl J Med 2001;345:1667–75.

[41] Pfeffer MA, McMurray JJV, Velazquez EJ, et al. Valsartan, captopril, or both in myocardial infarction complicated by heart failure, left ventricular dysfunction, or both. N Engl J Med 2003;349:1893–906.

[42] Granger CB, McMurray JJV, Yusuf S, et al. Effects of candesartan in patients with chronic heart failure and reduced left-ventricular systolic function intolerant to angiotensin-converting-enzyme inhibitors: the CHARM-Alternative trial. Lancet 2003; 362:772–6.

[43] McMurray JJV, Ostergren J, Swedberg K, et al. Effects of candesartan in patients with chronic heart failure and reduced left-ventricular systolic function taking angiotensin-converting-enzyme inhibitors: the CHARM-Added trial. Lancet 2003;362: 767–71.

[44] Yusuf S, Pfeffer MA, Swedberg K, et al. Effects of candesartan in patients with chronic heart failure and preserved left-ventricular ejection fraction: the CHARM-Preserved trial. Lancet 2003;362:777–81.

[45] Beta-Blocker Heart Attack Trial Research Group. A randomized trial of propranolol in patients with acute myocardial infarction. JAMA 1982;247:1707–14.

[46] Pedersen TR. Six-year follow-up of the Norwegian Multicentre Study on Timolol after acute myocardial infarction. N Engl J Med 1985;313:1055–8.

[47] Chadda K, Goldstein S, Byington R, et al. Effect of propranolol after acute myocardial infarction in patients with congestive heart failure. Circulation 1986;73:503–10.

[48] Kennedy HL, Brooks MM, Barker AH, et al. Beta-blocker therapy in the Cardiac Arrhythmia Suppression Trial. Am J Cardiol 1994;74:674–80.

[49] Aronow WS, Ahn C, Mercando AD, et al. Effect of propranolol versus no antiarrhythmic drug on sudden cardiac death, total cardiac death, and total death in patients ≥62 years of age with heart disease, complex ventricular arrhythmias, and left ventricular ejection fraction ≥40%. Am J Cardiol 1994;74:267–70.

[50] Aronow WS, Ahn C. Effect of beta blockers on incidence of new coronary events in older persons with prior myocardial infarction and diabetes mellitus. Am J Cardiol 2001;87: 780–1.

[51] Aronow WS, Ahn C. Effect of beta blockers on incidence of new coronary events in older persons with prior myocardial infarction and symptomatic peripheral arterial disease. Am J Cardiol 2001;87:1284–6.

[52] Furberg CD, Hawkins CM, Lichstein E. Effect of propranolol in postinfarction patients with mechanical or electrical complications. Circulation 1984;69:761–5.

[53] Packer M, Bristow MR, Cohn JN, et al. The effect of carvedilol on morbidity and mortality in patients with chronic heart failure. N Engl J Med 1996;334:1349–55.

[54] CIBIS-II Investigators and Committees. The Cardiac Insufficiency Bisoprolol Study II (CIBIS-II): a randomised trial. Lancet 1999;353:9–13.

[55] MERIT-HF Study Group. Effect of metoprolol CR/XL in chronic heart failure: Metoprolol CR/XL Randomised Intervention Trial in Congestive Heart Failure (MERIT-HF). Lancet 1999;353:2001–7.

[56] Packer M, Coats AJS, Fowler MB, et al. Effect of carvedilol on survival in chronic heart failure. N Engl J Med 2001;344:651–8.

[57] Flather MD, Shibata MC, Coats AJS, et al. Randomized trial to determine the effect of nebivolol on mortality and cardiovascular hospital admission in elderly patients with heart failure (SENIORS). Eur Heart J 2005;26:215–25.

[58] Mann DL, Deswal A, Bozkurt B, et al. New therapeutics for chronic heart failure. Annu Rev Med 2002;53:59–74.

[59] Ohtsuka T, Hamada M, Hiasa G, et al. Effect of beta-blockers on circulating levels of inflammatory and anti-inflammatory cytokines in patients with dilated cardiomyopathy. J Am Coll Cardiol 2001;37:412–7.

[60] Wiklund O, Hulthe J, Wikstrand J, et al. Effect of controlled release/extended release metoprolol on carotid intima-media thickness in patients with hypercholesterolemia: a 3-year randomized study. Stroke 2002;33:572–7.

[61] Moye L, Pfeffer M. Additional beneficial effects of beta-blockers to angiotensin-converting enzyme inhibitors in the Survival and Ventricular Enlargement (SAVE) Study. J Am Coll Cardiol 1997;29:229–36.

[62] Exner DV, Dries DL, Waclawiw MA, et al. Beta-adrenergic blocking agent use and mortality in patients with asymptomatic and symptomatic left ventricular systolic dysfunction: a post hoc analysis of the Studies of Left Ventricular Dysfunction. J Am Coll Cardiol 1999; 33:916–23.

[63] Task Force for the Diagnosis and Treatment of Chronic Heart Failure. Guidelines for the diagnosis and treatment of chronic heart failure. Eur Heart J 2001;22:1527–60.

[64] Pitt B, Zannad F, Remme WJ, et al. The effect of spironolactone on morbidity and mortality in patients with severe heart failure. N Engl J Med 1999;341:709–17.

[65] Pitt B, Remme W, Zannad F, et al. Eplerenone, a selective aldosterone blocker, in patients with left ventricular dysfunction after myocardial infarction. N Engl J Med 2003;348: 1309–21.

[66] Cohn JN, Archibald DG, Ziesche S, et al. Effect of vasodilator therapy on mortality in chronic congestive heart failure: results of a Veterans Administration Cooperative Study. N Engl J Med 1986;314:1547–52.

[67] The Digitalis Investigation Group. The effect of digoxin on mortality and morbidity in patients with heart failure. N Engl J Med 1997;336:525–33.

[68] Rich MW, McSherry F, Williford WO, et al. Effect of age on mortality, hospitalizations and response to digoxin in patients with heart failure: the DIG Study. J Am Coll Cardiol 2001; 38:806–13.

[69] Rathore SS, Wang Y, Krumholz HM. Sex-based differences in the effect of digoxin for the treatment of heart failure. N Engl J Med 2002;347:1403–11.

[70] Rathore SS, Curtis JP, Wang Y, et al. Association of serum digoxin concentration and outcomes in patients with heart failure. JAMA 2003;289:871–8.

[71] Ahmed A, Aban IB, Weaver MT, et al. Serum digoxin concentration and outcomes in women with heart failure: a bi-directional effect and a possible effect modification by ejection fraction. Eur J Heart Failure, accepted for publication.

[72] Aronow WS. Digoxin or angiotensin converting enzyme inhibitors for congestive heart failure in geriatric patients. Which is the preferred treatment? Drugs Aging 1991;1: 98–103.

[73] Packer M, Califf RM, Konstam MA, et al. Comparison of omapatrilat and enalapril in patients with chronic heart failure. The Omapatrilat Versus Enalapril Randomized Trial of Utility in Reducing Events (OVERTURE). Circulation 2002;106:920–6.

[74] Abraham WT, Ascheim D, Demarco T, et al. Effects of enrasentan, a nonselective endothelin receptor antagonist in class II to III heart failure: results of the Enrasentan Cooperative Randomized (ENCOR) Evaluation. J Am Coll Cardiol 2001;38:612.

[75] McMurray J, Pfeffer MA. New therapeutic options in congestive heart failure. Part II. Circulation 2002;105:2223–8.

[76] Gheorghiade M, Gattis WA, O'Connor CM, et al. Effects of tolvaptan, a vasopressin antagonist, in patients hospitalized with worsening heart failure: a randomized controlled trial. JAMA 2004;291:1963–71.

[77] Francis GS, Tang WHW. Vasopressin receptor antagonists. Will the "vaptans" fulfill their promise? JAMA 2004;291:2017–8.

[78] Elkayam U, Amin J, Mehra A, et al. A prospective, randomized, double-blind, crossover study to compare the efficacy and safety of chronic nifedipine therapy with that of

isosorbide dinitrate and their combination in the treatment of chronic congestive heart failure. Circulation 1990;82:1954–61.

[79] The Multicenter Diltiazem Postinfarction Trial Research Group. The effect of diltiazem on mortality and reinfarction after myocardial infarction. N Engl J Med 1988;319:385–92.

[80] Goldstein RE, Boccuzzi SJ, Cruess D, et al. Diltiazem increases late-onset congestive heart failure in postinfarction patients with early reduction in ejection fraction. Circulation 1991; 83:52–60.

[81] Packer M, O'Connor CM, Ghali JK, et al. Effect of amlodipine on morbidity and mortality in severe chronic heart failure. N Engl J Med 1996;335:1107–14.

[82] Cohn JN, Ziesche S, Smith R, et al. Effect of the calcium antagonist felodipine as suplementary vasodilator therapy in patients with chronic heart failure treated with enalapril. V-HeFT III. Circulation 1997;96:856–63.

[83] Aronow WS. CRT plus ICD in congestive heart failure. Use of cardiac resynchronization therapy and an implantable cardioverter-defibrillator in heart failure patients with abnormal left ventricular dysfunction. Geriatrics 2005;60(2):24–8.

[84] Young JB, Abraham WT, Smith AL, et al. Combined cardiac resynchronization and implantable cardioversion defibrillation in advanced chronic heart failure. The MIRACLE ICD trial. JAMA 2003;289:2685–94.

[85] Bristow MR, Saxon LA, Boehmer J, et al. Cardiac-resynchronization therapy with or without an implantable defibrillator in advanced chronic heart failure. N Engl J Med 2004;350: 2140–50.

[86] Cleland JGF, Daubert J-C, Erdmann E, et al. The effect of cardiac resynchronization on morbidity and mortality in heart failure. N Engl J Med 2005;352:1539–49.

[87] Bardy GH, Lee KL, Mark DB, et al. Amiodarone or an implantable cardioverter-defibrillator for congestive heart failure. N Engl J Med 2005;352:225–37.

[88] Packer M, Carver JR, Rodeheffer RJ, et al. Effect of oral milrinone on mortality in severe chronic heart failure. N Engl J Med 1991;325:1468–75.

[89] Packer M, Rouleau J, Swedberg K, et al. Effect of flosequinan on survival in chronic heart failure: preliminary results of the PROFILE study [abstract]. Circulation 1993;88(suppl I): I-301.

[90] Uretsky BF, Jessup F, Konstan MA, et al. Multicenter trial of oral enoximone in patients with moderate to moderately severe congestive heart failure. Circulation 1990;82:774–80.

[91] Cohn JN, Goldstein SO, Greenberg BH, et al. A dose-dependent increase in mortality with vesnarinone among patients with severe heart failure. N Engl J Med 1998;339:1810–6.

[92] Pimobendan in Congestive Heart Failure (PICO) Investigators. Effect of pimobendan on exercise capacity in patients with heart failure: main results from the Pimobendan in Congestive Heart Failure (PICO) Trial. Heart 1996;76:223–31.

[93] Xamoterol in Severe Heart Failure Study Group. Xamoterol in severe heart failure. Lancet 1990;336:1–6.

[94] Hampton JR, Van Veldhusien DJ, Kleber FX, et al. Randomized study of effect of ibopamine on survival in patients with advanced heart failure. Lancet 1997;349:971–7.

[95] O'Connor CM, Gattis WA, Uretsky BF, et al. Continuous intravenous dobutamine is associated with an increased risk of death in patients with advanced heart failure: insights from the Flolan International Randomized Survival Trial (FIRST). Am Heart J 2000; 138:78–86.

[96] Publication Committee for the VMAC Investigators. Intravenous nesiritide vs nitroglycerin for treatment of decompensated congestive heart failure. A randomized controlled trial. JAMA 2002;287:1531–40.

[97] Teerlink JR, Massie BM. Nesiritide and worsening of renal function. The emperor's new clothes? Circulation 2005;111:1459–61.

[98] Sackner-Bernstein JD, Skopicki HA, Aaronson KD. Risk of worsening renal function with nesiritide in patients with acutely decompensated heart failure. Circulation 2005;111: 1487–91.

[99] Sackner-Bernstein JD, Kowalski M, Fox M, et al. Short-term risk of death after treatment with nesiritide for decompensated heart failure. A pooled analysis of randomized controlled trials. JAMA 2005;293:1900–5.

[100] Athanasuleas CL, Stanley AW Jr, Buckberg GD, et al. Surgical anterior ventricular endo-cardial restoration (SAVER) in the dilated remodeled ventricle after anterior myocardial infarction. J Am Coll Cardiol 2001;37:1210–3.

[101] Rose EA, Gelijns AC, Moskowitz AJ, et al. Long-term use of a left ventricular assist device for end-stage heart failure. N Engl J Med 2001;345:1435–43.

CLINICS IN
GERIATRIC
MEDICINE

Clin Geriatr Med 23 (2007) 83–106

Diastolic Heart Failure in the Elderly

Dalane W. Kitzman, MD*, Kurt R. Daniel, DO

*Department of Internal Medicine, Wake Forest University Health Sciences Center,
Medical Center Boulevard, Winston-Salem, NC 27157, USA*

There has been growing recognition over the past two decades that a substantial proportion of patients who have heart failure (HF), particularly the elderly, have preserved systolic left ventricular (LV) function. This condition has been presumptively termed diastolic heart failure (DHF). This article discusses the pathophysiology, diagnosis, prognosis, and therapy of this important disorder in older people.

Epidemiology

In the population-based Olmsted Community project, records were reviewed from all patients during a 1-year period in whom an assessment of LV ejection fraction (EF) was obtained within 3 weeks of a new diagnosis of congestive heart failure (CHF) [1]. A normal EF was found in 43% of patients and this phenomenon increased with age (Fig. 1) [1]. This population was recently reassessed and it was found that the prevalence of DHF had increased mildly to 47%, whereas the prevalence of systolic heart failure (SHF) had decreased slightly [2]. Other large population-based reports, including the Framingham Study [3], the Cardiovascular Health Study (CHS) [4,5], the Strong Heart Study of American Indians [6], the Helsinki Ageing Study [7], and large Medicare studies [8,9], have found the prevalence of normal EF among those who have HF to be even higher, well over 50% [3–9].

There is a remarkable sex-related difference in DHF. In the cross-sectional analysis of CHS, 67% of elderly women who had prevalent CHF had a normal EF, whereas this finding was present in only 42% of men (Fig. 2) [4]. During the longitudinal analysis of 6-year follow-up in CHS,

Supported in part by National Institute on Aging Grant #R37 AG18915 and NIH Training Grant T32- -HL076132-02.

* Corresponding author. Section of Cardiology, Wake Forest University School of Medicine, Medical Center Boulevard, Winston-Salem, NC 27157-1045.

E-mail address: dkitzman@wfubmc.edu (D.W. Kitzman).

doi:10.1016/j.cger.2006.09.002   *geriatric.theclinics.com*

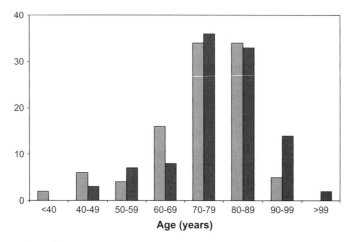

Fig. 1. Numbers of patients in Olmsted County, Minnesota hospitalized who had congestive heart failure in 1991 versus age with normal (*dark bars*) and reduced (*light bars*) ejection fraction. Note that CHF with a normal ejection fraction is absent in the youngest group (age <40 years) in contrast to the oldest group (age >99), where it comprises essentially all patients. (*Adapted from* Senni M, Tribouilloy CM, Rodeheffer RJ, et al. Congestive heart failure in the community: a study of all incident cases in Olmsted County, Minnesota, in 1991. Circulation 1998;98:2282–89.)

more than 90% of women who developed HF had normal systolic function [10]. Because women significantly outnumber men in the older population, the population-attributable risk for HF with reduced systolic function was relatively small compared with those who had HF and normal systolic function [10]. As a result, the typical community-dwelling patient who has

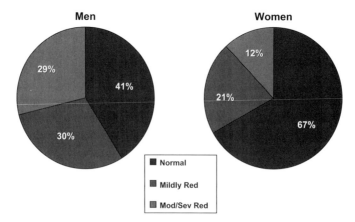

Fig. 2. LV ejection fraction by gender among community-dwelling elderly patients who have CHF in the Cardiovascular Health Study. (*Data from* Kitzman DW, Gardin JM, Gottdiener JS, et al. Importance of heart failure with preserved systolic function in patients ≥65 years of age. CHS Research Group. Cardiovascular Health Study. Am J Cardiol 2001;87:413–9.)

HF is an older woman who has normal systolic function and systolic hypertension. This profile contrasts sharply with the typical patients seen in referral HF clinics, who are middle-aged men who have severely reduced systolic function and ischemic heart disease. As one editorial declared, DHF is predominantly a disorder of older women [11].

Pathophysiology

Relatively few data are available regarding the pathophysiology of DHF. Both aging-related and sex-related differences in LV function may contribute. Among healthy normal subjects, older women tend to have higher left ventricular EFs, independent of their smaller chamber size, compared with men [12,13]. In addition, the female left ventricle in mammals has a distinctly different response to pressure load, such as is typical of systemic hypertension. In the HyperGen study, it was found that the deceleration time of early diastolic flow and isovolumic relaxation time were lengthened in women who had hypertension compared with men, independent of all other factors, indicating decreased myocardial relaxation [14]. In patients who had hypertension in the Framingham study the predominant pattern of hypertrophic remodeling in women was concentric, whereas in men it was eccentric, and this also has been reported in several other studies, including HyperGen [15] and LIFE.

Using aortic banding to create a model of chronic LV pressure overload in male and female rats, Douglas and colleagues [16] showed that male rats responded with LV dilation and modest wall thickening (eccentric hypertrophy) with resultant increased wall stress and decreased LV contractility. In contrast, the female rats increased their LV wall thickness and maintained a normal chamber size (concentric hypertrophy), and thereby enjoyed near-normal wall stress, and normal (even a trend toward supranormal) contractility. As a result, the female rats were able to continue to generate substantially higher systolic pressure, despite the excess afterload. Several other studies have shown similar overall results [17–19].

Large population-based studies have consistently shown that the strongest, most common risk factor for the development of HF is systolic hypertension. Combining this key point with the findings of the Douglas study provides a cohesive explanation for the divergent manifestations of HF in women versus men. The male LV is less able to tolerate pressure load, and in the presence of chronic systolic hypertension becomes dilated with thin walls and a depressed EF. The female LV is able to tolerate the pressure load better by developing concentric hypertrophy, allowing it to maintain normal LV size and EF. The long-term cost of this adaptation is impaired LV diastolic function. This phenomenon may help to explain the higher prevalence of DHF in women and why men tend to develop SHF whereas women tend to develop DHF. The above interplay between LV remodeling and pressure load has been shown in rodent models to be influenced substantially by estrogen and androgen, and to be related to gender differences in cardiac angiotensin-converting enzyme (ACE) expression [20].

In addition to these sex-related changes, there are several normal age-related changes in cardiovascular structure and function that are likely relevant to the development of DHF. These include increased arterial and myocardial stiffness, decreased diastolic myocardial relaxation, increased LV mass, decreased peak contractility, reduced myocardial and vascular responsiveness to β-adrenergic stimulation, decreased coronary flow reserve, and decreased mitochondrial response to increased demand for ATP production [21]. Consequently, insults from acute myocardial ischemia or infarction, poorly controlled hypertension, atrial fibrillation, iatrogenic volume overload, and pneumonia, which would be tolerated in younger patients, can cause acute CHF in older persons [21].

These normal age-related changes result in decreased cardiovascular reserve, which confers an approximately 1% per year decline in maximal exercise oxygen consumption [22]. In addition, women also have been shown to have different cardiovascular physiologic responses to exercise than men, particularly in heart rate and stroke volume independent of age and body size [22–24].

Exercise intolerance, manifested as exertional dyspnea and fatigue, is the primary symptom in chronic HF. Although the pathophysiology of exercise intolerance in SHF as it presents in middle-aged men has been intensively examined, few studies have examined the pathophysiology of exercise intolerance in DHF. In a recent study, maximal exercise testing with expired gas was performed in three groups of older subjects: SHF, DHF, and age-matched controls [25]. It was found that in comparison to the normal controls, peak exercise oxygen consumption, an objective measure of exercise capacity, was severely reduced in the patients who had DHF and to a similar degree as those who had SHF (Fig. 3) [25]. In addition, submaximal exercise capacity, as measured by the ventilatory anaerobic threshold, was similarly reduced in patients who had DHF versus SHF, and this was accompanied by reduced health-related quality of life [25].

Our laboratory has completed several studies that have examined the central (cardiac) and peripheral (vascular) components of the exercise response to determine the mechanisms of the severely reduced exercise capacity in DHF. In the first, using invasive cardiopulmonary exercise testing, it was demonstrated that severe exercise intolerance was related to an inability to increase stroke volume by way of the Frank-Starling mechanism despite severely increased LV filling pressure, indicating diastolic dysfunction (Fig. 4) [26]. This dysfunction resulted in severely reduced exercise cardiac output and early lactate formation that appeared responsible for the severely reduced exercise capacity and associated chronic exertional symptoms.

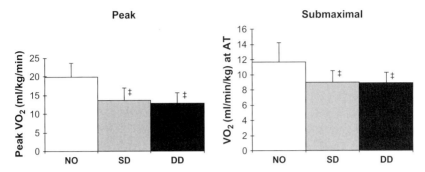

Fig. 3. Exercise oxygen consumption (VO₂) during peak exhaustive exercise (*left panel*) and during submaximal exercise at the ventilatory anaerobic threshold (*right panel*) in age-matched normal subjects (NO), elderly patients who have heart failure (HF) attributable to systolic dysfunction (SD), and elderly patients who have HF with normal systolic function, presumed diastolic dysfunction (DD). Exercise capacity is severely reduced in patients who have diastolic HF compared with normals ($P < .001$) and to a similar degree as in those who have systolic HF. (*Data from* Kitzman DW, Little WC, Brubaker PH, et al. Pathophysiologic characterization of isolated diastolic heart failure in comparison to systolic heart failure. JAMA 2002;288:2144–50.)

A relatively simple but overlooked contributor to exercise intolerance in older patients who have HF is chronotropic incompetence. Using the most standard definition of chronotropic incompetence, we recently showed that this was present in 20% to 25% of older patients who had HF, that the prevalence was similar in DHF compared with SHF, that the presence of chronotropic incompetence was a significant contributor to the degree of exercise intolerance, measured as maximal oxygen consumption, and that this was independent of medications, including beta-adrenergic antagonists [27]. This finding has therapeutic significance because it could be potentially addressable with rate-responsive atrioventricular synchronous pacing.

Another study indicated that decreased aortic distensibility, likely attributable to the combined effects of aging- and hypertension-induced thickening and remodeling of the thoracic aortic wall, may be an important contributor to exercise intolerance in chronic DHF. Magnetic resonance imaging and maximal exercise testing with expired gas analysis were performed in a group of elderly patients who had isolated DHF and in age-matched healthy subjects. The patients who had DHF had increased pulse pressure and thoracic aortic wall thickness and markedly decreased aortic distensibility, which correlated closely with their severely decreased exercise capacity (Fig. 5) [28].

As discussed previously, several lines of evidence suggest that systemic hypertension plays an important role in the genesis of DHF. In animal models, diastolic dysfunction develops early in systemic hypertension, and LV diastolic relaxation is sensitive to increased afterload [29–34]. Increased afterload may impair relaxation, leading to increased LV filling pressures, decreased stroke volume, and symptoms of dyspnea and congestion [32].

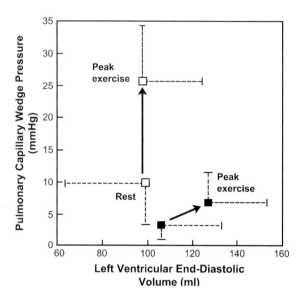

Fig. 4. LV diastolic function assessed by invasive cardiopulmonary exercise testing in patients who have heart failure and normal systolic function (*open boxes*) and age-matched normals (*closed boxes*). Pressure–volume relation was shifted upward and leftward at rest. In the patients with exercise, LV diastolic volume did not increase despite marked increase in diastolic (pulmonary wedge) pressure. Because of diastolic dysfunction, failure of the Frank-Starling mechanism resulted in severe exercise intolerance. (*From* Kitzman DW, Higginbotham MB, Cobb FR, et al. Exercise intolerance in patients with heart failure and preserved left ventricular systolic function: failure of the Frank-Startling mechanism. J Am Coll Cardiol 1991;17:1065–72; with permission.)

Nearly all (88%) DHF patients have a history of chronic systemic hypertension [4,35,36]. In addition, severe systolic hypertension usually is present during acute exacerbations (pulmonary edema) [37–39].

The role of ischemia in DHF is uncertain. It would seem likely that it is a significant contributor in many cases. It had been hypothesized that patients found to have a normal EF following an episode of CHF may merely have had transiently reduced systolic function or ischemia at the time of the acute exacerbation. To address this question, an echocardiogram was performed at the time of presentation in 38 consecutive patients who had acute hypertensive pulmonary edema and was repeated again about 3 days later after resolution of pulmonary edema and control of hypertension [39]. The left ventricular EF and wall motion score index at follow-up were similar to those found during the acute echocardiogram. Furthermore, of those who had LV EF of 50% or greater at follow-up (n = 18), all but two had LV EF of 50% or greater acutely, and in those two cases the LV EF was greater than 40%, above the level that would be expected to cause acute HF because of primary systolic dysfunction (Fig. 6). These data suggest that marked transient systolic dysfunction and overt ischemia do not play primary roles

Group	Young Normal	Old Normal	Elderly Diastolic HF
VO$_2$ Max (ml/kg/min)	28.6	22.6	12.7

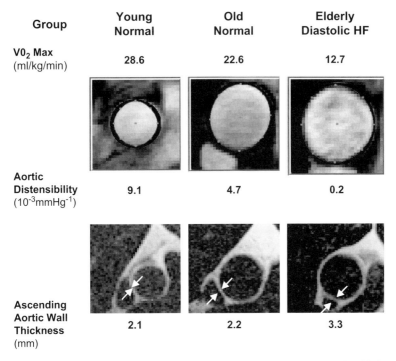

	Young Normal	Old Normal	Elderly Diastolic HF
Aortic Distensibility (10^{-3}mmHg^{-1})	9.1	4.7	0.2
Ascending Aortic Wall Thickness (mm)	2.1	2.2	3.3

Fig. 5. Data and images from representative subjects from healthy young, healthy elderly, and elderly patients who have diastolic heart failure (DHF). Maximal exercise oxygen consumption (VO$_2$max), aortic distensibility at rest, and left ventricular mass:volume ratio. Patients who have DHF have severely reduced exercise tolerance (VO$_2$max) and aortic distensibility and increased aortic wall thickness. (*Adapted from* Hundley WG, Kitzman DW, Morgan TM, et al. Cardiac cycle dependent changes in aortic area and aortic distensibility are reduced in older patients with isolated diastolic heart failure and correlate with exercise intolerance. J Am Coll Cardiol 2001;38:796–802; with permission.)

in most patients who present with acute CHF in the presence of severe systolic hypertension and are subsequently found to have a normal EF [39]. Further, the data support the concept that acute pulmonary edema in these patients most likely is because of an exacerbation of diastolic dysfunction caused by severe systolic hypertension. The data also suggest that the EF measurement from an echocardiogram performed in follow-up accurately reflects that during an episode of acute pulmonary edema [39].

In a related study, 3-year follow-up was performed in 46 patients who initially presented with acute hypertensive pulmonary edema [38]. Most patients had a normal EF. Of those who were referred clinically for coronary angiography (n = 38), 33 had obstructive epicardial coronary artery disease and 19 underwent revascularization. Of these 19, by 6-month follow-up, 9 had been hospitalized with recurrent pulmonary edema and 1 had died. Severe systolic hypertension was nearly uniformly present at the time of recurrent pulmonary edema [38]. These two studies suggest that

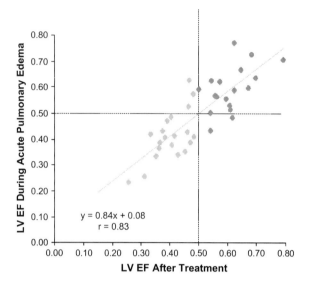

Fig. 6. Left ventricular ejection fraction (LVEF) measured during acute pulmonary edema and at follow-up, 1 to 3 days after treatment. Nearly all patients found to have normal EF ($> 50\%$) at follow-up also had normal EF during acute pulmonary edema. (*Adapted from* Gandhi SK, Powers JE, Fowle KM, et al. The pathogenesis of acute pulmonary edema associated with hypertension. N Engl J Med 2000;344:17–22; with permission. Copyright © 2000 Massachusetts Medical Society. All rights reserved.)

severe systolic hypertension may play a pivotal role in the pathogenesis of acute exacerbations of DHF.

Neurohormonal activation likely plays an important role in the pathophysiology of DHF as it does in patients who have SHF. In a group of patients who have primary DHF, Clarkson and colleagues [40] showed that atrial natriuretic peptide and brain natriuretic peptide were substantially increased and there was an exaggerated response during exercise, a pattern similar to that described in patients who have SHF. In the study described earlier [25], it was found that brain natriuretic peptide was significantly increased in patients who had DHF compared with normal controls, but not so severely as in those who had SHF. Norepinephrine, however, was increased to a similar degree as in SHF.

The role of genetic predisposition in the genesis of DHF in the elderly is not known. Diastolic LV relaxation is significantly modulated by beta-adrenergic stimulation by way of phospholamban and, to a lesser extent, cardiac troponin-I, both of which are substantially under genetic control. Furthermore, data from the HyperGen study have shown significant heritability of hypertension [41], LV mass [42], and Doppler diastolic filling [43], all factors that likely play a role in DHF in the elderly. The genetic basis of familial hypertrophic cardiomyopathy, which has substantial phenotypic similarities to isolated DHF in the elderly, has been described [44,45]. It is noteworthy that in that disorder the phenotype may not be expressed for 30 to 50 years.

Diagnosis and clinical features

The distinction between HF attributable to systolic dysfunction versus diastolic dysfunction usually cannot be made reliably at the bedside [46] and evaluation of new-onset HF in an elderly patient should include an imaging test, usually an echocardiogram [47]. This test not only assesses systolic function but also excludes unexpected but important diagnoses, such as aortic stenosis, severe valvular regurgitation, large pericardial effusion, hypertrophic obstructive cardiomyopathy, and cardiac amyloidosis. Unfortunately, a definitive noninvasive measure is not available for diastolic dysfunction. Doppler left ventricular diastolic filling indexes and particularly the newer tissue Doppler techniques [48] can provide helpful supplementary information, but their role in the clinical diagnosis of the DHF syndrome is unclear and their independent discriminatory power in unselected populations is not known.

Diagnostic criteria from the European Study Group on Diastolic Heart Failure [49] include: signs and symptoms of CHF, a normal or at most mildly reduced LV EF, and evidence of abnormal diastolic function. Subsequent work by Vasan [50] and Gandhi [39] suggest that DHF diagnosis usually can be made without the mandate for measurement of EF at the time of the acute event. Invasive measures of diastolic function are impractical and not feasible in most circumstances. Furthermore, two studies by Zile and co-workers [51,52] suggest that measures of diastolic function, invasive or otherwise, are not necessary for the diagnosis of DHF, because nearly all patients who meet the other criteria for DHF have diastolic dysfunction. The original European criteria thus have undergone substantial modification, primarily by simplification, as a result of the above progress in our understanding of the syndrome of DHF [53–55]. In addition to positive inclusion criteria, care should be taken to exclude other causes for the signs and symptoms suggesting HF [56]. Finally, patients who have HF, a normal EF, and no other explanation for their symptoms have the more pure diagnosis of isolated DHF. In CHS, this subgroup comprised 42% of the patients who had CHF and a normal EF [4]. Typical patients who have isolated DHF are women and often have high normal or super-normal EF (70% or more), normal or small left ventricular chamber size, thick walls with concentric hypertrophy, and no segmental wall motion abnormalities.

Because active myocardial ischemia can present as HF, particularly in the elderly, and has independent prognostic and therapeutic implications, a stress test is often indicated; in the case of concomitant severe or unstable angina, coronary angiography is indicated.

Rapid brain natriuretic peptide (BNP) assays can aid in the diagnosis of HF, particularly in the emergency setting, and may help in judging disease severity and prognosis [19]. The role of BNP assays in the routine evaluation and management of chronic, stable DHF patients is not well defined, however [19]. It is notable that among healthy subjects, both sex and age significantly affect ranges of BNP [57,58]. Further, because BNP seems to be increased in DHF and systolic failure [40] it may not be helpful in discriminating between these two disorders [25].

Prognosis

The severity of exercise intolerance and the frequency of hospitalization appear to be similar in patients who have systolic versus diastolic HF [25,59–62]. This high rate of hospitalization is associated with poor quality of life and high health care costs [63,64]. The annual mortality rate for diastolic HF in the Framingham Study was 8.9% per year, a rate about two-fold higher than nested case controls, although it was only half that reported for SHF (19.6%) [3]. Similar results were found in CHS [5]. In hospitalized patients, however, mortality is similar with diastolic and systolic HF (Fig. 7) [1,59,60,65,66]. This finding was recently confirmed in two large studies, which also showed that the mortality of DHF over the past 15 years is not decreasing [2,67,68]. An important observation in the Cardiovascular Health Study was that, given the higher prevalence among the elderly, the population-attributable mortality risk in patients who have DHF is actually higher than in those who have SHF, highlighting the public health implications of DHF in the elderly [5].

Predictors of prognosis are not as well defined in DHF as in SHF, but appear to include age, sex, and BNP levels [7,10,69].

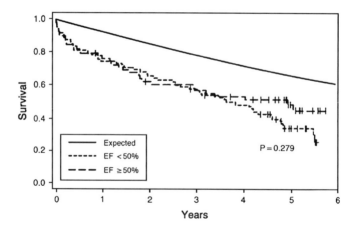

Fig. 7. Survival of patients admitted with congestive heart failure by ejection fraction. (*From* Senni M, Tribouilloy CM, Rodeheffer RJ, et al. Congestive heart failure in the community: a study of all incident cases in Olmsted County, Minnesota, in 1991. Circulation 1998; 98:2282–89.)

Management

Our literature base regarding therapy of DHF is embarrassingly scant [55,70,71]. In contrast to SHF, for which numerous studies in many thousands of patients have generated a rich evidence base to direct therapy, there is essentially only one large, multicenter trial in DHF. This is remarkable given the high prevalence, substantial morbidity, and significant mortality of DHF [55,71–73]. This situation is particularly regrettable for older patients who bear the greatest burden of DHF.

Considering the surprising reversals and seemingly paradoxic outcomes during the circuitous journey to definitive, evidence-based therapy for SHF during the past 3 decades, one should not expect a clear, easy path toward establishing effective evidence-based therapy for DHF. Several large trials are now in progress.

The absence of specific evidence-based data to guide therapy is reflected in the brief discussion of DHF in the recent American College of Cardiology/ American Heart Association 2005 Heart Failure Evaluation and Management Guidelines [74]. As discussed in the guidelines document, there are several empiric recommendations that can be provided [74].

General approach

The approach to the patient who has DHF should begin with a search for a primary cause. Most such patients are found to have hypertension as their main underlying condition [19]. Screening for ischemic heart disease with a noninvasive stress test or coronary angiography should be considered, especially in patients who have chest pain or flash pulmonary edema, to exclude severe coronary heart disease [19]. When found, manifest ischemia should be treated, including invasively if indicated [19], because ischemia is a therapeutic target in its own right and also strongly impairs diastolic relaxation. A small but important number of patients are found to have hypertrophic cardiomyopathy [75,76] with or without dynamic obstruction, undiagnosed valvular disease, or rarely amyloid heart disease [77].

Control of hypertension may be the single most important treatment strategy for DHF [78]. Chronic hypertension causes left ventricular hypertrophy and fibrosis, which impair diastolic chamber compliance. Acute hypertension significantly impairs diastolic relaxation. In addition, meta-analyses indicate that therapy for chronic, mild systolic hypertension in the elderly is a potent means of preventing the development of HF (Table 1), and it is likely that a major portion of cases prevented are attributable to DHF [78–82]. The ALLHAT study showed that the diuretic chlorthalidone was at least as effective for prevention of CHF as other antihypertensive medications [83].

Loss of atrial contraction is deleterious to LV filling, and atrial fibrillation with fast ventricular rate is a common precipitant to decompensated

Table 1
Effect of antihypertensive therapy on incident heart failure in the elderly

Trial	N	Age range (yrs)	Risk reduction (%)
European Working Party	840	>60	22
Coope and Warrender	884	60–79	32
Swedish Trial	1627	70–84	51
SHEP	4736	≥60	55
Syst-Eur	4695	≥60	36
STONE	1632	60–79	68

Adapted from Rich MW, Kitzman DW. Heart failure in octogenarians: a fundamentally different disease. Am J Geriatr Cardiol 2000;9(Suppl 5):97–111.

DHF. Sinus rhythm therefore should be maintained [19]. Achieving and maintaining sinus rhythm can be difficult in the elderly in whom the rate of atrial fibrillation is high. When sinus rhythm cannot be maintained, a more modest goal of rate control should be pursued.

Management goals in elders who have DHF include relief of symptoms, improvement in functional capacity and quality of life, prevention of acute exacerbations and related hospital admissions, and prolongation of survival. A systematic approach should comprise several elements: diagnosis and staging of disease, search for reversible cause, judicious use of medications, patient education, enhancement of self-management skills, coordination of care across disciplines, and effective follow-up. Every HF patient should have a scale, weigh regularly, and know what steps to take if weight increases beyond prespecified ranges. Diuretic adjustments can be performed by nurses over the telephone and in some cases by patients themselves. There must be easy access to health care providers so that problems can be addressed early to avoid decompensation with periodic telephone calls, frequent follow-up appointments, and monitoring programs using telephone and the internet [19,84].

There is now undisputed evidence of the efficacy of a multidisciplinary approach to care in reducing acute exacerbations leading to rehospitalization, improving quality of life, reducing total costs, and increasing survival [85–88]. Notably, many of these studies included significant numbers of patients who had normal EF [86]. Elders and women who have HF often have severe deconditioning and severe exercise intolerance and they should be encouraged to undertake regular moderate physical activity.

The association between alcohol intake and HF is controversial; one recent study suggested that moderate alcohol intake had a mild protective effect for HF in the elderly [89].

Pharmacologic therapy

Despite the fact that numerous randomized, controlled trials have shown a marked decrease in development of HF in patients treated for systolic hypertension (Table 1) [79–82], community surveys consistently show undertreatment of hypertension. Adequate treatment of systemic hypertension is a potent means for prevention of DHF.

Diuretics

Diuretics are indispensable for rapid relief of pulmonary congestion and peripheral edema and are necessary in most patients who have moderate to severe HF to mitigate volume overload. They may accelerate activation of the renin-angiotensin system and cause renal insufficiency and electrolyte disturbances, however. The lowest dose capable of maintaining euvolemia should be used. Although some patients who have mild DHF can be treated effectively with a thiazide diuretic for some time, usually a loop diuretic is eventually required to maintain euvolemia.

Most patients who have HF have an intrinsic diuretic threshold below which minimal diuresis occurs, even when repeated doses are administered. Multiple daily doses thus are not usually necessary and are inconvenient particularly in older women in whom they can exacerbate urinary incontinence [56]. Usually, a single morning oral dose somewhat greater than the diuretic threshold provides effective control of salt and fluid retention. Nonsteroidal anti-inflammatory medications, frequently used in older patients, can cause relative diuretic resistance and should be discontinued if possible. During active diuresis, careful monitoring and replacement of electrolytes, particularly potassium and magnesium, are important; fluid restriction may be needed to avoid or alleviate hyponatremia [90].

Digoxin

Because most inotropes enhance early diastolic relaxation, digoxin might theoretically have a similar effect. In a recent report from the Digitalis Investigation Group Trial (DIG), in the large subset of ambulatory elderly patients who had mild to moderate symptomatic DHF and normal sinus rhythm, digoxin had no net positive or negative effect when assessed as either overall mortality or all-cause or cardiovascular hospitalizations (Fig. 8) [91]. Contrary to prior, small anecdotal reports, digoxin does not increase overall mortality and need not be avoided if indicated for other reasons in DHF patients.

Angiotensin-converting enzyme inhibitors

ACE inhibitors (ACEI) and angiotensin receptor blockers (ARBs) are attractive as therapy for patients who have DHF. They are the cornerstone of systolic HF therapy because they reduce mortality and hospital admissions and improve exercise tolerance and symptoms. As discussed previously, patients who have DHF also appear to have neuroendocrine activation, increased left ventricular filling pressure, and decreased stroke volume similar to those who have systolic failure [25,26,40]. ACE inhibition reduces blood pressure and LVH and improves left ventricular relaxation and aortic distensibility [92–96].

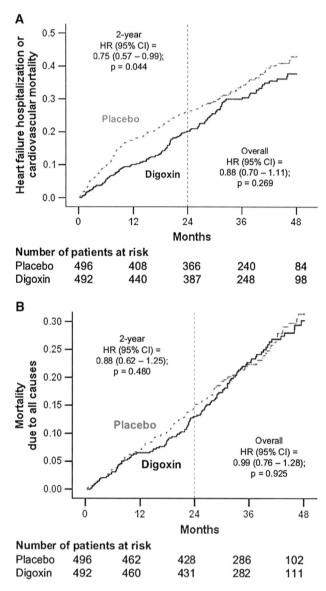

Fig. 8. Effect of digoxin on heart failure hospitalization and cardiovascular mortality (*A*) and all cause mortality (*B*) in patients who have heart failure and normal ejection fraction in the DIG trial. (*From* Ahmed A, Rich MW, Fleg JL, et al. Effects of digoxin on morbidity and mortality in diastolic heart failure. The Ancillary Digitalis Investigation Group Trial. Circulation 2006;114:397–403; with permission.)

Aronow and colleagues [97] showed in a group of New York Heart Association class III HF patients who had presumed diastolic dysfunction (EF > 50%) that enalapril significantly improved functional class, exercise duration, EF, diastolic filling, and left ventricular mass. In an observational study of 1402 patients admitted to 10 community hospitals, ACEI use in DHF patients was associated with substantially reduced all-cause mortality (odds ratio 0.61) and CHF death (odds ratio 0.55) [98,99]. The European trial PEP-CHF is assessing the effect of the ACEI perindopril in elderly (age > 70 years) patients who have HF with an LV EF 40% or greater on death, HF admission, quality of life, and 6-minute walk distance [100].

Angiotensin receptor blockers

In a blinded, randomized, controlled, crossover trial of 20 elderly patients who had diastolic dysfunction and an exaggerated blood pressure response to exercise, the ARB losartan substantially improved exercise capacity and quality of life [101]. The CHARM-Preserved trial assessed the effect of candesartan on death and hospital admission in patients who had HF with EF > 40% [102]. This study included a substantial number of women and elderly. Over a median follow-up of 36 months, cardiovascular death did not differ from placebo; however, fewer patients in the candesartan group than in the placebo group (230 versus 279, $P = .017$) were admitted to the hospital for new episodes of CHF. The ongoing I-PRESERVE trial is assessing the effect of the ARB irbesartan compared with placebo, is recruiting a larger number of DHF patients, and is using more specific inclusion criteria.

Calcium channel antagonists

Calcium channel antagonists often have been suggested for DHF. In hypertrophic cardiomyopathy, a disorder in which diastolic dysfunction is common, verapamil seems to improve symptoms and objectively measured exercise capacity [103–106]. In laboratory animal models calcium antagonists, particularly dihydropyridines, prevent ischemia-induced increases in LV diastolic stiffness [107] and improve diastolic performance in pacing-induced HF [108–110]. Negative inotropic calcium antagonists significantly impair early relaxation, however [110–114], and in general have shown a tendency toward adverse outcome in patients who have systolic HF [110]. Setaro and coworkers [115] examined 22 men (mean age 65) who had clinical HF despite EF greater than 45% in a randomized, double-blind, placebo-controlled crossover trial of verapamil. There was a 33% improvement in exercise time and significant improvements in clinicoradiographic HF scoring and peak filling rate.

In a randomized, crossover, blinded trial, Little and colleagues [116] compared the calcium channel antagonist verapamil to the angiotensin receptor antagonist candesartan with the outcomes of peak exercise blood pressure, exercise time, and quality of life. Although both agents blunted the peak systolic blood pressure response to exercise, only candesartan, and not verapamil, improved exercise time and quality of life (Fig. 9) [116].

Beta-adrenergic antagonists

Beta-adrenergic antagonists also have been successful as therapy for hypertrophic obstructive cardiomyopathy [117]. In addition, they substantially improve mortality in SHF patients. Furthermore, they reduce blood pressure, assist in the regression of ventricular hypertrophy, and increase the ischemic threshold, all of hypothetical importance in DHF [29,31,35,118,119].

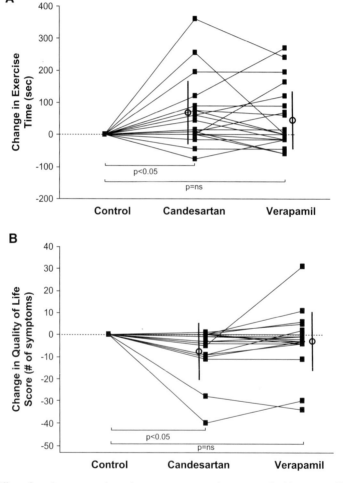

Fig. 9. Effect of candesartan angiotensin receptor antagonist compared with verapamil calcium channel blocker on exercise time (*A*) and quality of life (*B*) in patients who have diastolic dysfunction. (*From* Little WC, Wesley-Farrington DJ, Hoyle J et al. Effects of candesartan and verapamil on exercise tolerance in diastolic dysfunction. J Cardiovasc Pharmacol 2004;43(2):288–93; with permission.)

Cheng and coworkers and others have shown that early diastolic relaxation is impaired by beta-adrenergic blockade, however [120,121]. Delineating the role of beta-blockers in DHF will require large, well-designed clinical trials.

Aldosterone antagonists

The addition of low-dose spironolactone (12.5 to 50 mg daily) to standard therapy has been shown to reduce mortality 30% in patients who have severe SHF [122]. Aldosterone antagonism has numerous potential benefits in patients who have DHF, including LV remodeling, reversal of myocardial fibrosis, and improved LV diastolic function and vascular function [123–125]. Few data are presently available regarding aldosterone antagonism in DHF, however. In one small study, low-dose spironolactone was well tolerated and appeared to improve exercise capacity and quality of life in older women who had isolated DHF [126]. In another, spironolactone improved measures of myocardial function in hypertensive patients who had DHF [127]. Notably, spironolactone is much better tolerated in women, who have lower rates of mastodynia than men [122]. Spironolactone and eplerenone are contraindicated in patients who have advanced renal dysfunction or pre-existing hyperkalemia. Delineation of the role of this potentially promising strategy will need to await results of clinical trials [55]. The National Heart, Lung, and Blood Institute is sponsoring a large, multicenter, randomized, placebo-controlled trial of spironolactone in older patients who have DHF, which is in the process of launching at the time of this writing.

Novel agents

Glucose cross-links increase with aging and diabetes, and cause increased vascular and myocardial stiffness. Alagebrium, a novel cross-link breaker, improved vascular and LV stiffness in dogs. In a small, open-label, 4-month trial of this agent in elderly patients, LV mass, quality of life, and tissue Doppler diastolic function indexes improved, but there were no significant improvements in exercise capacity or aortic distensibility, the primary outcomes of the trial [128]. Various other agents and strategies currently are being evaluated or under consideration for this syndrome, including a selective endothelin antagonist.

References

[1] Senni M, Tribouilloy CM, Rodeheffer RJ, et al. Congestive heart failure in the community: a study of all incident cases in Olmsted County, Minnesota, in 1991. Circulation 1998; 98(21):2282–9.

[2] Owan TE, Hodge DO, Herges RM, et al. Trends in prevalence and outcome of heart failure with preserved ejection fraction. N Engl J Med 2006;355(3):251–9.

[3] Ramachandran S, Vasan RS, Larson MG, et al. Congestive heart failure in subjects with normal versus reduced left ventricular ejection fraction. J Am Coll Cardiol 1999;33(7): 1948–55.

[4] Kitzman DW, Gardin JM, Gottdiener JS, et al. Importance of heart failure with preserved systolic function in patients ≥65 Years of Age. CHS Research Group. Cardiovascular Health Study. Am J Cardiol 2001;87(4):413–9.

[5] Gottdiener JS, McClelland R, Marshall RJ, et al. Outcome of congestive heart failure in elderly persons: Influence of left ventricular systolic function. The Cardiovascular Health Study. Ann Intern Med 2002;137(8):631–9.

[6] Devereux RB, Roman MJ, Liu JE, et al. Congestive heart failure despite normal left ventricular systolic function in a population-based sample: the Strong Heart Study. Am J Cardiol 2000;86(10):1090–6.

[7] Kupari M, Lindroos M, Iivanainen AM, et al. Congestive heart failure in old age: prevalence, mechanisms and 4-year prognosis in the Helsinki Ageing Study. J Intern Med 1997;241:387–94.

[8] Masoudi FA, Havranek EP, Smith G, et al. Gender, age, and heart failure with preserved left ventricular systolic function. J Am Coll Cardiol 2003;41(2):217–23.

[9] Havranek EP, Masoudi FA, Westfall KA, et al. Spectrum of heart failure in older patients: results from the National Heart Failure project. Am Heart J 2002;143(3):412–7.

[10] Gottdiener JS, Arnold AM, Aurigemma GP, et al. Predictors of congestive heart failure in the elderly: the Cardiovascular Health Study. J Am Coll Cardiol 2000;35(6):1628–37.

[11] Samuel RS, Hausdorff JM, Wei JY. Congestive heart failure with preserved systolic function: Is it a woman's disease? Womens Health Issue 1999;9:219–22.

[12] Gerdts E, Zabalgoitia M, Bjornstad H, et al. Gender differences in systolic left ventricular function in hypertensive patients with electrocardiographic left ventricular hypertrophy (the LIFE study). Am J Cardiol 2001;87(8):980–3.

[13] Kane GC, Hauser MF, Behrenbeck TR, et al. Impact of gender on rest Tc-99m sestamibi-gated left ventricular ejection fraction. Am J Cardiol 2002;89(10):1238–41.

[14] Bella JN, Palmieri V, Kitzman DW, et al. Gender difference in diastolic function in hypertension (the HyperGEN study). Am J Cardiol 2002;89(9):1052–6.

[15] Bella JN, Wachtell K, Palmieri V, et al. Relation of left ventricular geometry and function to systemic hemodynamics in hypertension: the LIFE Study. Losartan Intervention For Endpoint Reduction in Hypertension Study. J Hypertens 2001;19(1):127–34.

[16] Douglas PS, Katz SE, Weinberg EO, et al. Hypertrophic remodeling: gender differences in the early response to left ventricular pressure overload. J Am Coll Cardiol 1998;32(4):1118–25.

[17] Aurigemma GP, Silver KH, McLaughlin M, et al. Impact of chamber geometry and gender on left ventricular systolic function in patients >60 years of age with aortic stenosis. Am J Cardiol 1994;74(8):794–8.

[18] Aurigemma GP, Gaasch WH, McLaughlin M, et al. Reduced left ventricular systolic pump performance and depressed myocardial contractile function in patients >65 years of age with normal ejection fraction and a high relative wall thickness. Am J Cardiol 1995;76(10):702–5.

[19] Mendes LA, Davidoff R, Cupples LA, et al. Congestive heart failure in patients with coronary artery disease: the gender paradox. Am Heart J 1997;134(2 Pt 1):207–12.

[20] Freshour JR, Chase SE, Vikstrom KL. Gender differences in cardiac ACE expression are normalized in androgen-deprived male mice. Am J Physiol Heart Circ Physiol 2002;283(5):H1997–2003.

[21] Rich MW, Kitzman DW. Heart failure in octogenarians: a fundamentally different disease. Am J Geriatr Cardiol 2000;9(Suppl 5):97–104.

[22] Ogawa T, Spina RJ, Martin WH, et al. Effect of aging, sex, and physical training on cardiovacular responses to exercise. Circulation 1992;86:494–503.

[23] Spina RJ, Ogawa T, Miller TR, et al. Effect of exercise training on left ventricular performance in older women free of cardiopulmonary disease. Am J Cardiol 1993;71:99–194.

[24] Sullivan M, Cobb FR, Knight JD, et al. Stroke volume increases by similar mechanisms in men and women. Am J Cardiol 1991;67:1405–12.

[25] Kitzman DW, Little WC, Brubaker PH, et al. Pathophysiological characterization of isolated diastolic heart failure in comparison to systolic heart failure. JAMA 2002;288(17): 2144–50.

[26] Kitzman DW, Higginbotham MB, Cobb FR, et al. Exercise intolerance in patients with heart failure and preserved left ventricular systolic function: failure of the Frank-Starling mechanism. J Am Coll Cardiol 1991;17:1065–72.

[27] Brubaker PH, Joo KC, Stewart KP, et al. Chronotropic incompetence and its contribution to exercise intolerance in older heart failure patients. J Cardiopulm Rehabil 2006;26(2): 86–9.

[28] Hundley WG, Kitzman DW, Morgan TM, et al. Cardiac cycle dependent changes in aortic area and aortic distensibility are reduced in older patients with isolated diastolic heart failure and correlate with exercise intolerance. J Am Coll Cardiol 2001;38(3):796–802.

[29] Little WC. Enhanced load dependence of relaxation in heart failure: clinical implications. Circulation 1992;85(6):2326–8.

[30] Gelpi RJ. Changes in diastolic cardiac function in developing and stable perinephritic hypertension in conscious dogs. Circ Res 1991;68:555–67.

[31] Shannon RP, Komamura K, Gelpi RJ, et al. Altered load: an important component of impaired diastolic function in hypertension and heart failure. In: Lorell BH, Grossman W, editors. Diastolic relaxation of the heart. Norwell, Massachusetts: Kluwer Academic Publishers; 1994. p. 177–85.

[32] Little WC. Assessment of normal and abnormal cardiac function. In: Braunwald E, Zipes DP, Libby P, editors. Heart disease. Philadelphia: W.B. Saunders Company; 2001. p. 479–502.

[33] Hoit BD, Walsh RA. Diastolic dysfunction in hypertensive heart disease. In: Gaasch WH, LeWinter MM, editors. Left ventricular diastolic dysfunction and heart failure. Philadelphia: Lea & Febiger; 1994. p. 354–72.

[34] Little WC, Ohno M, Kitzman DW, et al. Determination of left ventricular chamber stiffness from the time for deceleration of early left ventricular filling. Circulation 1995;92: 1933–9.

[35] Iriarte M, Murga N, Morillas M, et al. Congestive heart failure from left ventricular diastolic dysfunction in systemic hypertension. Am J Cardiol 1993;71:308–12.

[36] Iriarte MM, Perez OJ, Sagastagoitia D, et al. Congestive heart failure due to hypertensive ventricular diastolic dysfunction. Am J Cardiol 1995;76(13):43D–7D.

[37] Cohen-Solal A, Desnos M, Delahaye F, et al, for the Myocardiopathy and Heart Failure Working Group of the French Society of Cardiology tNCoGHCatFGS. A national survey of heart failure in French hospitals. Eur Heart J 2000;21:763–9.

[38] Kramer K, Kirkman P, Kitzman DW, et al. Flash pulmonary edema: association with hypertension, recurrence despite coronary revascularization. Am Heart J 2000;140(3): 451–5.

[39] Gandhi SK, Powers JE, Fowle KM, et al. The pathogenesis of acute pulmonary edema associated with hypertension. N Engl J Med 2000;344(1):17–22.

[40] Clarkson PBM, Wheeldon NM, MacFadyen RJ, et al. Effects of brain natriuretic peptide on exercise hemodynamics and neurohormones in isolated diastolic heart failure. Circulation 1996;93:2037–42.

[41] Bella JN, Palmieri V, Liu JE, et al. Relationship between left ventricular diastolic relaxation and systolic function in hypertension: the hypertension genetic epidemiology network (hypergen) study. Hypertension 2001;38(3):424–8.

[42] Arnett DK, Hong Y, Bella J, et al. Sibling correlation of left ventricular mass and geometry in hypertensive African Americans and whites: the HyperGEN Study. Am J Hypertens 2001;14(12):1226–30.

[43] Tang W, Arnett DK, Devereux RB, et al. Linkage of left ventricular diastolic peak filling velocity to chromosome 5 in hypertensive African Americans: the HyperGEN echocardiography study. Am J Hypertens 2002;15(7 Pt 1):621–7.

[44] Vikstrom KL, Leinwand LA. The molecular genetic basis of familial hypertrophic cardiomyopathy. Heart Fail 1995;11(1):5–14.

[45] Webster KA, Bishopric NH. Molecular aspects and gene therapy prospects for diastolic failure. Cardiol Clin 2000;18(3):621–35.

[46] Ghali JK, Kadakia S, Cooper R, et al. Bedside diagnosis of preserved versus impaired left ventricular systolic function in heart failure. Am J Cardiol 1991;67:1002–6.

[47] Aronow WS, Ahn C, Kronzon I. Normal left ventricular ejection fraction in older persons with congestive heart failure. Chest 1998;113(4):867–9.

[48] Nagueh SF, Middleton KJ, Kopelen HA, et al. Doppler tissue imaging: a noninvasive technique for evaluation of left ventricular relaxation and estimation of filling pressures. J Am Coll Cardiol 1997;30(6):1527–33.

[49] European Study Group on Diastolic Heart Failure. How to diagnose diastolic heart failure. Eur Heart J 1998;19:990–1003.

[50] Vasan RS, Levy D. Defining diastolic heart failure: a call for standardized diagnostic criteria. Circulation 2000;101(17):2118–21.

[51] Zile MR, Gaasch WH, Carroll JD, et al. Heart failure with a normal ejection fraction: is measurement of diastolic function necessary to make the diagnosis of diastolic heart failure? Circulation 2001;104(7):779–82.

[52] Zile MR, Baicu CF, Gaasch WH. Diastolic heart failure–abnormalities in active relaxation and passive stiffness of the left ventricle. N Engl J Med 2004;350(19):1953–9.

[53] Zile MR, Brutsaert DL. New concepts in diastolic dysfunction and diastolic heart failure: Part I: diagnosis, prognosis, and measurements of diastolic function. Circulation 2002; 105(11):1387–93.

[54] Zile MR, Brutsaert DL. New concepts in diastolic dysfunction and diastolic heart failure: Part II: causal mechanisms and treatment. Circulation 2002;105(12):1503–8.

[55] Redfield MM. Understanding "diastolic" heart failure. N Engl J Med 2004;350(19):1930–1.

[56] Kitzman DW. Heart failure and cardiomyopathy. In: Abrams WB, Beers MH, Berkow B, editors. The Merck manual of geriatrics. Whitehouse Station, N.J.: Merck Research Laboratories; 2000. p. 900–14.

[57] Redfield MM, Rodeheffer RJ, Jacobsen SJ, et al. Plasma brain natriuretic peptide concentration: impact of age and gender. J Am Coll Cardiol 2002;40(5):976–82.

[58] Davis KM, Fish LC, Minaker KL, et al. Atrial natriuretic peptide levels in the elderly: differentiating normal aging changes from disease. J Gerontol 1996;51A:M95–101.

[59] Pernenkil R, Vinson JM, Shah AS, et al. Course and prognosis in patients ≥ 70 years of age with congestive heart failure and normal versus abnormal left ventricular ejection fraction. Am J Cardiol 1997;79(2):216–9.

[60] Vinson JM, Rich MW, Sperry JC, et al. Early readmission of elderly patients with congestive heart failure. J Am Geriatr Soc 1990;38:1290–5.

[61] Rich MW, Vinson JM, Sperry JC, et al. Prevention of readmission in elderly patients with congestive heart failure: results of a prospective, randomized pilot study. J Gen Intern Med 1993;8:585–90.

[62] Kitzman DW. Heart failure in the elderly: systolic and diastolic dysfunction. Am J Geriatr Cardiol 1995;5:20–6.

[63] Schocken DD, Arrieta MI, Leaverton PE, et al. Prevalence and mortality rate of congestive heart failure in the United States. J Am Coll Cardiol 1992;20:301–6.

[64] Senni M, Tribouilloy CM, Rodeheffer RJ, et al. Congestive heart failure in the community: trends in incidence and survival in a 10-year period. Arch Intern Med 1999;159(1):29–34 [see comments].

[65] Taffet GE, Teasdale TA, Bleyer AJ, et al. Survival of elderly men with congestive heart failure. Age Ageing 1992;21:49–55.

[66] Aronow WS, Ahn C, Kronzon I. Prognosis of congestive heart failure in elderly patients with normal versus abnormal left ventricular systolic function associated with coronary artery disease. Am J Cardiol 1990;66:1257–9.

[67] Bhatia RS, Tu JV, Lee DS, et al. Outcome of heart failure with preserved ejection fraction in a population-based study. N Engl J Med 2006;355(3):260–9.

[68] Aurigemma GP. Diastolic heart failure—a common and lethal condition by any name. N Engl J Med 2006;355(3):308–10.

[69] Opasich C, Tavazzi L, Lucci D, et al. Comparison of one-year outcome in women versus men with chronic congestive heart failure. Am J Cardiol 2000;86(3):353–7.

[70] Kitzman DW. Therapy for diastolic heart failure: on the road from myths to multicenter trials. J Card Fail 2001;7(3):229–31.

[71] Vasan RS, Benjamin EJ. Diastolic heart failure—no time to relax. N Engl J Med 2001; 344(1):56–9.

[72] Tresch DD, McGough MF. Heart failure with normal systolic function: a common disorder in older people. J Am Geriatr Soc 1995;43:1035–42.

[73] Dauterman K, Massie BM, Gheorghiade M. Heart failure associated with preserved systolic function: a common and costly clinical entity. Am Heart J 1998;135(6 Pt 2):S310–7.

[74] Hunt SA, Abraham WT, Chin MH, et al. ACC/AHA 2005 guidelines for the diagnosis and management of chronic heart failure in the adult. A report of the American College of Cardiology/American Heart Association Task Force on Practice Guidelines (Committee to revise the 2001 Guidelines for the Evaluation and Management of Heart Failure). J Am Coll Cardiol 2005;46(6):e1–82.

[75] Lewis JF, Maron BJ. Clinical and morphologic expression of hypertrophic cardiomyopathy in patients ≥ 65 years of age. Am J Cardiol 1994;73:1105–11.

[76] Lewis JF, Maron BJ. Elderly patients with hypertrophic cardiomyopathy: a subset with distinctive left ventricular morphology and progressive clinical course late in life. J Am Coll Cardiol 1989;13:36–45.

[77] Olson LJ, Gertz MA, Edwards WD, et al. Senile cardiac amyloidosis with myocardial dysfunction. Diagnosis by endomyocardial biopsy and immunohistochemistry. N Engl J Med 1987;317:738–42.

[78] Moser M, Hebert PR. Prevention of disease progression, left ventricular hypertrophy and congestive heart failure in hypertension treatment trials. J Am Coll Cardiol 1996;27: 1214–8.

[79] Amery A, Birkenhager W, Brixko P, et al. Mortality and morbidity results from the European Working Party on High Blood Pressure in the Elderly Trial. Lancet 1985;I(8442): 1349–54.

[80] Dahlof B, Lindholm L, Hannson L, et al. Morbidity and mortality in the Swedish Trial in Old Patients with Hypertension (STOP-Hypertension). Lancet 1991;338:1281–5.

[81] Stassen JA, Fagard R, Thijs L, et al. Randomised double-blind comparison of placebo and active treatment for older patients with isolated systolic hypertension. Lancet 1997;350: 757–64.

[82] Gong LS, Zhang W, Zhu Y. Shanghai Trial of Nifedipine in the Elderly (STONE). J Hypertens 2001;14:1237–45.

[83] Major outcomes in high-risk hypertensive patients randomized to angiotensin-converting enzyme inhibitor or calcium channel blocker vs diuretic: The Antihypertensive and Lipid-Lowering Treatment to Prevent Heart Attack Trial (ALLHAT). JAMA 2002; 288(23):2981–97.

[84] Kitzman DW. Diastolic dysfunction in the elderly: genesis and diagnostic and therapeutic implications. In: Kovacs SJ, editor. Cardiology Clinics of North America—Diastolic Function. Philadelphia: W.B. Saunders; 2000. p. 597–617.

[85] Stewart S, Marley JE, Horowitz JD. Effects of a multidisciplinary, home-based intervention on unplanned readmissions and survival among patients with chronic congestive heart failure: a randomised controlled study. Lancet 1999;354(9184):1077–83.

[86] Rich MW, Beckham V, Wittenberg C, et al. A multidisciplinary intervention to prevent the readmission of elderly patients with congestive heart failure. N Engl J Med 1995;333: 1190–5.

[87] Stewart S, Vanderheyden M, Pearson S, et al. Prolonged beneficial effects of a home-based intervention on unplanned readmissions and mortality among patients with congestive heart failure. Arch Intern Med 1999;159(3):257–61.

[88] Tsuyuki RT, McKelvie RS, Arnold JM, et al. Acute precipitants of congestive heart failure exacerbations. Arch Intern Med 2001;161(19):2337–42.

[89] Bryson CL, Mukamal KJ, Mittleman M, et al. The association between alcohol consumption and incident heart failure: the Cardiovascular Health Study. J Am Coll Cardiol 2006; 48:305–11.

[90] Leier CV, Dei Cas L, Metra M. Clinical relevance and management of the major electrolyte abnormalities in congestive heart failure: hyponatremia, hypokalemia, and hypomagnesemia. Am Heart J 1994;128:564–74.

[91] Ahmed A, Rich MW, Fleg JL, et al. Effects of digoxin on morbidity and mortality in diastolic heart failure. The Ancillary Digitalis Investigation Group Trial. Circulation 2006; 114:397–403.

[92] Lorell BH, Grossman W. Cardiac hypertrophy: the consequences for diastole. J Am Coll Cardiol 1987;9:1189–93.

[93] Lorell BH. Cardiac renin-angiotensin system in cardiac hypertrophy and failure. In: Lorell BH, Grossman W, editors. Diastolic relaxation of the heart. 2nd edition. Norwell, Massachusetts: Kluwer Academic Publishers; 1996. p. 91–9.

[94] Oren S, Grossman E, Frohlich ED. Reduction in left ventricular mass in patients with systemic hypertension treated with Enalapril, Lisinopril, or Fosinopril. Am J Cardiol 1996;77: 93–6.

[95] Friedrich SP, Lorell BH, Douglas PS, et al. Intracardiac ACE inhibition improves diastolic distensibility in patients with left ventricular hypertrophy due to aortic stenosis. Circulation 1992;86(suppl I):I-119.

[96] Lakatta E. Cardiovascular aging research: The next horizons. J Am Geriatr Soc 1999;47: 613–25.

[97] Aronow WS, Kronzon I. Effect of enalapril on congestive heart failure treated with diuretics in elderly patients with prior myocardial infarction and normal left ventricular ejection fraction. Am J Cardiol 1993;71:602–4.

[98] Philbin EF, Rocco TA. Use of angiotensin-converting enzyme inhibitors in heart failure with preserved left ventricular systolic function. Am Heart J 1997;134(2):188–95.

[99] Philbin EF, Rocco TA Jr, Lindenmuth NW, et al. Clinical outcomes in heart failure: report from a community hospital-based registry. Am J Med 1999;107(6):549–55.

[100] Cleland JG, Tendera M, Adamus J, et al. Perindopril for elderly people with chronic heart failure: the PEP-CHF study. The PEP investigators. Eur J Heart Fail 1999;1(3):211–7 [see comments].

[101] Abraham TP, Kon ND, Nomeir AM, et al. Accuracy of transesophageal echocardiography in preoperative determination of aortic anulus size during valve replacement. J Am Soc Echocardiogr 1997;10:149–54.

[102] Yusuf S, Pfeffer MA, Swedberg K, et al. Effects of candesartan in patients with chronic heart failure and preserved left-ventricular ejection fraction: the CHARM-Preserved Trial. Lancet 2003;362(9386):777–81.

[103] Vandenberg VF, Rath LS, Stuhlmuller P, et al. Estimation of left ventricular cavity area with on-line, semiautomated echocardiographic edge detection system. Circulation 1992; 86:159–66.

[104] Bonow RO, Leon MB, Rosing DR, et al. Effects of verapamil and propranolol on left ventricular systolic function and diatsolic filling in patients with coronary artery disease: radionuclide angiographic studies at rest and during exercise. Circulation 1981;65: 1337–50.

[105] Bonow RO, Dilsizian V, Rosing DR, et al. Verapamil-induced improvement in left ventricular diastolic filling and increased exercise tolerance in patients with hypertrophic cardiomyopathy: short- and long-term effects. Circulation 1985;72:853–64.

[106] Udelson J, Bonow RO. Left ventricular diastolic function and calcium channel blockers in hypertrophic cardiomyopathy. In: Gaasch WH, editor. Left ventricular diastolic dysfunction and heart failure. Malvern, Pennsylvania: Lea & Febiger; 1996. p. 465–89.

[107] Serizawa T, Shin-Ichi M, Nagai Y, et al. Diastolic abnormalities in low-flow and pacing tachycardia-induced ischemia in isolated rat hearts-modification by calcium antagonists. In: Lorell BH, Grossman W, editors. Diastolic relaxation of the heart. Norwell, Massachusetts: Kluwer Academic Publishers; 1996. p. 266–74.

[108] Cheng CP, Pettersson K, Little WC. Effects of felodipine on left ventricular systolic and diastolic performance in congestive heart failure. J Pharma and Exper Thera 1994;271: 1409–17.

[109] Cheng CP, Noda T, Ohno M, et al. Differential effects of enalaprilat and felodipine on diastolic function during exercise in dogs with congestive heart failure. Circulation 1993;88(4) I–294.

[110] Little WC, Cheng CP, Elvelin L, et al. Vascular selective calcium entry blockers in the treatment of cardiovascular disorders: focus on felodipine. Cardiovasc Drugs Ther 1995;9(5): 657–63.

[111] Ten Cate FJ, Serruys PW, Mey S, et al. Effects of short-term administration of verapamil on left ventricular filling dynamics measured by a combined hemodynamic-ultrasonic technique in patients with hypertrophic cardiomyopathy. Circulation 1983;68(6):1274–9.

[112] Hess OM, Murakami T, Krayenbuehl HP. Does verapamil improve left ventricular relaxation in patients with myocardial hypertrophy? Circulation 1996;74:530–43.

[113] Brutsaert DL, Rademakers F, Sys SU, et al. Analysis of relaxation in the evaluation of ventricular function of the heart. Prog Cardiovasc Dis 1985;28:143–63.

[114] Brutsaert DL, Sys SU, Gillebert TC. Diastolic failure: pathophysiology and therapeutic implications. J Am Coll Cardiol 1993;22:318–25.

[115] Setaro JF, Zaret BL, Schulman DS, et al. Usefulness of verapamil for congestive heart failure associated with abnormal left ventricular diastolic filling and normal left ventricular systolic performance. Am J Cardiol 1990;66:981–6.

[116] Little WC, Wesley-Farrington DJ, Hoyle J, et al. Effect of candesartan and verapamil on exercise tolerance in diastolic dysfunction. J Cardiovasc Pharmacol 2004;43(2):288–93.

[117] Sasayama S, Asanoi H, Ishizaka S, et al. Diastolic dysfunction in experimental heart failure. In: Lorell BH, Grossman W, editors. Diastolic relaxation of the heart. Norwell, Massachusetts: Kluwer Academic Publishers; 1994. p. 195–202.

[118] Copeland JL, Consitt LA, Tremblay MS. Hormonal responses to endurance and resistance exercise in females aged 19–69 years. J Gerontol A Biol Sci Med Sci 2002;57(4): B158–65.

[119] Udelson J, Bonow RO. Left ventricular diastolic function and calcium channel blockers in hypertrophic cardiomyopathy. In: Gaasch WH, LeWinter MM, editors. Left ventricular diastolic dysfunction and heart failure. Philadelphia: Lea & Febiger; 1994. p. 462–89.

[120] Cheng CP, Igarashi Y, Little WC. Mechanism of augmented rate of left ventricle filling during exercise. Circ Res 1992;70:9–19.

[121] Cheng CP, Noda T, Nozawa T, et al. Effect of heart failure on the mechanism of exercise induced augmentation of mitral valve flow. Circ Res 1993;72:795–806.

[122] Pitt B, Zannad F, Remme WJ, et al. The effect of spironolactone on morbidity and mortality in patients with severe heart failure. N Engl J Med 1999;341(10):709–17.

[123] Pitt B, Reichek N, Willenbrock R, et al. Effects of eplerenone, enalapril, and eplerenone/ enalapril in patients with essential hypertension and left ventricular hypertrophy: the 4E-left ventricular hypertrophy study. Circulation 2003;108(15):1831–8.

[124] Rajagopalan S, Pitt B. Aldosterone as a target in congestive heart failure. Med Clin North Am 2003;87(2):441–57.

[125] Zannad F, Alla F, Dousset B, et al. Limitation of excessive extracellular matrix turnover may contribute to survival benefit of spironolactone therapy in patients with congestive heart failure: insights from the randomized Aldactone evaluation study (RALES). Rales Investigators. Circulation 2000;102(22):2700–6.

[126] Daniel KR, Wells GL, Fray B, et al. The effect of spironolactone on exercise tolerance and quality of life in elderly women with diastolic heart failure. Am.J.Geriatr. Cardiol 2003; 12(2):131.

[127] Mottram PM, Haluska B, Leano R, et al. Effect of aldosterone antagonism on myocardial dysfunction in hypertensive patients with diastolic heart failure. Circulation 2004;110(5): 558–65.

[128] Little WC, Zile MR, Kitzman DW, et al. The effect of alagebrium chloride (ALT-711), a novel glucose cross-link breaker, in the treatment of elderly patients with diastolic heart failure. J Card Fail 2005;11(3):191–5.

ELSEVIER
SAUNDERS

CLINICS IN
GERIATRIC
MEDICINE

Clin Geriatr Med 23 (2007) 107–121

Use of Diuretics in the Treatment of Heart Failure in the Elderly

Domenic A. Sica, MD[a], Todd W.B. Gehr, MD[a],
William H. Frishman, MD[b,*]

[a]Division of Nephrology, Virginia Commonwealth University Health System,
Richmond, VA, USA
[b]Department of Medicine, New York Medical College/Westchester Medical Center,
Valhalla, NY, USA

Most therapies used in the contemporary management of heart failure (HF) have been rigorously evaluated in large-scale clinical trials to assess their beneficial effects on quality of life and prognosis. Such therapies include angiotensin-converting enzyme (ACE) inhibitors, angiotensin-receptor blockers, β-blockers, and aldosterone receptor antagonists (ARAs). Diuretics are the most commonly prescribed class of drugs in HF patients and in the short term they remain the most effective treatment for relief from fluid congestion. Diuretic therapy in the HF patient often is as much an art as a science. Moreover, as a class of drugs, diuretics are fairly heterogeneous in their effects. Diuretic therapy in HF should always be accompanied by dietary sodium restriction. Important considerations in defining diuretic effect include issues of dose amount, frequency of dosing, concomitant medications, blood pressure, and, most importantly, the degree to which cardiac function is compromised. Diuretic combinations are often quite effective in the more advanced stages of HF. Diuretic-related electrolyte side effects are common and require ongoing vigilance both to detect their occurrence as well as to track their correction.

Diuretics are tools of considerable therapeutic importance. First, they effectively reduce blood pressure, while at the same time decreasing the morbidity and mortality associated with hypertension. The Joint National Committee on Prevention, Detection, Evaluation, and Treatment of Hypertension recommends diuretics as first-line therapy for the treatment of hypertension [1]. In addition, they remain an important component of HF

* Corresponding author.
E-mail address: William_Frishman@nymc.edu (W.H. Frishman).

0749-0690/07/$ - see front matter © 2006 Elsevier Inc. All rights reserved.
doi:10.1016/j.cger.2006.08.006
geriatric.theclinics.com

therapy, in that they improve the symptoms of congestion, which typify the more advanced stages of HF [2–5]. This article reviews the mode of action of the various diuretic classes and the physiologic adaptations that follow and sets up the basis for their use in the treatment of volume-retaining states particularly as applies to the elderly. In addition, the article reviews the common side effects related to diuretics.

Overview

Guideline-promulgating committees have positioned diuretics as necessary adjuncts in the medical therapy for HF when symptoms of volume overload exist [2–5]. Diuretics are typically used first for the acute relief of congestion and thereafter for achieving and maintaining a target or "dry" weight. Diuretic doses are typically higher in the case of congestion relief and can generally be scaled back in the chronic treatment phase of HF. Diuretic therapy typically results in rapid improvement of dyspnea and increased exercise tolerance [6]. No controlled randomized trials have assessed the effect on symptoms or survival of diuretics and they should always be administered in combination with ACE inhibitors and β-blockers if tolerated.

The relation of systolic to diastolic HF is clearly shifted toward diastolic HF in elderly patients, especially in women [7]. Mortality increases with systolic dysfunction in elderly patients compared with younger HF patients [8]. Mortality is less with diastolic dysfunction, but still higher compared with elderly without HF [9]. In addition, morbidity is increased both with diastolic and systolic HF in elderly patients. Drug therapy for systolic HF in elderly is similar to younger patients although guideline recommendations for drug therapy are based in most cases on studies conducted in younger systolic HF patients. However, when administering drug therapy for systolic HF in the elderly, clinicians should be mindful of the physiologic decrease in renal function with age and the more frequent renal impairment that occurs in elderly patients receiving diuretics for HF management [10]. In addition, loop diuretic treatment of any HF patient should always be at the lowest effective dose. This is particularly so in the elderly patient with HF because the hypercalciuria, produced in a dose-dependent manner by loop diuretics [11], increases the bone-fracture rate, a finding not observed with thiazide-type diuretics [12].

Treatment algorithm for diuretic use in heart failure

A diuretic treatment algorithm for the treatment of HF can become extremely complicated. No one such algorithm can ever meet the treatment needs of all patients, particularly elderly patients. In cases involving the elderly, negative effects of excessive diuresis on blood pressure and renal function often have an impact on decisions related to diuretic dose and frequency. Table 1 offers some guidance on the order of medication choice

Table 1
Diuretic treatment in heart failure

Treatment situation	Comments
Initial treatment given with a loop or a thiazide diuretic in conjunction with an ACE inhibitor.	Severity of volume overload and level of heart failure dictate initial choice and whether drug is given orally or intravenously.
Higher total doses given as needed.	Higher total doses can be given by increasing the individual dose amount, by giving the diuretic more frequently, or both. If diuretic doses need to be titrated upwards, excessive dietary sodium intake needs to be considered as a factor contributing to the change in dose.
Single diuretic therapy fails to produce the desired response.	Factors that may reduce diuretic response, such as insufficient blood pressure, poor diuretic absorption, suboptimal neurohumoral blockade, or use of nonsteroidal anti-inflammatory drugs, should be considered before moving to combination therapy.
Single diuretic therapy fails to produce the desired response and combination therapy is started.	Metolazone can be added to a loop diuretic but is poorly absorbed. Poor absorption needs to be considered in determining the timing of its dosing. Metolazone has a very long half-life and may not need to be given on a daily basis.
Potassium-sparing diuretics are started at varying times in the overall treatment.	These drugs are used to facilitate treatment of diuretic-related hypokalemia or hypomagnesemia. Serum potassium needs to be regularly measured until it is stable.
Once a dry weight is established and maintained, some consideration can be given to reducing the amount of diuretic being given.	Optimizing neurohumoral blockade with ACE inhibition and β-blockade will often allow lowering or sometimes discontinuation of diuretics.

and the basis for such choices. Loop diuretics offer short-term benefits in HF because of symptomatic relief. However, in the long term, they have the potential to adversely influence outcome due to electrolyte changes or excessive neurohumoral activation [13–15]. Consequently, in the long term, diuretic withdrawal or dosage reduction is desirable [16]. Diuretic withdrawal (or interruption) is facilitated by adherence to a low-sodium (low-Na^+) diet. Such withdrawal is typically better tolerated in patients requiring lower diuretic doses, a patient subset characterized by having both smaller ventricles and a higher left ventricular ejection fraction [16].

Individual classes of diuretics

Inter- and intraclass differences exist for all diuretic classes. The diuretic classes of note include carbonic anhydrase inhibitors, loop and distal tubular diuretics, and potassium (K^+)-sparing agents [17].

Carbonic anhydrase inhibitors

Acetazolamide is the only carbonic anhydrase inhibitor with relevant diuretic effects. Acetazolamide is readily absorbed and undergoes renal elimination predominantly by tubular secretion. Its administration is ordinarily accompanied by a brisk alkaline diuresis. Although carbonic anhydrase inhibitors are proximal tubular diuretics (where the bulk of Na^+ reabsorption occurs), their net diuretic effect is modest, since Na^+ reabsorption in more distal nephron segments offsets proximal Na^+ losses. Acetazolamide use is constrained by both its transient action as well as the development of metabolic acidosis with its prolonged administration. Alternatively, acetazolamide (250–500 mg daily) can correct the metabolic or contraction alkalosis that on occasion occurs with aggressive thiazide or loop diuretic therapy [18].

Loop diuretics

Loop diuretics act predominantly at the apical membrane in the thick ascending limb of the loop of Henle, where they compete with chloride (Cl^-) for binding to the $Na^+/K^+/2Cl^-$ cotransporter, thereby inhibiting both Na^+ and Cl^- reabsorption [19]. Loop diuretics also affect Na^+ reabsorption within other nephron segments. However, these effects are qualitatively minor compared with their action at the thick ascending limb. Other clinically important effects of loop diuretics include a decrease in both free water excretion during water loading and free water absorption during dehydration, about a 30% increase in fractional calcium (Ca^{++}) excretion, a significant increase in magnesium (Mg^{++}) excretion, and a decrease in uric acid excretion.

The available loop diuretics include bumetanide, ethacrynic acid, furosemide, and torsemide. These compounds are typically highly protein-bound. To gain access to the tubular lumen (site of action), they must undergo secretion. The same applies to thiazide-type diuretics. Tubular secretion is by way of probenecid-sensitive organic anion transporters localized to the proximal tubule and may be appreciably slowed in the aged kidney [20]. The pharmacologic characteristics of all loop diuretics are similar. Therefore, a lack of response to adequate doses of one loop diuretic reasons against the administration of another loop diuretic. Instead, combinations of diuretics with different sites of action should be given if aggressive diuresis is truly needed.

The rate of diuretic excretion approximates drug delivery to the medullary thick ascending limb and corresponds to the observed natriuretic response [17,20]. The relationship between the urinary loop diuretic excretion rate and the natriuretic effect is described by a sigmoidal curve and can be distorted (downward and rightward shifted) by a variety of circumstances, ranging from volume depletion ("braking phenomenon") and the use of nonsteroidal anti-inflammatory agents (NSAIDs), to HF or nephrotic syndrome (disease-state alterations) [21].

Furosemide is the most widely used diuretic in this class. However, its use in the elderly (and probably in all subjects) is confused by extremely erratic absorption with a bioavailability range of 12% to 112% [22]. The coefficient of variation for absorption varies from 25% to 43% for different furosemide products. Thus, exchanging one furosemide formulation for another will not standardize patient absorption (and thus response) to oral furosemide [22]. Bumetanide and especially torsemide are more predictably absorbed than furosemide. The consistency of torsemide's absorption and its longer duration of action are pharmacologic features to consider when loop diuretic therapy is called for in the elderly HF patient [23].

Thiazide diuretics

The main site of action for thiazide-type diuretics is the early distal convoluted tubule where the coupled reabsorption of Na^+ and Cl^- is inhibited. Besides effects on Na^+ excretion, thiazide diuretics also impair urinary diluting capacity (while preserving urinary concentrating mechanisms and thus the greater likelihood of their causing diuretic-related hyponatremia), reduce Ca^{++} and uric acid excretion, and increase Mg^{++} excretion. The latter is especially the case with long-acting thiazide-type diuretics, such as chlorthalidone [24].

Hydrochlorothiazide is the most widely used thiazide-type diuretic in the United States and is given mainly for its blood-pressure–reducing properties. Hydrochlorothiazide is little used in HF because of its variable absorption, short duration of action, and limited potency. However, metolazone, chlorthalidone, and other thiazide-type diuretics with much longer durations of action can be safely and effectively used in the earlier stages of HF [25]. In addition, chlorthalidone therapy has been shown to be superior to calcium channel blockers and, at least in the short term, ACE inhibitors in preventing HF in hypertensive individuals [26].

Metolazone is a quinazoline diuretic with chief site of action in the distal tubule and a minor inhibitory effect on proximal Na^+ reabsorption through a carbonic-anhydrase–independent mechanism. Metolazone is lipid soluble and has a wide volume of distribution, which plays a role in its extended duration of action in the setting of either renal insufficiency or diuretic-resistant situations when being given together with a loop diuretic [21,25]. Oral metolazone is absorbed slowly and fairly unpredictably, which can confuse the diagnosis of "diuretic-resistance" in a volume overloaded HF patient. Diuretic-resistance, the failure to respond to a diuretic regimen, is usually taken to signify a worsening of the primary volume-retaining state, but with metolazone, it can be a consequence of failure to absorb sufficient amounts of drug in a timely manner to effect a diuresis [21,25].

Distal K^+-sparing diuretics

There are two classes of K^+-sparing diuretics: competitive antagonists of aldosterone, such as spironolactone and eplerenone, and compounds, such as amiloride and triamterene, that act independent of aldosterone. The large majority of the treatment experience with K^+-sparing diuretics in HF is with the ARA spironolactone and eplerenone. Spironolactone is a highly protein-bound and well-absorbed, lipid-soluble compound with a 20-hour half-life. The onset of action for spironolactone is characteristically slow, with a peak diuretic response at times 48 hours or more after the first dose. 7α-Thiomethylspirolactone and canrenone are two metabolites of spironolactone that are responsible for much of its antimineralocorticoid activity [27]. Eplerenone, a highly selective ARA compound (reduced affinity for androgen and progesterone receptors), is associated with fewer endocrine side effects than occur with spironolactone [28].

ARAs are used in the HF patient, elderly or otherwise, for three primary reasons: for their diuretic effect, to reduce K^+ or Mg^{++} losses produced by non–K^+-sparing diuretics, and to improve the morbidity and mortality of HF. First, drugs in this class work by way of inhibiting active Na^+ absorption in the late distal tubule and the collecting duct. Typically, eplerenone has a mild diuretic effect, which may relate to its having a short half-life and no active metabolites [29]. Conversely, spironolactone can generate a more significant diuretic response in HF, particularly when used in combination with a loop diuretic and an ACE inhibitor [30]. Spironolactone can remain active as a diuretic in states of reduced renal function because it gains access to its tubular site of action independent of the glomerular filtration rate.

Spironolactone and eplerenone both have a propensity to cause hyperkalemia, which limits use in many elderly patients with HF or chronic kidney disease [28,31,32]. Conversely, these compounds are effective in attenuating diuretic-related K^+ or Mg^{++} losses [33]. Spironolactone and eplerenone both have also been shown to improve the morbidity and mortality associated with various forms of HF [34–36]. In this regard, the Randomized Aldactone Evaluation Study showed that, when added to standard treatment (including an ACE inhibitor), a 25-mg dose of the ARA spironolactone reduced the risk of death by 30% over an average follow-up period of 2 years among carefully selected patients with current or recent HF of New York Heart Association functional class IV [35]. Also, in the Eplerenone Post–Acute Myocardial Infarction HF Efficacy and Survival Study, the addition of 50 mg of eplerenone to standard medical therapy significantly improved mortality and morbidity within 30 days of randomization in patients with left ventricular systolic dysfunction and clinical evidence of HF following acute myocardial infarction [34,36]. These positive survival benefits with ARA therapy in HF are independent of patient age and have been suggested (but not proved) to relate to any of a number of processes, including positive vascular, immunologic, cellular, and electrolyte changes that follow from ARA therapy [37–39].

Special considerations in diuretic therapy

A range of common variables, which are, in general, age-independent, can unfavorably influence the response to diuretic therapy. Such variables include body position, dietary Na^+ intake, blood pressure, the pattern of diuretic absorption, the use of NSAIDs, and the braking phenomenon. These are important factors to identify because otherwise patients are incorrectly viewed as being diuretic resistant, which is a much worse prognostic category [40].

Bed rest is a useful ancillary treatment measure when patients are being actively diuresed [41]. This may be particularly so in the elderly patient, where excessive orthostatic changes in blood pressure and posturally induced neurohumoral activation may serve to attenuate the response to a diuretic. Noncompliance with prescribed Na^+ and fluid intake is a major cause of apparent diuretic resistance and an important precipitant of HF exacerbations [42]. An excessive Na^+ intake as a cause of apparent diuretic resistance can be established by the measurement of 24-hour Na^+ excretion in the steady state. In volume-expanded subjects receiving diuretic therapy, dietary noncompliance can be presumed when daily Na^+ excretion is high (> 100 mmol/d) without concurrent weight loss.

For a diuretic to work effectively, blood pressure must be sufficient to allow for drug delivery into the intratubular space and filtrate to be produced. What constitutes an effective blood pressure for diuretic action is highly variable in HF but, in general, is a systolic value above 100 to 110 mm Hg [43]. Atheromatous disease is commonly seen in many elderly patients. This disease, if present in the renal vascular bed, often dictates that even higher systemic blood pressure values be maintained for diuretic action. Also, conventional doses of an ACE inhibitor, such as captopril, can inhibit the natriuretic and diuretic responses to furosemide if systemic blood pressure is excessively reduced or glomerular hemodynamics are adversely affected [44]. On a practical note, separating the administration of each drug by several hours can minimize this interaction between an ACE inhibitor and a loop diuretic.

For the best natriuretic response to a loop diuretic, urinary drug delivery must be timed precisely and take into account many potential variables that influence the rate of delivery. Absorption and subsequent urinary delivery of orally administered loop diuretics must occur at a rate sufficient to exceed a response threshold. Disease states, such as HF, which slow diuretic absorption and thereby the rate of urinary delivery, can influence the response to a diuretic solely by slow absorption [45]. This is even more apparent when diuretic absorption is inherently erratic, as is the case with furosemide, and low doses of drug are used (eg, furosemide 40–80 mg) [22]. Such difficulties can be minimized by choosing a diuretic, such as torsemide, with an absorptive profile that is rapid and complete and thus more compatible with the pharmacologic needs of HF [46]. The use of NSAIDs is a major cause of apparent diuretic resistance. These drugs interfere with prostaglandin synthesis by inhibiting cyclooxygenase and thereby antagonize the natriuretic response to loop diuretics. Consumption of NSAIDs is associated with an increased risk of hospital admission because of HF in patients with pre-existing HF [47].

Pharmacodynamic alterations presenting as "apparent" resistance to the effects of a diuretic frequently surface with repetitive administration of diuretics. This tolerance evolves sequentially, and commences abruptly at the time of the first dose of a diuretic. This braking phenomenon or "post-diuretic sodium retention" ultimately determines the influence of a diuretic on net Na^+ balance [48]. The braking phenomenon involves a complex series of counterbalancing changes that ultimately serve to stimulate Na^+ and water absorption at tubular sites, which are proximal and distal to the site of action of the particular diuretic in question [21]. The braking phenomenon can be attenuated by the more frequent administration of a diuretic or, on occasion, by the judicious use of multiple-site diuretic combinations such as hydrochlorothiazide and furosemide, or metolazone and furosemide [25]. Diuretics active at the distal tubule, such as the thiazide diuretics, not only block this increase in Na^+ reabsorption but may also prevent the development of cellular hypertrophy at this location [49]. These structural adaptations in the nephron may contribute to postdiuretic Na^+ retention and to diuretic tolerance in humans. The adaptations may also cause persistent Na^+ retention occurring up to 2 weeks after discontinuation of diuretic therapy [50].

Neurohumoral responses to diuretics

Neurohumoral activation by diuretics remains an important consideration in the sustained effectiveness of diuretic therapy in HF. The neurohumoral response to a diuretic is dependent on both its route of administration and the level of drug exposure. Intravenous loop diuretics have an immediate (within minutes) stimulatory effect on the renin-angiotensin-aldosterone system that is independent of volume depletion. This may diminish the effectiveness of a diuretic for a short time. A second-phase response is initiated within 15 minutes of intravenous loop diuretic administration, which is the result of an increase in the renal production of prostaglandins. This second response offers a probable explanation for the reduction in preload and ventricular filling pressures that takes place shortly after intravenous loop diuretic administration. The next stage of neurohumoral activation occurs with excess volume removal, and can occur with either intravenous or oral diuretics. Volume removal can chronically activate the renin-angiotensin-aldosterone system and increase circulating concentrations of both angiotensin-II and aldosterone, which, in turn, can promote Na^+ absorption in proximal and distal tubular locations, respectively [21].

Adverse effects of diuretics

Diuretic-related side effects can be separated into several categories including those with well worked out mechanisms, such as electrolyte defects or metabolic abnormalities, and occurrences that are less well understood mechanistically, such as impotence. In addition, various drug–drug interactions are recognized to occur with diuretics. Diuretic-related side effects are dose-dependent as well as being more common and of greater intensity with loop diuretics. Thiazide-related side effects tend to be more common with longer-acting compounds, such as chlorthalidone and metolazone [51].

Hyponatremia

Mild hyponatremia is not uncommon in untreated HF and can either improve or worsen with diuretic therapy. Thiazide diuretics are more likely to cause hyponatremia than are loop diuretics. Loop diuretics inhibit Na^+ transport in the renal medulla and preclude the generation of a maximal osmotic gradient. Thus, urinary concentrating ability is impaired with loop diuretics. Alternatively, thiazide-type diuretics increase Na^+ excretion and prevent maximal urine dilution while preserving the kidney's innate concentrating capacity. Diuretic-related hyponatremia is of little immediate clinical consequence if serum Na^+ values are ≥ 130 mEq/L. However, HF management becomes more complex in that both diuretic therapy and free water intake must be at least temporarily reduced [51]. Heretofore, serum Na^+ values < 130 mEq/L in diuretic-treated HF patients were especially difficult to treat. Therapy of such patients may be simplified soon with the availability of orally administered selective vasopressin-receptor antagonists [52].

Acid–base changes

Mild metabolic alkalosis is not uncommon with thiazide-type diuretic therapy.

Severe metabolic alkalosis is much less frequent and, when it occurs, it does so in association with the use of loop diuretics. The generation of a metabolic alkalosis with diuretic therapy is primarily due to contraction of the extracellular fluid space caused by urinary losses of a relatively bicarbonate-free fluid. Diuretic-induced metabolic alkalosis is best managed by administration of K^+ or Na^+ chloride, although the latter is oftentimes ill-advised in HF patients. In such cases, a carbonic anhydrase inhibitor, such as acetazolamide, may be considered. Metabolic alkalosis also impairs the natriuretic response to loop diuretics and may contribute to diuretic resistance in the HF patient [53]. All K^+-sparing diuretics can cause hyperkalemic metabolic acidosis, which in elderly patients, especially those with HF, can represent a serious complication [54].

Hyperuricemia

Xanthine oxidoreductase activity is up-regulated in patients with HF, leading to increased free radicals and hyperuricemia, independent of renal impairment or the effects of diuretics. A beneficial effect of targeted inhibition of xanthine oxidoreductase with allopurinol, and hence reduction of free radical load and uric acid production, has been suggested in a number of studies [55]. In fact, in patients with mild-to-moderate HF, hyperuricemia predicts exercise intolerance and inflammatory activation and is strongly and independently related to a worse prognosis [56]. If a gouty attack occurs in a diuretic-treated patient (unusual unless serum urate concentrations exceed 12 mg/dL), the diuretic should be at least temporarily discontinued. If diuretic discontinuation is not practical, then the lowest effective dose should be given with careful attention to maintaining an euvolemic state. An additional alternative in the gouty patient requiring diuretic therapy is the use of the xanthine oxidase inhibitor, allopurinol [57]. Allopurinol should be used cautiously (dose-adjusted according to level of renal function) in patients receiving a thiazide-type diuretic (and probably a loop diuretic as well), since allopurinol hypersensitivity reactions are more frequent with this combination than with allopurinol alone.

Hypokalemia and hyperkalemia

A serum K^+ value of <3.5 mEq/L, which is the most common criterion for a diagnosis of hypokalemia, is not uncommon in HF patients treated with loop or thiazide diuretics [58]. It is unusual, however, for serum K^+ values to remain <3.0 mEq/L in diuretic-treated outpatients unless there is a high dietary Na^+ intake, high-dose diuretic therapy is in play, or hypomagnesemia is present. Mechanisms that contribute to the onset of hypokalemia during diuretic use include increased flow-dependent distal nephron K^+ secretion (more commonly observed with a high Na^+ intake), a fall in distal tubule luminal Cl^- concentration, metabolic alkalosis, or secondary hyperaldosteronism [59].

The risk from diuretic-related hypokalemia is most apparent in patients with left ventricular hypertrophy, HF, or myocardial ischemia, particularly when they become acutely ill and require hospitalization [59,60]. Logically, arrhythmia-related event rates should be coupled to the degree of hypokalemia. However, this is in no way a clear-cut relationship, at least in the outpatient setting. Several factors complicate the relationship. These factors include the variable correlation between serum K^+ concentrations and total body K^+ deficits in the setting of diuretic therapy. The range of serum K^+ values most commonly associated with increased ventricular ectopy is narrow, typically between 3.0 and 3.5 mEq/L. Uncertainty continues to surround the issue of whether hypokalemia caused by transcellular shifts of K^+ bears the same risk as a value seen on the basis of body losses [59].

K^+-sparing diuretics (such as triamterene and amiloride) and ARAs (such as spironolactone and eplerenone) may treat diuretic-related hypokalemia just as well as they cause significant hyperkalemia [61]. Hyperkalemia is more likely to develop in K^+-sparing diuretic-treated patients in the setting of a reduction in the glomerular filtration rate (especially the elderly); in patients also receiving K^+ chloride supplements or salt substitutes (60 mEq/teaspoonful); in patients on an ACE inhibitor, an angiotensin receptor blocker, or an NSAID; or in other situations that predispose to hyperkalemia, such as metabolic acidosis, hyporeninemic hypoaldosteronism, or heparin therapy (including subcutaneous heparin regimens) [61].

Hypomagnesemia

Both thiazide and loop diuretics increase urine Mg^{++} excretion. Conversely, all K^+-sparing diuretics reduce urinary Mg^{++} losses. Prolonged therapy with thiazide or loop diuretics decreases plasma Mg^{++} concentration on average by 5% to 10%, although some patients can develop more severe hypomagnesemia. Cellular Mg^{++} depletion occurs in up to 50% of patients during diuretic therapy, and can be present regardless of normal serum Mg^{++} concentrations. Hypomagnesemia occurs more often in the elderly and in those receiving continuous high-dose diuretic therapy, as is the case for HF patients.

While a low serum Mg^{++} level is helpful in making the diagnosis, and is in general indicative of low intracellular stores, normal serum Mg^{++} values can still be observed in the face of a significant body deficiency of Mg^{++}. Thus, serum Mg^{++} determinations are an unreliable measure of total body Mg^{++} balance. Hypomagnesemia often coexists with hyponatremia and hypokalemia, with one study finding 42% of patients with hypokalemia to also have low serum Mg^{++} concentrations [62]. Hypokalemia or hypocalcemia occurring in the presence of hypomagnesemia typically cannot be corrected until the underlying Mg^{++} deficit is put right.

Diuretic-related hypomagnesemia should be treated (beyond simple empiric correction to normalize a laboratory value) for several theoretical reasons. Such treatment can lead, for example, to improved control of blood pressure, fewer arrhythmias, or resolution of co-existing electrolyte or neuromuscular symptoms. Mg^{++} deficiency should be sought and treated in patients with HF, ischemic heart disease, or an established arrhythmia patterns [63]. In mild-deficiency states, Mg^{++} balance can often be reestablished by simply controlling the contributing factors (eg, by limiting diuretic use and Na^+ intake) and allowing dietary Mg^{++} to correct the deficit. Parenteral Mg^{++}, however, is the most efficient way to correct hypomagnesemia and should always be the mode of administration when replacement is more urgent. Total body Mg^{++} deficits are typically in the order of 1 to 2 mEq/kg body weight in the depleted patient.

A variety of Mg^{++} salts are available for oral use. Mg^{++} oxide is a commonly employed Mg^{++} salt, but is not very water-soluble and has a major cathartic effect. Thus, its use can unpredictably influence Mg^{++} concentrations. Mg^{++} gluconate is the preferred therapy for oral use. This salt form is very soluble and causes minimal diarrhea. Mg^{++} carbonate is also not very water-soluble and is not as effective as the gluconate salt in correcting hypomagnesemia.

Summary

Diuretic therapy remains a cornerstone of HF therapy. In the treatment of volume-overloaded patients, diuretics clearly improve symptoms and quality of life. Despite the acceptance of diuretic therapy for treatment of symptoms, considerable debate has ensued for many decades about the impact of this class of agent on mortality, cardiac function, and disease progression. Accordingly, diuretics should be used judiciously in the HF patient, at the minimum effective dose, with careful monitoring of electrolyte balance, and continued only if there is a demonstrable ongoing clinical need. ARAs should be distinguished from both loop and thiazide-type diuretics in that outcomes data support their routine use in advanced systolic HF and in post–myocardial infarction patients with clinical HF symptoms and a left ventricular ejection fraction $<40\%$.

References

[1] Chobanian AV, Bakris GL, Black HR, et al. Seventh report of the Joint National Committee on Prevention, Detection, Evaluation, and Treatment of High Blood Pressure. Hypertension 2003;42:1206–52.
[2] HFSA 2006 comprehensive heart failure practice guidelines. Executive summary. J Card Fail 2006;12:10–38.
[3] Arnold JM, Liu P, Demers C, et al. Canadian Cardiovascular Society consensus conference recommendations on heart failure 2006: diagnosis and management. Can J Cardiol 2006;22: 23–45.
[4] Swedberg K, Cleland J, Dargie H, et al. Guidelines for the diagnosis and treatment of chronic heart failure (update 2005). Eur Heart J 2005;26:1115–41.
[5] Hunt SA, Abraham WT, Chin MH, et al. ACC/AHA 2005 guideline update for the diagnosis and management of chronic heart failure in the adult. A report of the American College of Cardiology/American Heart Association Task Force on Practice Guidelines (Writing Committee to Update the 2001 Guidelines for the Evaluation and Management of Heart Failure). J Am Coll Cardiol 2005;46(6):1116–43.
[6] Faris R, Flather MD, Purcell H, et al. Diuretics for heart failure. Cochrane Database Syst Rev 2006;1:CD003838.
[7] Aurigemma GP, Gottdiener JS, Shemanski L, et al. Predictive value of systolic and diastolic function for incident congestive heart failure in the elderly: the cardiovascular health study. J Am Coll Cardiol 2001;37:1042–8.
[8] de Giuli F, Khaw KT, Cowie MR, et al. Incidence and outcome of persons with a clinical diagnosis of heart failure in a general practice population of 696,884 in the United Kingdom. Eur J Heart Fail 2005;7:295–302.

 [9] Kitzman DW. Diastolic heart failure in the elderly. Heart Fail Rev 2002;7:17–27.
[10] Sun WY, Reiser IW, Chou SY. Risk factors for acute renal insufficiency induced by diuretics in patients with congestive heart failure. Am J Kidney Dis 2006;47:798–808.
[11] Rejnmark L, Vestergaard P, Mosekilde L. Fracture risk in patients treated with loop diuretics. J Intern Med 2006;259:117–24.
[12] Rejnmark L, Vestergaard P, Mosekilde L. Reduced fracture risk in users of thiazide diuretics. Calcif Tissue Int 2005;76:167–75.
[13] Eshaghian S, Horwich TB, Fonarow GC. Relation of loop diuretic dose to mortality in advanced heart failure. Am J Cardiol 2006;97:1759–64.
[14] Krum H, Cameron P. Diuretics in the treatment of heart failure: mainstay of therapy or potential hazard? J Card Fail 2006;12:333–5.
[15] Domanski M, Tian X, Haigney M, et al. Diuretic use, progressive heart failure, and death in patients in the DIG study. J Card Fail 2006;12:327–32.
[16] Galve E, Mallol A, Catalan R, et al. Clinical and neurohumoral consequences of diuretic withdrawal in patients with chronic, stabilized heart failure and systolic dysfunction. Eur J Heart Fail 2005;7:892–8.
[17] Brater DC. Diuretic therapy. N Engl J Med 1998;339:387–95.
[18] Mazur JE, Devlin JW, Peters MJ, et al. Single versus multiple doses of acetazolamide for metabolic alkalosis in critically ill medical patients: a randomized, double-blind trial. Crit Care Med 1999;27:1257–61.
[19] Shankar SS, Brater DC. Loop diuretics: from the Na-K-2Cl transporter to clinical use. Am J Physiol Renal Physiol 2003;284:F11–21.
[20] Andreasen F, Hansen U, Husted SE, et al. The pharmacokinetics of frusemide are influenced by age. Br J Clin Pharmacol 1983;16:391–7.
[21] Sica DA, Gehr TWB. Diuretic combinations in refractory edema states: pharmacokinetic-pharmacodynamic relationships. Clin Pharmacokinet 1996;30:229–49.
[22] Murray MD, Haag KM, Black PK, et al. Variable furosemide absorption and poor predictability of response in elderly patients. Pharmacotherapy 1997;17:98–106.
[23] Vargo DL, Kramer WG, Black PK, et al. Bioavailability, pharmacokinetics, and pharmacodynamics of torsemide and furosemide in patients with congestive heart failure. Clin Pharmacol Ther 1995;57:601–9.
[24] Cocco G, Iselin HU, Strozzi C, et al. Magnesium depletion in patients on long-term chlorthalidone therapy for essential hypertension. Eur J Clin Pharmacol 1987;32:335–8.
[25] Sica DA. Metolazone and its role in edema management. Cong Heart Fail 2003;9:100–5.
[26] Davis BR, Piller LB, Cutler JA, et al. Antihypertensive and Lipid-Lowering Treatment to Prevent Heart Attack Trial Collaborative Research Group. Role of diuretics in the prevention of heart failure: the Antihypertensive and Lipid-Lowering Treatment to Prevent Heart Attack Trial. Circulation 2006;113:2201–10.
[27] Gardiner P, Schrode K, Quinlan D, et al. Spironolactone metabolism: steady-state serum levels of the sulfur-containing metabolites. J Clin Pharmacol 1989;29:342–7.
[28] Sica DA. Pharmacokinetics and pharmacodynamics of mineralocorticoid blocking agents and their effects on potassium homeostasis. Heart Fail Rev 2005;10:23–9.
[29] Ravis WR, Reid S, Sica DA, et al. Pharmacokinetics of eplerenone after single and multiple dosing in subjects with and without renal impairment. J Clin Pharmacol 2005;45: 810–21.
[30] van Vliet AA, Donker AJ, Nauta JJ, et al. Spironolactone in congestive heart failure refractory to high-dose loop diuretic and low-dose angiotensin-converting enzyme inhibitor. Am J Cardiol 1993;71:21A–8A.
[31] Masoudi FA, Gross CP, Wang Y, et al. Adoption of spironolactone therapy for older patients with heart failure and left ventricular systolic dysfunction in the United States, 1998–2001. Circulation 2005;112:39–47.
[32] Dinsdale C, Wani M, Steward J, et al. Tolerability of spironolactone as adjunctive treatment for heart failure in patients over 75 years of age. Age Ageing 2005;34:395–8.

[33] Soberman JE, Weber KT. Spironolactone in congestive heart failure. Curr Hypertens Rep 2000;2:451–6.

[34] Pitt B, Remme W, Zannad F, et al. Eplerenone, a selective aldosterone blocker, in patients with left ventricular dysfunction after myocardial infarction. N Engl J Med 2003;348: 1309–21.

[35] Pitt B, Zannad F, Remme WJ, et al. The effect of spironolactone on morbidity and mortality in patients with severe heart failure. N Engl J Med 1999;341:709–17.

[36] Pitt B, White H, Nicolau J, et al. Eplerenone reduces mortality 30 days after randomization following acute myocardial infarction in patients with left ventricular systolic dysfunction and heart failure. J Am Coll Cardiol 2005;46:425–31.

[37] Pitt B, Reichek N, Willenbrock R, et al. Effects of eplerenone, enalapril, and eplerenone/ena-lapril in patients with essential hypertension and left ventricular hypertrophy: the 4E-left ventricular hypertrophy study. Circulation 2003;108:1831–8.

[38] Bianchi S, Bigazzi R, Campese VM. Antagonists of aldosterone and proteinuria in patients with CKD: an uncontrolled pilot study. Am J Kidney Dis 2005;46:45–51.

[39] Tang WH, Parameswaran AC, Maroo AP, et al. Aldosterone receptor antagonists in the medical management of chronic heart failure. Mayo Clin Proc 2005;80:1623–30.

[40] Neuberg GW, Miller AB, O'Connor CM, et al. Diuretic resistance predicts mortality in pa-tients with advanced heart failure. Am Heart J 2002;144:31–8.

[41] Abildgaard U, Aldershvile J, Ring-Larsen H, et al. Bed rest and increased diuretic treatment in chronic congestive heart failure. Eur Heart J 1985;6:1040–6.

[42] Tsuyuki RT, McKelvie RS, Arnold JM, et al. Acute precipitants of congestive heart failure exacerbations. Arch Intern Med 2001;161:2337–42.

[43] De Pasquale CG, Dunne JS, Minson RB, et al. Hypotension is associated with diuretic re-sistance in severe chronic heart failure, independent of renal function. Eur J Heart Fail 2005;7:888–91.

[44] McLay JS, McMurray JJ, Bridges AB, et al. Acute effects of captopril on the renal actions of furosemide in patients with chronic heart failure. Am Heart J 1993;126:879–86.

[45] Sica DA. Drug absorption in the management of congestive heart failure: loop diuretics. Congest Heart Fail 2003;9:287–92.

[46] Bleske BE, Welage LS, Kramer WG, et al. Pharmacokinetics of torsemide in patients with decompensated and compensated congestive heart failure. J Clin Pharmacol 1998;38: 708–14.

[47] Feenstra J, Heerdinck ER, Grobbee DE, et al. Association of nonsteroidal anti-inflammatory drugs with first occurrence of heart failure and with relapsing heart failure. Arch Intern Med 2002;162:262–70.

[48] Kelly RA, Wilcox CS, Mitch WE, et al. Response of the kidney to furosemide. II. Effect of captopril on sodium balance. Kidney Int 1983;24:233–9.

[49] Ellison DH, Velazquez H, Wright FS. Adaptation of the distal convoluted tubule of the rat. Structural and functional effects of dietary salt intake and chronic diuretic infusion. J Clin Invest 1989;83:113–26.

[50] Loon NR, Wilcox CS, Unwin RJ. Mechanism of impaired natriuretic response to furose-mide during prolonged therapy. Kidney Int 1989;36:682–9.

[51] Sica DA. Diuretic-related side effects: development and treatment. J Clin Hypertens (Green-wich) 2004;6:532–40.

[52] Gheorghiade M. The clinical effects of vasopressin receptor antagonists in heart failure. Cleve Clin J Med 2006;73(Suppl 2):S24–9.

[53] Loon NR, Wilcox CS. Mild metabolic alkalosis impairs the natriuretic response to bumeta-nide in normal human subjects. Clin Sci (Lond) 1998;94:287–92.

[54] O'Connell JE, Colledge NR. Type IV renal tubular acidosis and spironolactone therapy in the elderly. Postgrad Med J 1993;69:887–9.

[55] Cappola TP, Kass DA, Nelson GS, et al. Allopurinol improves myocardial efficiency in patients with idiopathic dilated cardiomyopathy. Circulation 2001;104:2407–11.

[56] Niizeki T, Takeishi Y, Arimoto T, et al. Hyperuricemia associated with high cardiac event rates in the elderly with chronic heart failure. J Cardiol 2006;47:219–28.

[57] Gurwitz JH, Kalish SC, Bohn RL, et al. Thiazide diuretics and the initiation of anti-gout therapy. J Clin Epidemiol 1997;50:953–9.

[58] Morgan DB, Davidson C. Hypokalemia and diuretics: an analysis of publications. BMJ 1980;280:905–8.

[59] Sica DA, Struthers AD, Cushman WC, et al. Importance of potassium in cardiovascular disease. J Clin Hypertens 2003;4:198–206.

[60] Macdonald JE, Struthers AD. What is the optimal serum potassium level in cardiovascular patients? J Am Coll Cardiol 2004;43:155–61.

[61] Sica DA, Hess M. Aldosterone receptor antagonism: interface with hyperkalemia in heart failure. Congest Heart Fail 2004;10:259–64.

[62] Whang R, Oei TO, Aikawa JK, et al. Predictors of clinical hypomagnesemia. Hypokalemia, hypophosphatemia, hyponatremia, and hypocalcemia. Arch Intern Med 1984;144:1794–6.

[63] Sica DA, Frishman WH, Cavusoglu E. Magnesium, potassium, and calcium as potential cardiovascular disease therapies. In: Frishman W, Sonnenblick E, Sica DA, editors. Cardiovascular pharmacotherapeutics. New York: McGraw-Hill; 2003. p. 177–90.

ELSEVIER
SAUNDERS

CLINICS IN
GERIATRIC
MEDICINE

Clin Geriatr Med 23 (2007) 123–139

Heart-Failure–Complicating Acute Myocardial Infarction

Wilbert S. Aronow, MD

*Department of Medicine, Divisions of Cardiology, Geriatrics, and Pulmonary/Critical Care,
Westchester Medical Center, New York Medical College, Macy Pavilion, Room 138,
Valhalla, NY 10595, USA*

Factors predisposing the older person with acute myocardial infarction (MI) to develop congestive heart failure (CHF) include an increased prevalence of prior MI and multivessel coronary artery disease, decreased left ventricular (LV) contractile reserve, impairment of LV diastolic relaxation, and an increased prevalence of hypertension, LV hypertrophy, diabetes mellitus, valvular heart disease, and renal insufficiency [1–4]. Women with acute MI are more likely to be older and to develop CHF than men with acute MI [5–8]. Prior CHF was present in 12% of 124 patients younger than 70 years of age and in 17% of 137 patients 70 years of age and older with acute MI [5]. CHF occurred during acute MI in 33% of the 124 patients younger than 70 years of age and in 56% of the 137 patients 70 years of age and older [5]. Dyspnea due to CHF was the initial clinical manifestation of acute MI in 35% of 110 patients older than 62 years of age (mean age: 82 years) with acute MI [9].

CHF-complicating acute MI is associated with a high mortality [10]. CHF occurred during acute MI in 40% of 30 patients who died at 1-year follow-up and in 9% of 202 patients who were alive at 1-year follow-up [5]. In the Multicenter Postinfarction Program, the 1-year mortality rate was 28% in 123 patients with pulmonary congestion occurring during acute MI versus 5.5% in 744 patients with no pulmonary congestion occurring during acute MI [11]. An analysis of 790 surviving patients from the Multicenter Postinfarction Program and 1060 placebo-treated patients from the Multicenter Diltiazem Postinfarction Trial showed at 2-year follow-up that the cardiac mortality hazard ratios were 1.43 for patients with mild or moderate pulmonary congestion occurring during acute MI and 4.20 for patients with severe pulmonary congestion during acute MI [12].

E-mail address: WSAronow@aol.com

Pulmonary venous hypertension with pulmonary congestion and a low cardiac output may complicate acute MI. Pulmonary congestion occurs when the pulmonary capillary wedge pressure exceeds 18 mm Hg [13]. Peripheral hypoperfusion occurs when the cardiac index falls below 2.2 $L/min/m^2$ [13]. The greater the extent of injury to the left ventricle, the lower the LV ejection fraction and the higher the incidence of clinical manifestations of CHF. At follow-up, a low LV ejection fraction is an independent predictor of mortality in patients with CHF associated with acute MI [5,12,14].

Older patients with prior MI and CHF have a higher mortality at follow-up if they have an abnormal LV ejection fraction than if they have a normal LV ejection fraction [15,16]. Table 1 shows the mortality rates in older men and in older women with prior MI and CHF at 1-year, 2-year, 3-year, 4-year, and 5-year follow-up [16]. The mortality rates were similar in men versus women with normal or abnormal LV ejection fraction [16]. Older patients with an abnormal LV ejection fraction had a 2.2 times higher mortality rate than older patients with a normal LV ejection fraction after controlling other prognostic variables [16].

General measures

In general, management of CHF-complicating acute MI is similar in older and younger patients. Underlying causes of CHF should be treated when possible [17,18]. Precipitating factors of CHF should be identified and treated [17,18]. The LV ejection fraction must be measured in patients with CHF associated with acute MI to guide therapy [17]. Echocardiography with Doppler may be helpful in determining the presence and severity of valvular heart disease, such as aortic stenosis or mitral regurgitation, LV diastolic dysfunction due to LV hypertrophy, LV wall-motion abnormalities caused by acute myocardial ischemia, and complications of acute MI, including ventricular rupture, ventricular septal rupture, papillary muscle rupture, ruptured chordae tendineae, papillary muscle dysfunction, LV aneurysm, intracardiac thrombi, pericardial effusion with and without cardiac tamponade, and right ventricular infarction [5,18–22].

Table 1
Mortality rates in older men and women with CHF and prior MI

Mortality	Normal LV ejection fraction (n = 276)	Abnormal LV ejection fraction (n = 340)
1 year	19%	41%
2 years	39%	65%
3 years	49%	78%
4 years	56%	86%
5 years	74%	92%

Data from Aronow WS, Ahn C, Kronzon I. Prognosis of congestive heart failure after prior myocardial infarction in older men and women with abnormal versus normal left ventricular ejection fraction. Am J Cardiol 2000;85:1382–4.

Hemodynamic monitoring

Invasive hemodynamic monitoring may be necessary to guide the therapy of some patients with acute MI and a pulmonary capillary wedge pressure >18 mm Hg or a cardiac index <2.2 L/min/m^2. The American College of Cardiology/American Heart Association (ACC/AHA) guidelines state that class-I indications for balloon flotation right-heart catheter monitoring during acute MI include (1) severe or progressive CHF or pulmonary edema, (2) progressive hypotension when unresponsive to fluid administration or when fluid administration may be contraindicated, and (3) suspected mechanical complications of acute MI, such as ventricular septal defect, papillary muscle rupture, or pericardial tamponade if an echocardiogram has not been performed [23].

Oxygen

Experimental data have shown that breathing oxygen may limit ischemic myocardial injury [24]. Patients with acute MI and CHF may have hypoxemia due to pulmonary vascular congestion, pulmonary interstitial edema, and ventilation–perfusion mismatch [25]. Respiratory depression from narcotic analgesics can also contribute to hypoxemia. The ACC/AHA guidelines state that the class-I indications for using oxygen during acute MI are (1) overt pulmonary congestion or (2) arterial oxygen desaturation (oxygen saturation $<90\%$) [23].

Supplemental oxygen administered by nasal prongs may not correct significant hypoxemia in patients with severe CHF, pulmonary edema, or a mechanical complication of acute MI. Continuous positive-pressure breathing or endotracheal intubation and mechanical ventilation is often needed in these patients [26]. The preferred modes of administering oxygen in these patients who are capable of initiating spontaneous ventilation are intermittent mandatory ventilation, assist control, or pressure-support ventilation [27]. If wheezing complicates pulmonary congestion, bronchodilators that act primarily on β_2-adrenoceptors, such as albuterol, are preferable to bronchodilators, such as isoproterenol, which can increase myocardial ischemia by increasing myocardial oxygen demand.

Morphine

Intravenous morphine should be used to treat acute pulmonary edema associated with acute MI. Intravenous morphine provides beneficial effects in pulmonary edema by decreasing systemic vascular resistance, by increasing venodilation, and by reducing the work of breathing through inducing central nervous system euphoria [28,29]. Morphine should be avoided in patients with bronchospastic pulmonary disease or hypotension. The initial intravenous dose of morphine is 2 to 4 mg. This dose should be repeated every 10 to 15 minutes as necessary. The blood pressure should be checked before each dose because morphine can cause significant hypotension.

Diuretics

Older persons with CHF associated with acute MI should be treated with a loop diuretic, such as furosemide. These persons should not take nonsteroidal anti-inflammatory drugs because they may inhibit the induction of diuresis by furosemide. If severe CHF is present, furosemide should be administered intravenously initially in a dose of 20 to 40 mg with the dose doubled if there is no significant clinical improvement [30]. In addition to its diuretic effect, intravenous furosemide causes venodilation with a clinical benefit occurring within several minutes [31,32]. Older persons with severe CHF or concomitant renal insufficiency may need the addition of metolazone to the loop diuretic. Continuous intravenous infusion of furosemide may be necessary in some patients with severe CHF.

Older patients with CHF treated with diuretics need close monitoring of serum electrolytes. Hypokalemia and hypomagnesemia may occur, both of which may precipitate ventricular arrhythmias and digitalis toxicity. Hyponatremia with activation of the renin-angiotensin-aldosterone system may develop [17].

Older patients with CHF are especially sensitive to volume depletion. Dehydration and prerenal azotemia may develop if excessive doses of diuretics are given. Therefore, the minimum effective dose of diuretics should be administered. Older patients with CHF and abnormal LV ejection fraction tolerate higher doses of diuretics than do older patients with CHF and normal LV ejection fraction. Older patients with CHF associated with LV diastolic dysfunction with normal LV ejection fraction often need high LV filling pressures to maintain an adequate stroke volume and cardiac output and cannot tolerate intravascular depletion [17]. The use of diuretics in the treatment of patients with CHF is discussed extensively the article by Sica and colleagues elsewhere in this issue.

Nitroglycerin

In patients with acute MI, intravenous nitroglycerin reduces LV filling pressure and systemic vascular resistance [33]. Intravenous nitroglycerin is principally a venodilator at infusion rates of less than 50 μg/min and causes more balanced venous and arterial dilating effects at higher infusion rates [33]. Intravenous nitroglycerin improves LV hemodynamics, LV geometry, and myocardial blood flow and perfusion in patients with acute MI [34].

In 5124 patients older than 70 years of age in the *Gruppo Italiano per lo Studio della Sopravvivenza nell'Infarcto Miocardico* (GISSI-3) trial, administration of transdermal nitroglycerin within 24 hours of symptom onset was associated with an 11% insignificant reduction in 6-week mortality and with a 9% insignificant decrease in the 6-week combined endpoint of death, heart failure, or severe LV dysfunction [14]. When data from all randomized control trials of nitrate use in the treatment of acute MI are combined, there is a 6% significant decrease in mortality, with 4 lives saved per 1000 patients treated [23,35]. The ACC/AHA guidelines state that class-I indications for using intravenous nitroglycerin in patients with acute MI are (1) for relief of ongoing ischemic discomfort, (2) for control of hypertension, or (3) for managing pulmonary congestion [23].

Nitroglycerin should not be used if the systolic blood pressure is <90 mm Hg or if marked bradycardia (<50 beats/min) or tachycardia is present [36]. Nitroglycerin should also be avoided in patients with right ventricular infarction [37].

Long-acting oral nitrate preparations should not be used in the management of acute MI [23]. Sublingual or transdermal nitroglycerin can be used [23]. However, intravenous infusion of nitroglycerin is preferred because of its rapid onset and offset of action. Intravenous nitroglycerin can be titrated by frequent measurements of cuff blood pressure and heart rate. However, invasive hemodynamic monitoring should be used if high doses of vasodilators are administered, if there is an unstable blood pressure, or if there is doubt about the LV filling pressure [38].

A bolus injection of 12.5 to 25.0 μg of intravenous nitroglycerin should be administered with a pump-controlled infusion of 10 to 20 μg/min and the dosage increased by 5 to 10 μg every 5 to 10 minutes [23]. The endpoints are control of clinical symptoms or reduction in mean arterial pressure of 10% in normotensive patients or 30% in hypertensive patients, an increase in heart rate > 10 beats/min, or reduction in pulmonary artery end-diastolic pressure of 10% to 30% [23]. The systolic blood pressure should not be allowed to fall below 90 mm Hg or the heart rate to exceed 110 beats/min [23]. The nitroglycerin infusion should be slowed or temporarily discontinued if the systolic blood pressure falls below 90 mm Hg. The maximum dose infused should not exceed 200 μg/min.

Angiotensin-converting enzyme inhibitors

Angiotensin-converting enzyme (ACE) inhibitors should not be administered intravenously early in the course of acute MI [39]. The Cooperative New Scandinavian Enalapril Survival Study II was stopped due to a higher frequency of adverse outcomes in patients receiving enalapril [39]. Patients over 70 years of age in this study also had an increased incidence of serious hypotension [39].

However, all randomized trials investigating the use of oral ACE inhibitors early in the course of acute MI showed that ACE inhibitors reduced mortality [14,35,40–44]. Small but statistically significant decreases in mortality were reported in patients treated with captopril [35] or lisinopril [14] within 24 hours of onset of acute MI in the Fourth International Study of

Infarct Survival [35] and in the GISSI-3 trial [14]. Patients aged 70 years and older treated with lisinopril in the GISSI-3 trial had a 14% significant decrease in the combined endpoint of death or severe LV dysfunction at 6-month follow-up [45].

In the Acute Infarction Ramipril Efficacy Study, 2006 patients with acute MI and CHF were randomized to ramipril or placebo on day 3 to 10 after acute MI [44]. At 15-month follow-up, compared with placebo, ramipril 5 mg twice daily significantly reduced mortality by 27% overall and by 36% in persons 65 years of age and older [44]. At 42-month follow-up in the Survival and Ventricular Enlargement Trial, asymptomatic patients with a LV ejection fraction ≤40% treated with captopril 3 to 16 days after MI had, compared with placebo, a 19% decrease in mortality, a 21% reduction in death from cardiovascular causes, a 37% decrease in development of severe CHF, a 22% reduction in the development of CHF requiring hospitalization, and a 25% decrease in recurrent MI [46]. Captopril reduced mortality 8% in patients 55 years of age and younger, 13% in patients aged 56 to 64 years, and 25% in patients aged 65 years and older [46].

An observational prospective study was performed in 477 patients (mean age: 79 years) with prior MI and a low LV ejection fraction (mean LV ejection fraction: 31%) [47]. Compared with no ACE inhibitor or β-blocker therapy, at 34-month follow-up, ACE inhibitors alone significantly reduced new coronary events by 17% and new CHF by 32% [47]. Compared with no ACE inhibitor or β-blocker therapy, ACE inhibitors plus β-blockers significantly reduced new coronary events by 37% and new CHF by 61% [47].

The ACC/AHA guidelines state that class-I indications for the use of ACE inhibitors during acute MI are (1) patients within the first 24 hours of a suspected acute MI with ST-segment elevation in two or more anterior precordial leads or with clinical heart failure in the absence of significant hypotension or known contraindications to the use of ACE inhibitors or (2) patients with MI and a LV ejection fraction <40% or patients with clinical heart failure on the basis of systolic pump dysfunction during and after convalescence from acute MI [48].

ACE inhibitors should be started within the first 24 hours in patients with acute MI and CHF after the blood pressure has stabilized [23,48]. ACE inhibitors should not be used if the systolic blood pressure is <100 mm Hg if renal failure is present, if there is a history of bilateral renal artery stenosis, or if there is known allergy to ACE inhibitors [23,48]. The initial dose should be low, such as captopril 6.25 mg, and the dose gradually increased to achieve a maintenance dose within 24 to 48 hours [23,48]. The patient's blood pressure, renal function, and serum potassium level should be monitored closely. Intravenous ACE inhibitors should be avoided, especially in elderly patients [49].

The ACC/AHA guidelines recommend administering ACE inhibitors to all patients after MI without contraindications to their use and continuing their use indefinitely [23]. ACE inhibitors are effective in the treatment of postinfarction patients with CHF associated with abnormal LV ejection fraction [40,41,50,51] or normal LV ejection fraction [52,53].

Asymptomatic hypotension (systolic blood pressure 80–90 mm Hg) and a small increase in serum creatinine to a level of <2.5 mg/dL are side effects of ACE-inhibitor therapy that should not necessarily cause cessation of therapy in postinfarction patients with CHF, but should cause the physician to reduce the dose of diuretics, if the jugular venous pressure is normal, and to consider decreasing the dose of ACE inhibitor [17]. Symptomatic hypotension, progressive azotemia, intolerable cough, angioneurotic edema, hyperkalemia, and rash are contraindications to treatment with ACE inhibitors.

Angiotensin II receptor blockers

Angiotensin II receptor blockers (ARBs) should be used for treating CHF with a class-I indication if the patient cannot tolerate ACE inhibitors because of cough, angioneurotic edema, rash, or altered taste sensation [54–60]. ARBs are reasonable to use as an alternative to ACE inhibitors in patients with mild-to-moderate CHF and reduced LV ejection fraction, especially in patients taking ARBs for other reasons, with a class-IIa indication [54].

Spironolactone

Patients with severe CHF associated with an abnormal LV ejection fraction treated with diuretics, ACE inhibitors, and digoxin who received spironolactone 25 mg daily instead of placebo had a 30% significant reduction in mortality and a 35% significant decrease in hospitalization for CHF at 2-year follow-up [61]. At 16-month follow-up of 6632 patients (mean age: 64 years) with acute MI complicated by CHF and a low LV ejection fraction treated with diuretics, ACE inhibitors, and 75% with β-blockers, eplerenone 50 mg daily significantly reduced mortality 15% and death from cardiovascular causes or hospitalization for cardiovascular events by 13% [62].

The ACC/AHA guidelines recommend with a class-I indication the addition of an aldosterone antagonist in selected patients with moderately severe to severe symptoms of CHF and reduced LV ejection fraction who can be carefully monitored for preserved renal function and normal serum potassium concentration [54]. Patients should have a serum creatinine ≤2.5 mg/dL in men and 2.0 mg/dL in women, and the serum potassium should be <5.0 mEq/L [54].

β-blockers

In the Göteborg Metoprolol Trial, intravenous metoprolol was given within 48 hours of acute MI and followed by therapy with oral metoprolol for 90 days [63]. In the Metoprolol in Acute Myocardial Infarction Trial, intravenous metoprolol was administered within 24 hours of acute MI and followed by treatment with oral metoprolol for 15 days [64]. In the First International Study of Infarct Survival, intravenous atenolol was given within 12 hours of acute MI and followed by treatment with oral atenolol for 7 days [65]. If the results of these three studies in which thrombolytic therapy was not used are pooled, the younger persons had a 5% nonsignificant decrease in mortality, and the older persons had a 23% significant reduction in mortality. Data from the Thrombolysis in Myocardial Infarction II-B Study [66] and the Global Utilization of Streptokinase and Tissue Plasminogen Activator for Occluded Coronary Arteries (GUSTO-I) Trial [67] support the use of early intravenous β-blockade in patients with acute MI treated with thrombolytic therapy.

In the Göteborg Metoprolol Trial, 262 of 1395 randomized patients had mild-to-moderate CHF before randomization [68]. The 1-year mortality was significantly reduced in patients treated with metoprolol (14%) compared with patients treated with placebo (27%) [68].

The ACC/AHA class-I indications for use of early intravenous β-blockade in patients with acute MI are (1) patients without a contraindication to β-blockers who can be treated within 12 hours of onset of MI, (2) patients with continuing or recurrent ischemic pain, and (3) patients with tachyarrhythmias, such as atrial fibrillation with a rapid ventricular rate, or hypertension [23,48]. Intravenous β-blockers should not be administered to older patients with severe CHF-complicating acute MI, and the dose should be reduced in older patients with mild-to-moderate CHF.

Intravenous atenolol and metoprolol are the two β-blockers that have been approved by the US Food and Drug Administration for use in patients with acute MI. The dose of atenolol used in the First International Study of Infarct Survival was 5 mg intravenously given twice at 10-minute intervals followed by oral atenolol 50 mg every 12 hours [65]. The dose of metoprolol used in the studies cited was 5 mg administered intravenously at 5-minute intervals for 3 doses followed by oral metoprolol 50 mg every 6 hours with 100 mg given twice daily after 24 to 48 hours [63,64,66–68]. Lower doses may need to be used in older persons.

An analysis of 55 randomized controlled trials investigating the use of β-blockers after MI demonstrated that β-blockers caused a 19% significant decrease in mortality [69]. High-risk survivors of acute MI at 12 Norwegian hospitals randomized to treatment with propranolol for 1 year had a 52% significant reduction in sudden cardiac death [70].

At 17-month follow-up in the Norwegian Multicenter Study, timolol administered in a dose of 10 mg twice daily, compared with placebo, caused a 31% significant decrease in mortality in persons younger than 65 years of age and a 43% significant reduction in mortality in persons aged 65 to 74 years [71]. At 61-month follow-up in this study, timolol caused a 13% nonsignificant decrease in mortality in persons younger than 65 years of age and a 19% significant reduction in mortality in persons aged 65 to 74 years [72]. At 25-month follow-up in the Beta Blocker Heart Attack Trial, propranolol administered in a dose of 80 mg three times daily caused a 19% nonsignificant decrease in mortality in persons younger than 60 years of age and a 33% significant reduction in mortality in persons aged 60 to 69 years old [73]. A retrospective cohort study also showed that persons aged 60 to 89 years treated after MI with metoprolol had an age-adjusted mortality decrease of 76% compared with a control group that did not receive β-blockers [74].

In the Beta Blocker Heart Attack Trial, propranolol caused a 27% significant reduction in mortality and a 47% significant decrease in sudden cardiac death in patients with a history of CHF [75]. In the Beta Blocker Pooling Project, data from nine studies involving 3519 patients with CHF at the time of acute MI demonstrated that β-blockers caused a 25% significant decrease in mortality [76]. β-blockers have also been shown to reduce mortality in patients with CHF due to coronary artery disease associated with a LV ejection fraction ≤35% [77–80] or ≥40% [81].

In a prospective study of 158 persons (mean age: 81 years) with CHF, prior MI, and a LV ejection fraction ≥40% treated with diuretics plus ACE inhibitors, persons randomized to treatment with propranolol had a 35% significant reduction in mortality at 32-month follow-up [81]. The reduction in mortality in persons treated with propranolol was similar in women and men and in persons older and younger than 80 years [81].

A retrospective analysis of the use of after MI found that persons aged 65 years and older treated with β-blockers after MI had a 43% significant decrease in 2-year mortality and a 22% significant reduction in 2-year cardiac hospital readmissions than older persons who were not receiving β-blockers [82]. Use of a calcium channel blocker instead of a β-blocker after MI doubled the risk of mortality in this elderly population [82]. β-blockers were associated with a significant decrease in mortality after MI in persons aged 65 to 74 years, aged 75 to 84 years, and 85 years of age and older [82].

In 477 patients (mean age: 79 years) with prior MI and a low LV ejection fraction, compared with no ACE inhibitor or β-blocker therapy, at 34-month follow-up, β-blockers alone significantly reduced new coronary events by 25% and new CHF by 41% [47]. Compared with no ACE inhibitor or β-blocker therapy, β-blockers plus ACE inhibitors significantly reduced new coronary events by 37% and new CHF by 61% [47].

A meta-analysis of trials also showed that the use of β-blockers after non-Q-wave MI was likely to reduce mortality and recurrent MI by 25% [83]. All older patients with Q-wave MI or non-Q-wave MI, with or without CHF, and without contraindications to β-blockers should be treated with β-blockers indefinitely after MI. Propranolol, metoprolol, timolol, and carvedilol have been approved by the US Food and Drug Administration for long-term treatment after acute MI.

The ACC/AHA guidelines recommend that persons without contraindications to β-blockers should receive β-blockers within a few days of acute

MI (if not initiated acutely) and continue them indefinitely [23,48]. Contra-indications to the use of β-blockers for long-term treatment after MI include severe CHF, severe peripheral arterial disease with the threat of gangrene, greater than first-degree atrioventricular block, hypotension, severe brady-cardia, lung disease with bronchospasm, and bronchial asthma.

Calcium channel blockers and magnesium

The ACC/AHA guidelines state that there are no class-I indications for using calcium channel blockers or magnesium during acute MI [23,48]. These guidelines also state that there are no class-I indications for using cal-cium channel blockers after MI [23,48].

On the basis of the available data, calcium channel blockers should not be used in treating patients during or after MI [69,82,84–87] or in treating patients with CHF associated with an abnormal LV ejection fraction [75,85,88]. However, the author would treat postinfarction patients who have persistent angina pectoris despite nitrates and β-blockers and who are not candidates for coronary revascularization with verapamil or diltia-zem if the LV ejection fraction is normal, and with amlodipine or felodipine if the LV ejection fraction is abnormall.

Digoxin

Although mortality is higher in patients treated with digoxin after MI, it is not clear whether this increase in mortality is due to digoxin [89]. In the Digitalis Investigation Group trial, a recent MI was an exclusion criterion [90]. Although the overall trial showed at 37-month follow-up a similar mor-tality in patients treated with digoxin or placebo, there was a reduction in deaths due to CHF but a trend toward increased deaths due to presumed arrhythmia or MI in the digoxin-treated group [90]. Digitalis toxicity increased with age [91].

Digoxin may be used together with β-blockers in treating supraventricu-lar tachyarrhythmias, such as atrial fibrillation with a rapid ventricular rate during and after acute MI. To reduce hospitalization for CHF with a class-IIa indication, a low dose of digoxin (0.125 mg daily in elderly patients) may be given to postinfarction patients with sinus rhythm and with persistent CHF associated with an abnormal LV ejection fraction despite diuretics plus ACE inhibitors plus β-blockers [17,54]. Elderly persons are at increased risk for developing digitalis toxicity [89,91].

Positive inotropic drugs

If patients with acute MI have CHF associated with severe LV systolic dysfunction and a low cardiac output with marked hypotension, intravenous norepinephrine should be administered until the systolic arterial pressure increases to at least 80 mm Hg [23,48]. These patients need balloon flotation right-heart catheter monitoring. Intravenous dopamine may then be administered in a dose of 5 to 15 µg/kg/min [23,48]. After the systolic arterial pressure increases to 90 mm Hg, intravenous dobutamine may be given simultaneously in an attempt to reduce the dosages of the norepinephrine and dopamine infusions [23,48] Intravenous milrinone administered in a dose of 0.25 to 0.75 µg/kg/min is reserved for patients who do not respond to catecholamines or who have significant arrhythmias, tachycardia, or ischemia induced by catecholamines [23,48].

Arrhythmic events are common in older persons with CHF receiving intravenous dobutamine [92]. Patients needing intravenous inotropic support should receive these drugs for as short a time as possible [23,48]. Whenever possible, afterload-reducing drugs and intra-aortic balloon pumping should be substituted for positive inotropic drugs [23,48]. Long-term intermittent therapy with intravenous dobutamine has been associated with increased ventricular arrhythmias and mortality [93,94].

Treatment of arrhythmias

Patients with acute MI and CHF who develop ventricular fibrillation or sustained ventricular tachycardia should be treated with direct-current electric shock [23,48]. β-blockers reduce mortality in postinfarction patients with complex ventricular arrhythmias and a LV ejection fraction ≤40% [95] or ≥40% [96] and should be administered to postinfarction patients with complex ventricular arrhythmias and no contraindications to β-blockers.

Patients with acute MI and CHF who develop bradyarrhythmias may need temporary pacing [23,48]. The ACC/AHA has developed recommendations for permanent pacing after acute MI [97].

When CHF occurs during acute MI because of a rapid ventricular rate or loss of atrial contraction associated with atrial fibrillation, immediate direct-current cardioversion should be performed [23,48,98]. Heparin should be given. In treating postinfarction patients with chronic atrial fibrillation, the author prefers long-term warfarin therapy plus ventricular rate control with a β-blocker plus digoxin, adding verapamil or diltiazem if necessary to slow the ventricular rate during exercise [98]. The dose of oral warfarin administered should achieve an International Normalized Ratio of 2.0 to 3.0 [98].

Mechanical complications

Sudden or progressive hemodynamic deterioration with low cardiac output or pulmonary edema in patients with acute MI may be due to acute mitral valve regurgitation, postinfarction ventricular septal defect, LV free-wall rupture, or ventricular aneurysm [23,48,99–102]. Transthoracic or transesophageal echocardiography can usually establish the diagnosis.

A balloon flotation catheter is helpful for the diagnosis and monitoring of therapy. Coronary angiography to detect the presence of surgically correctable coronary artery disease should be performed unless the patient is severely unstable hemodynamically from the mechanical defect alone [23,48]. Insertion of an intra-aortic balloon pump can help stabilize the patient.

Prompt surgical repair of these mechanical defects is usually indicated because medical treatment alone is associated with a 90% mortality [23,48,100]. The ACC/AHA guidelines state that class-I indications for emergent or urgent cardiac repair of mechanical defects caused by an acute MI are (1) papillary muscle rupture with severe acute mitral insufficiency (emergent), (2) postinfarction ventricular septal defect or free-wall rupture and pulmonary edema or cardiogenic shock (emergent or urgent), and (3) postinfarction ventricular aneurysm associated with intractable ventricular tachyarrhythmias or pump failure (urgent) [23,48]. Surgical repair may be deferred in patients with postinfarction ventricular septal defect if they are hemodynamically stable [23,48].

Cardiac resynchronization therapy and implantable cardioverter defibrillators

See the article by Kron and Conti elsewhere in this issue for a discussion of class-I indications for using cardiac resynchronization therapy to treat post-MI patients with CHF [54,103,104]. Class-I indications for using implantable cardioverter defibrillators in treating post-MI patients with CHF is addressed in the article by Goldenberg and Moss elsewhere in this issue [54,105].

References

[1] Aronow WS. Epidemiology, pathophysiology, prognosis, and treatment of systolic and diastolic heart failure in elderly patients. Heart Dis 2003;5:279–94.
[2] Aronow WS, Ahn C, Kronzon I. Normal left ventricular ejection fraction in older persons with congestive heart failure. Chest 1998;113:867–9.
[3] Aronow WS, Ahn C. Incidence of heart failure in 2,737 older persons with and without diabetes mellitus. Chest 1999;115:867–8.
[4] Aronow WS, Ahn C, Kronzon I. Comparison of incidences of congestive heart failure in older African-Americans, Hispanics, and whites. Am J Cardiol 1999;84:611–2.
[5] Rich MW, Bosner MS, Chung MK, et al. Is age an independent predictor of early and late mortality in patients with acute myocardial infarction? Am J Med 1992;92:7–13.
[6] Bueno H, Vidan MT, Almazan A, et al. Influence of sex on the short-term outcome of elderly patients with a first acute myocardial infarction. Circulation 1995;92:1133–40.
[7] Kober L, Torp-Pedersen C, Ottesen M, et al. Influence of gender on short- and long-term mortality after acute myocardial infarction. Am J Cardiol 1996;77:1052–6.
[8] Weaver WD, White HD, Wilcox RG, et al. Comparisons of characteristics and outcomes among women and men with acute myocardial infarction treated with thrombolytic therapy. JAMA 1996;275:777–82.

[9] Aronow WS. Prevalence of presenting symptoms of recognized acute myocardial infarction and of unrecognized healed myocardial infarction in elderly patients. Am J Cardiol 1987;60: 1182.

[10] Wolk MJ, Scheidt S, Killip T. Heart failure complicating acute myocardial infarction. Circulation 1972;45:1125–38.

[11] Dwyer EM Jr, Greenberg HM, Steinberg G, et al. Clinical characteristics and natural history of survivors of pulmonary congestion during acute myocardial infarction. Am J Cardiol 1989;63:1423–8.

[12] Gottlieb S, Moss AJ, McDermott M, et al. Interrelation of left ventricular ejection fraction, pulmonary congestion and outcome in acute myocardial infarction. Am J Cardiol 1992;69: 977–84.

[13] Forrester J, Diamond G, Chatterjee K, et al. Medical therapy of acute myocardial infarction by the application of hemodynamic subsets. N Engl J Med 1976;295:1356–62.

[14] Gruppo Italiano per lo Studio della Sopravvivenza nell' Infarto Miocardico: GISSI-3: effects of lisinopril and transdermal glyceryl trinitrate singly and together on 6-week mortality and ventricular function after acute myocardial infarction. Lancet 1994;343:1115–22.

[15] Aronow WS, Ahn C, Kronzon I. Prognosis of congestive heart failure in elderly patients with normal versus abnormal left ventricular systolic function associated with coronary artery disease. Am J Cardiol 1990;66:1257–9.

[16] Aronow WS, Ahn C, Kronzon I. Prognosis of congestive heart failure after prior myocardial infarction in older men and women with abnormal versus normal left ventricular ejection fraction. Am J Cardiol 2000;85:1382–4.

[17] Aronow WS. Treatment of systolic and diastolic heart failure in elderly persons. J Gerontol: Med Sci 2006;60A:1597–605.

[18] Rich MW. Therapy of acute myocardial infarction. In: Aronow WS, Fleg JL, editors. Cardiovascular disease in the elderly. 3rd edition. New York: Marcel Dekker; 2004. p. 297–327.

[19] Aronow WS. Echo in the elderly. Cardio 1990;8:81–90.

[20] Harrison MR, MacPhail B, Gurley JC, et al. Usefulness of color Doppler flow imaging to distinguish ventricular septal defect from acute mitral regurgitation complicating acute myocardial infarction. Am J Cardiol 1989;64:697–701.

[21] Butman S, Olson HG, Aronow WS. Remote right ventricular infarction mimicking pericardial constriction. Am Heart J 1982;103:912–4.

[22] Smyllie JH, Sutherland GR, Geuskens R, et al. Doppler color flow mapping in the diagnosis of ventricular septal rupture and acute mitral regurgitation after myocardial infarction. J Am Coll Cardiol 1990;15:1449–55.

[23] Antman EM, Anbe DT, Armstrong PW, et al. ACC/AHA guidelines for the management of patients with ST-elevation myocardial infarction—executive summary. J Am Coll Cardiol 2004;44:671–719.

[24] Maroko PR, Radvany P, Braunwald E, et al. Reduction of infarct size by oxygen inhalation following acute coronary occlusion. Circulation 1975;52:360–8.

[25] Fillmore SJ, Shapiro M, Killip T. Arterial oxygen tension in acute myocardial infarction: serial analysis of clinical state and blood gas changes. Am Heart J 1970;79:620–9.

[26] Aubier M, Trippenbach T, Roussos C. Respiratory muscle fatigue during cardiogenic shock. J Appl Physiol 1981;51:499–508.

[27] Hyzy R, Popovich J. Mechanical ventilation and weaning. In: Carlson RW, Geheb MA, editors. Principles and practice of medical intensive care. Philadelphia: WB Saunders; 1993. p. 924–33.

[28] Zelis R, Mansour EJ, Capone RJ, et al. The cardiovascular effects of morphine: the peripheral capacitance and resistance vessels in human subjects. J Clin Invest 1974;54:1247–58.

[29] Vismara LA, Leaman DM, Zelis R. The effects of morphine on venous tone in patients with acute pulmonary edema. Circulation 1976;54:335–7.

[30] Butman S, Aronow WS. Updated treatment for left ventricular failure and acute cardiogenic pulmonary edema. ER Reports 1981;2:53–8.

[31] Biddle TL, Yu PN. Effect of furosemide on hemodynamics and lung water in acute pulmonary edema secondary to myocardial infarction. Am J Cardiol 1973;43:86–90.

[32] Dikshit K, Vyden MB, Forrester JS, et al. Renal and extrarenal hemodynamic effects of furosemide in congestive heart failure after acute myocardial infarction. N Engl J Med 1973;288:1087–90.

[33] Flaherty JT. Role of nitrates in acute myocardial infarction. Am J Cardiol 1992;70: 73B–81B.

[34] Jugdutt BI. Role of nitrates after acute myocardial infarction. Am J Cardiol 1992;70:82B–7B.

[35] ISIS-4 (Fourth International Study of Infarct Survival) Collaborative Group. ISIS-4: a randomised factorial trial assessing early oral captopril, oral mononitrate, and intravenous magnesium sulphate in 58,050 patients with suspected acute myocardial infarction. Lancet 1995;345:669–85.

[36] Come PC, Pitt B. Nitroglycerin-induced severe hypotension and bradycardia in patients with acute myocardial infarction. Circulation 1976;54:624–8.

[37] Kinch JW, Ryan TJ. Right ventricular infarction. N Engl J Med 1994;330:1211–7.

[38] Gunnar RM, Lambrew CT, Abrams W, et al. Task force IV: pharmacologic interventions. Emergency cardiac care. Am J Cardiol 1982;50:393–408.

[39] Swedberg K, Held P, Kjekhus J, et al. Effects of the early administration of enalapril on mortality in patients with myocardial infarction. N Engl J Med 1992;327:678–84.

[40] Cohn JN, Johnson G, Ziesche S, et al. A comparison of enalapril with hydralazine-isosorbide dinitrate in the treatment of chronic congestive heart failure. N Engl J Med 1991;325: 303–10.

[41] The Acute Infarction Ramipril Efficacy (AIRE) Study Investigators. Effect of ramipril on mortality and morbidity of survivors of acute myocardial infarction with clinical evidence of heart failure. Lancet 1993;342:821–8.

[42] Ambrosioni E, Borghi C, Magnani B, et al. The effect of the angiotensin-converting-enzyme inhibitor zofenopril on mortality and morbidity after anterior myocardial infarction. N Engl J Med 1995;332:80–5.

[43] Kober L, Torp-Pedersen C, Carlsen JE, et al. A clinical trial of the angiotensin-converting-enzyme inhibitor trandolapril in patients with left ventricular dysfunction after myocardial infarction. N Engl J Med 1995;333:1670–6.

[44] Lisheng L, Liu LS, Wang W, et al. Oral captopril versus placebo among 13,364 patients with suspected acute myocardial infarction: interim report from the Chinese Cardiac Study (CCS-1). Lancet 1995;345:686–7.

[45] Gruppo Italiano per lo Studio della Sopravvivenza nell' Infarto Miocardico: six-month effects of early treatment with lisinopril and transdermal glyceryl trinitrate singly and together withdrawn six-weeks after acute myocardial infarction: the GISSI-3 trial. J Am Coll Cardiol 1996;27:337–44.

[46] Pfeffer MA, Braunwald E, Moye LA, et al. Effect of captopril on mortality and morbidity in patients with left ventricular dysfunction after myocardial infarction. Results of the Survival and Ventricular Enlargement Trial. N Engl J Med 1992;327:669–77.

[47] Aronow WS, Ahn C, Kronzon I. Effect of beta blockers alone, of angiotensin-converting enzyme inhibitors alone, and of beta blockers plus angiotensin-converting enzyme inhibitors on new coronary events and on congestive heart failure in older persons with healed myocardial infarcts and asymptomatic left ventricular systolic dysfunction. Am J Cardiol 2001;88:1298–300.

[48] Ryan TJ, Anderson JL, Antman EM, et al. ACC/AHA guidelines for the management of patients with acute myocardial infarction. A report of the American College of Cardiology/ American Heart Association Task Force on Practice Guidelines (Committee on Management of Acute Myocardial Infarction). J Am Coll Cardiol 1996;28:1328–428.

[49] Sigurdsson A, Swedberg K. Left ventricular remodelling, neurohormonal activation and early treatment with enalapril (CONSENSUS II) following myocardial infarction. Eur Heart J 1994;15(Suppl B):14–9.

[50] The CONSENSUS Trial Study Group. Effect of enalapril on mortality in severe congestive heart failure: results of the Cooperative North Scandinavian Enalapril Survival Study (CONSENSUS). N Engl J Med 1987;316:1429–35.

[51] The SOLVD Investigators. Effect of enalapril on survival in patients with reduced left ventricular ejection fractions and congestive heart failure. N Engl J Med 1991;325:293–302.

[52] Aronow WS, Kronzon I. Effect of enalapril on congestive heart failure treated with diuretics in elderly patients with prior myocardial infarction and normal left ventricular ejection fraction. Am J Cardiol 1993;71:602–4.

[53] Philbin EF, Rocco TA Jr, Lindenmuth NW, et al. Systolic versus diastolic heart failure in community practice: clinical features, outcomes, and the use of angiotensin-converting enzyme inhibitors. Am J Med 2000;109:605–13.

[54] Hunt SA, Abraham WT, Chin MH, et al. ACC/AHA 2005 guideline update for the diagnosis and management of chronic heart failure in the adult—summary article. Circulation 2005;112:1825–52.

[55] Pitt B, Poole-Wilson PA, Segal R, et al. Effect of losartan compared with captopril on mortality in patients with symptomatic heart failure: randomised trial—the Losartan Heart Failure Survival Study ELITE II. Lancet 2000;355:1582–7.

[56] Cohn JN, Tognoni G. A randomized trial of the angiotensin-receptor blocker valsartan in chronic heart failure. N Engl J Med 2001;345:1667–75.

[57] Pfeffer MA, McMurray JJV, Velazquez EJ, et al. Valsartan, captopril, or both in myocardial infarction complicated by heart failure, left ventricular dysfunction, or both. N Engl J Med 2003;349:1893–906.

[58] Granger CB, McMurray JJV, Yusuf S, et al. Effects of candesartan in patients with chronic heart failure and reduced left-ventricular systolic function intolerant to angiotensin-converting-enzyme inhibitors: the CHARM-Alternative trial. Lancet 2003;362:772–6.

[59] McMurray JJV, Ostergren J, Swedberg K, et al. Effects of candesartan in patients with chronic heart failure and reduced left-ventricular systolic function taking angiotensin-converting-enzyme inhibitors: the CHARM-Added trial. Lancet 2003;362:767–71.

[60] Yusuf S, Pfeffer MA, Swedberg K, et al. Effects of candesartan in patients with chronic heart failure and preserved left-ventricular ejection fraction: the CHARM-Preserved trial. Lancet 2003;362:777–81.

[61] Pitt B, Zannad F, Remme WJ, et al. The effect of spironolactone on morbidity and mortality in patients with severe heart failure. N Engl J Med 1999;341:709–17.

[62] Pitt B, Remme W, Zannad F, et al. Eplerenone, a selective aldosterone blocker, in patients with left ventricular dysfunction after myocardial infarction. N Engl J Med 2003;348:1309–21.

[63] Hjalmarson A, Elmfeldt D, Herlitz J, et al. Effect on mortality of metoprolol in acute myocardial infarction. Lancet 1981;2:823–7.

[64] MIAMI Trial Research Group. Metoprolol in acute myocardial infarction (MIAMI): a randomised placebo-controlled international trial. Eur Heart J 1985;6:199–226.

[65] ISIS-1 (First International Study of Infarct Survival) Collaborative Group. Randomised trial of intravenous atenolol among 16,027 cases of suspected acute myocardial infarction. Lancet 1986;2:57–66.

[66] Roberts R, Rogers WJ, Mueller HS, et al. Immediate versus deferred β-blockade following thrombolytic therapy in patients with acute myocardial infarction. Results of the Thrombolysis in Myocardial Infarction (TIMI) II-B Study. Circulation 1991;83:422–37.

[67] Smith SC Jr. Drug treatment after acute myocardial infarction: is treatment the same for the elderly as in the young patient? Am J Geriatr Cardiol 1998;7:60–4.

[68] Herlitz J, Waagstein F, Lindqvist J, et al. Effect of metoprolol on the prognosis for patients with suspected acute myocardial infarction and indirect signs of congestive heart failure (a subgroup analysis of the Goteborg Metoprolol Trial). Am J Cardiol 1997;80:40J–4J.

[69] Teo KK, Yusuf S, Furberg CD. Effects of prophylactic antiarrhythmic drug therapy in acute myocardial infarction. An overview of results from randomized controlled trials. JAMA 1993;270:1589–95.

[70] Hansteen V. Beta blockade after myocardial infarction: the Norwegian Propranolol Study in high-risk patients. Circulation 1983;67(suppl I):I-57–I-60.

[71] Gundersen T, Abrahamsen AM, Kjekshus J, et al. Timolol-related reduction in mortality and reinfarction in patients ages 65–75 years surviving acute myocardial infarction. Circulation 1982;66:1179–84.

[72] Pedersen TR. Six-year follow-up of the Norwegian Multicentre Study on Timolol after acute myocardial infarction. N Engl J Med 1985;313:1055–8.

[73] Beta-Blocker Heart Attack Trial Research Group. A randomized trial of propranolol in patients with acute myocardial infarction. JAMA 1982;247:1707–14.

[74] Park KC, Forman DE, Wei JY. Utility of beta-blockade treatment for older postinfarction patients. J Am Geriatr Soc 1995;43:751–5.

[75] Chadda K, Goldstein S, Byington R, et al. Effect of propranolol after acute myocardial infarction in patients with congestive heart failure. Circulation 1986;73:503–10.

[76] The Beta-Blocker Pooling Project Research Group. The Beta-Blocker Pooling Project (BBPP): subgroup findings from randomised trials in post-infarction patients. Eur Heart J 1988;9:8–16.

[77] Packer M, Bristow MR, Cohn JN, et al. The effect of carvedilol on morbidity and mortality in patients with chronic heart failure. N Engl J Med 1996;334:1349–55.

[78] CIBIS-II Investigators and Committees. The Cardiac Insufficiency Bisoprolol Study II (CIBIS-II): a randomised trial. Lancet 1999;353:9–13.

[79] MERIT-HF Study Group. Effect of metoprolol CR/XL in chronic heart failure: Metoprolol CR/XL Randomised Intervention Trial in Congestive Heart Failure (MERIT-HF). Lancet 1999;353:2001–7.

[80] Packer M, Coats AJS, Fowler MB, et al. Effect of carvedilol on survival in chronic heart failure. N Engl J Med 2001;344:651–8.

[81] Aronow WS, Ahn C, Kronzon I. Effect of propranolol versus no propranolol on total mortality plus nonfatal myocardial infarction in older patients with prior myocardial infarction, congestive heart failure, and left ventricular ejection fraction $\geq 40\%$ treated with diuretics plus angiotensin-converting-enzyme inhibitors. Am J Cardiol 1997;80: 207–9.

[82] Soumerai SB, McLaughlin TJ, Spiegelman D, et al. Adverse outcomes of underuse of beta-blockers in elderly survivors of acute myocardial infarction. JAMA 1997;277:115–21.

[83] Yusuf S, Wittes J, Probstfield J. Evaluating effects of treatment subgroups of patients within a clinical trial: the case of non-Q-wave myocardial infarction and beta blockers. Am J Cardiol 1990;60:220–2.

[84] The Multicenter Diltiazem Postinfarction Trial Research Group. The effect of diltiazem on mortality and reinfarction after myocardial infarction. N Engl J Med 1988;319:385–92.

[85] Goldstein RE, Boccuzzi SJ, Cruess D, et al. Diltiazem increases late-onset congestive heart failure in postinfarction patients with early reduction in ejection fraction. Circulation 1991; 83:52–60.

[86] Furberg CD, Psaty BM, Meyer JV. Nifedipine: dose-related increase in mortality in patients with coronary heart disease. Circulation 1995;92:1321–6.

[87] Yusuf S, Held P, Furberg C. Update of effects of calcium antagonists in myocardial infarction or angina in light of the second Danish Verapamil Infarction Trial (DAVIT-II) and other recent studies. Am J Cardiol 1991;67:1295–7.

[88] Elkayam U, Amin J, Mehra A, et al. A prospective, randomized, double-blind, crossover study to compare the efficacy and safety of chronic nifedipine therapy with that of isosorbide dinitrate and their combination in the treatment of chronic congestive heart failure. Circulation 1990;82:1954–61.

[89] Aronow WS. Digoxin or angiotensin converting enzyme inhibitors for congestive heart failure in geriatric patients. Which is the preferred treatment? Drugs Aging 1991;1:98–103.

[90] The Digitalis Investigation Group. The effect of digoxin on mortality and morbidity in patients with heart failure. N Engl J Med 1997;336:525–33.

[91] Rich MW, McSherry F, Williford WO, et al. Effect of age on mortality, hospitalizations and response to digoxin in patients with heart failure: the DIG Study. J Am Coll Cardiol 2001; 38:806–13.

[92] Rich MW, Woods WL, Davila-Roman VG, et al. A randomized comparison of intravenous amrinone versus dobutamine in older patients with decompensated congestive heart failure. J Am Geriatr Soc 1995;43:271–4.

[93] Dies F, Krell MJ, Whitlow P, et al. Intermittent dobutamine in ambulatory out-patients with chronic cardiac failure [abstract]. Circulation 1986;74(suppl II):II-38.

[94] O'Connor CM, Gattis WA, Uretsky BF, et al. Continuous intravenous dobutamine is associated with an increased risk of death in patients with advanced heart failure: insights from the Flolan International Randomized Survival Trial (FIRST). Am Heart J 2000;138: 78–86.

[95] Kennedy HL, Brooks MM, Barker AH, et al. Beta-blocker therapy in the Cardiac Arrhythmia Suppression Trial. Am J Cardiol 1994;74:674–80.

[96] Aronow WS, Ahn C, Mercando AD, et al. Effect of propranolol versus no antiarrhythmic drug on sudden cardiac death, total cardiac death, and total death in patients ≥62 years of age with heart disease, complex ventricular arrhythmias, and left ventricular ejection fraction ≥40%. Am J Cardiol 1994;74:267–70.

[97] Gregoratos G, Abrams J, Epstein AE, et al. ACC/AHA/NASPE guideline update for implantation of cardiac pacemakers and antiarrhythmia devices: summary article. Circulation 2002;106:2145–61.

[98] Aronow WS. Management of the older person with atrial fibrillation. J Gerontol: Med Sci 2002;57A:M352–63.

[99] Nunez L, de La Llana R, Lopez Sendon J, et al. Diagnosis of treatment of subacute free wall ventricular rupture after infarction. Ann Thorac Surg 1983;35:525–9.

[100] Labovitz AJ, Miller LW, Kennedy HL. Mechanical complications of acute myocardial infarction. Cardiovasc Rev Rep 1984;5:948–52.

[101] Bolooki H. Surgical treatment of complications of acute myocardial infarction. JAMA 1990;263:1237–40.

[102] Lemery R, Smith HC, Giuliani ER, et al. Prognosis in rupture of the ventricular septum after acute myocardial infarction and role of early surgical intervention. Am J Cardiol 1992;70:147–51.

[103] Aronow WS. CRT plus ICD in congestive heart failure. Use of cardiac resynchronization therapy and an implantable cardioverter-defibrillator in heart failure patients with abnormal left ventricular dysfunction. Geriatrics 2005;60(2):24–8.

[104] Cleland JGF, Daubert J-C, Erdmann E, et al. The effect of cardiac resynchronization on morbidity and mortality in heart failure. N Engl J Med 2005;352:1539–49.

[105] Bardy GH, Lee KL, Mark DB, et al. Amiodarone or an implantable cardioverter-defibrillator for congestive heart failure. N Engl J Med 2005;352:225–37.

CLINICS IN
GERIATRIC
MEDICINE

Clin Geriatr Med 23 (2007) 141–153

Inotropic Drugs and Neurohormonal Antagonists in the Treatment of HF in the Elderly

Christopher M. O'Connor, MD[a,b,*],
Pradeep Arumugham, MD[a]

[a]*Division of Clinical Pharmacology, Duke University Medical Center,
2400 Pratt Street, Durham, NC 27710, USA*
[b]*Duke HF Program, Duke Heart Center, PO Box 3356, Durham, NC 27710, USA*

Introduction

HF (HF) is the most common reason for hospital admission among individuals over age 65 years and results in more than 1 million admissions each year [1]. HF incidence is 10 out of 1000 for patients over age 65. The overall annual death rate for HF is approximately 20%. For 2006, the estimated cost of HF is $29.6 billion, of which $15.4 billion or 52% is attributable to hospitalization [1]. HF results from decreased contractile function of the heart, and neurohormonal dysregulation plays a major part in the morbidity and mortality of the heart [2]. The purpose of this article is to review recent studies on inotropic drugs and neurohormonal antagonists used in the treatment of patients who have HF, especially the elderly.

Inotropic drugs

Inotropic drugs have been shown to improve hemodynamics in patients who have HF [3,4]. Many randomized clinical trials have been conducted to measure the clinical impact of these drugs on HF. The decision to use inotropic drugs and the choice of inotropic drug should depend on the clinical situation.

---

* Corresponding author. Duke University Medical Center, Division of Cardiology, Department of Medicine, Room 7401-A Duke North, Box 3356, Durham, NC 27710-0001.
E-mail address: oconn002@mc.duke.edu (C.M. O'Connor).

0749-0690/07/$ - see front matter © 2006 Elsevier Inc. All rights reserved.
doi:10.1016/j.cger.2006.09.001   *geriatric.theclinics.com*

Cardiac glycosides

Digoxin

Digoxin, a cardiac glycoside, works by inhibiting Na^+/K^+-ATPase (adenosine triphosphatase) resulting in the net availability of cytosolic Ca^{++} during systole, thus increasing contractility.

Digoxin was evaluated in a large, randomized controlled trial completed in 1997. The Digitalis Investigation Group (DIG) study evaluated the effect of digoxin on mortality and hospitalization in 7788 patients who had HF and a mean age of 63 who were randomized to placebo and digoxin. Although digoxin did not reduce mortality it did reduce hospitalization attributable to HF in patients who had an ejection fraction (EF) of 45% or less. In patients who had an EF greater than 45%, digoxin did not reduce mortality or hospitalization [5]. This finding is especially important because studies with other inotropic drugs have consistently shown increased mortality. A post hoc analysis was performed on a small subgroup of DIG patients (n = 1687) who had digoxin levels drawn 6 hours after their digoxin dose. These patients were divided into low serum digoxin concentration (SDC) (0.5–0.9 ng/mL) or high SDC (≥ 1.0 ng/mL) and their digoxin levels were compared with matched patients in the placebo group. All-cause mortality was reduced by 3.6% and HF mortality was decreased by 3.3% in the low SDC group. In contrast, all-cause mortality was increased by 8.8% and HF mortality was increased by 1.5% in the high SDC group. Rates of hospitalization followed a similar trend [6]. This finding is consistent with other studies demonstrating increased mortality with increased digoxin levels [7]. Further digoxin withdrawal studies, the Randomized Assessment of Digoxin and Inhibitors of Angiotensin-Converting Enzyme and the Prospective Randomized Study of Ventricular Function and Efficacy of Digoxin, showed increased mortality associated with the withdrawal of digoxin [8,9].

These trials support the use of digoxin in patients who have left ventricular (LV) dysfunction and sinus rhythm. A subgroup analysis on the DIG patients showed increased mortality in patients who had diastolic dysfunction and in elderly women. Digoxin should be avoided in women and men who have diastolic dysfunction. Digoxin should be considered in all patients who have atrial fibrillation and HF in which ventricular slowing is required. Because of the frequent coexistence of renal dysfunction in elderly patients, digoxin levels should be closely monitored and the SDC level kept in the range of 0.5 to 0.9 ng/mL.

Adrenergic agonists

The adrenergic agonists stimulate the heart through the autonomic nervous system pathway. Most adrenergic agonists (dopamine, epinephrine, isoproterenol, norepinephrine, and phenylephrine) are not used routinely in the treatment of HF because of their vasoconstrictive and proarrhythmic properties. Dobutamine is the only adrenergic agonist that is used routinely for HF.

Dobutamine

Dobutamine stimulates beta-1– and beta-2–adrenergic receptor subtypes, thus increasing contractility through its beta-1 effect and vasodilation because of its beta-2 effect. At higher doses, dobutamine stimulates alpha-1 and causes vasoconstriction.

Dobutamine has been evaluated in clinical trials [10–18]. Continuous use of dobutamine causes desensitization and tolerance. The Dobutamine Infusion in Severe HF (DICE) trial [15] was designed to evaluate intermittent low-dose dobutamine. In the DICE trial, 38 patients with an average age of 65 ± 2 years were randomized to two groups: optimized oral therapy and intermittent ambulatory low-dose dobutamine, or optimized oral therapy alone. The addition of dobutamine did not improve functional status and did not increase mortality. Hospitalization for all causes and worsening congestive HF (CHF) were fewer. Insights from the Flolan International Randomized Survival Trial [16] evaluated continuous intravenous dobutamine and found that it increases mortality and major morbidity.

Some studies in the elderly have shown improved well being and cardiac function [17,18], but large-scale randomized trials on long-term mortality and functional status are lacking. Because dobutamine works through the beta adrenergic pathway the use of beta blockers, which has become the standard of care, in such patients can attenuate the action of dobutamine [19,20].

Phosphodiesterase inhibitors

The phosphodiesterase III (PDE III) enzyme is present in the cardiac muscle closely associated with the sarcoplasmic reticulum. This enzyme degrades cyclic adenosine monophosphate (cAMP) to adenosine monophosphate (AMP) and is involved in the release of calcium. PDE III inhibition in low doses results in increasing contractility without increasing heart rate. PDE III also is present in vascular smooth muscle and its inhibition enhances vasodilation through nitric oxide–dependent pathways. This inotrope-vasodilator property of PDE increases contractility, reduces preload, and reduces afterload, which are all beneficial effects for the failing heart.

Milrinone

Milrinone increases cardiac output and reduces systemic vascular resistance and pulmonary capillary wedge pressure; it rarely causes thrombocytopenia [22]. The Outcomes of a Prospective Trial of Intravenous Milrinone for Exacerbations of Chronic HF (OPTIME-CHF) [23] was designed to evaluate the use of milrinone in acute decompensated HF. Milrinone did not show any improvement in symptoms, dosing of angiotensin-converting enzyme (ACE) inhibitors, or duration of hospitalization. The Acute

Decompensated Heart Failure National Registry (ADHERE) [24] also showed increased mortality compared with nesiritide and nitroglycerin. Long-term therapy with oral milrinone for chronic HF increases mortality as evidenced by the Prospective Randomized Milrinone Survival Evaluation [25], in which there was a 28% increase in all-cause mortality and a 34% increase in cardiovascular mortality.

Enoximone

Enoximone is highly specific for PDE III. It is approved for intravenous use in Europe. In the United States, studies are ongoing for low-dose oral enoximone [26]. Enoximone was tested initially with high doses resulting in increased mortality [27]. Low-dose enoximone has been shown to increase exercise capacity in patients who have HF [28]. The results of the enoximone clinical trials program will help determine the clinical use of enoximone in heart failure.

Amrinone

Because amrinone causes thrombocytopenia and rapid tolerance, it is no longer used in treating HF [21].

Phosphodiesterase inhibitors with calcium sensitization

The inotropic actions of PDE inhibitors with calcium sensitization are believed to be primarily attributable to calcium sensitization [29]. These drugs stabilize the conformational change in troponin-C when it binds to calcium. They are more effective in systole when calcium is abundant and less effective in diastole; hence, they do not affect relaxation. The inotropic effects also are attributable to its PDE III inhibition at higher concentrations. Because these drugs increase contractility without increasing calcium concentration their arrhythmogenic potential is low. They are potent vasodilators and also increase coronary blood flow. Vasodilation is attributable to activation of ATP-sensitive potassium channels.

Pimobendan

Pimobendan has weak calcium sensitization action and its major inotropic activity is attributable to PDE III inhibition. Pimobendan was evaluated in the Pimobendan in Congestive HF trial [30], however, and showed increased mortality. Its development has been halted.

Levosimendan

Levosimendan has been evaluated in two large-scale randomized control trials: Randomized Multicenter Evaluation of Intravenous Levosimendan Efficacy versus Placebo in the Short-term Treatment of Acute HF (REVIVE) II and Survival of Patients with Acute HF in Need of Intravenous Inotropic Support (SURVIVE). In REVIVE II [31], levosimendan was shown to have a superior effect on the composite primary outcome compared with placebo. In SURVIVE [31], there was no significant difference in long-term outcome between dobutamine and levosimendan. There is still some concern with sustained hypotension, proarrhythmic activity, and a trend toward a higher mortality.

Summary

Most studies of inotropic drugs have been conducted in patients with a mean age of 65 years; hence, the results of these studies can be extrapolated to use in elderly patients. Although all inotropes, except digoxin, have been shown to be detrimental for long-term outcome in heart failure [13,25,30,32], there are special situations in HF in which inotropes are important.

Inpatient settings

- Cardiogenic shock—Dobutamine lowers systemic vascular resistance and increases contractility. Milrinone should be used only when blood pressure is high enough to tolerate vasodilation. Milrinone might be a better choice in patients using beta blockers.
- Tide over potentially reversible conditions (eg, arrhythmia, noncardiac surgery).
- CHF with low perfusion—The ADHERE studies suggest more benefit from vasodilator therapy than from inotropic drugs. In special circumstances in which blood pressure will not tolerate vasodilation, inotropic drugs might be a better choice.
- CHF with acute renal failure.

Outpatient settings

- Bridge to transplant.
- HF refractory to conventional management.
- Palliative care—in end-stage heart failure.

Neurohormonal antagonists

Neurohormonal activation in patients who have HF results in adverse outcomes. Inhibition of this activation results in improvement of heart failure.

Renin angiotensin aldosterone system

Angiotensin-converting enzyme inhibitors

ACE inhibitor agents act by inhibiting the production of angiotensin II using the angiotensin-converting enzyme.

ACE inhibitors improve symptoms, quality of life (QOL), exercise toler-ance [33–35], mortality [25,36], and hospitalization [36] in patients who have heart failure. Few studies have been conducted to evaluate the use of ACE inhibitors in the elderly. Elderly patients are underrepresented in clinical tri-als on HF [37]. A meta-analysis of five large trials revealed a mean age of less than 65 years for patients in these trials [38]. Because of the high prev-alence of diastolic HF in the elderly [39–41], especially in older women, in whom the prevalence might be higher than that attributable to systolic dys-function [41], trials conducted in younger patients may not be appropriate. One study done on the effect of ACE inhibitors or angiotensin receptor blockers (ARBs) on patients at least 65 years old who have preserved sys-tolic function showed improved 1-year mortality [40]. Although multiple studies have shown improvement in HF, ACE inhibitors are still underused in patients who have HF [42,43]. Prescription rates for ACE inhibitors vary from 40% to 60% of patients who have HF [42–44].

ACE inhibitors should be started at low doses in elderly patients and renal function should be monitored frequently to detect increases in blood urea nitrogen and serum creatinine. Chronic renal insufficiency (CRI) at baseline should not be a contraindication for ACE-inhibitor therapy, espe-cially because ACE inhibitors have been shown to benefit renal function in CRI in patients who have diabetes [45,46] and patients who do not have di-abetes [47,48]. Potassium-sparing diuretics should be used carefully with ACE inhibitors as they can cause hyperkalemia. Dry cough is the most com-mon adverse effect and the most common reason for discontinuing ACE-inhibitor therapy. Angioneurotic edema does occur because of increased bradykinin production.

Combined use of ACE inhibitors and aspirin tends to attenuate the effects of ACE inhibitors on mortality and morbidity [49,50]. There are no recommendations for this because there is no good evidence either way.

Angiotensin receptor blockers

Angiotensin receptor blockers (ARBs) act by blocking the angiotensin II receptor. Because maximal doses of ACE inhibitors did not eliminate the levels of angiotensin II [51], the logical next step was to design an angioten-sin receptor blocker.

Similar to the ACE inhibitors, ARBs have been shown to improve symp-toms [52], QOL, exercise tolerance [52], mortality, and hospitalization [53]. They also have been shown to be beneficial in patients intolerant to ACE inhibitors [54,55] and in patients who have preserved systolic function [56].

ARBs have a reduced incidence of cough compared with ACE inhibitors. The Losartan HF Survival Study [13] was designed to test whether losartan was superior to captopril. There was no significant improvement in mortal-ity. Other studies have shown similar results [57].

Combination therapy with ACE inhibitors and ARBs was shown to have a synergistic effect in the Valsartan Heart Failure Trial [53]. The trial revealed a reduction in HF hospitalizations in the elderly patients.

Aldosterone antagonists
Spironolactone. The Randomized Aldactone Evaluation Study (RALES) was conducted to evaluate the effect of spironolactone at a dose of 25 mg on all-cause mortality for patients who had severe systolic HF receiving standard therapy. A total of 1663 patients with mean age of 65 years were randomized to spironolactone or placebo. There was a 30% reduction in the risk for death in the spironolactone group and the study was terminated early. Reduction in mortality was attributed to the reduction in deaths attributable to HF and sudden death. Symptoms also were improved.

The RALES study did not evaluate the effect of spironolactone in patients who had diastolic heart failure. Small studies conducted to evaluate the effect of spironolactone on patients who have diastolic heart failure indicate benefit [58,59], specifically in the elderly [59].

Spironolactone has been associated with gynecomastia, impotence, and menstrual irregularities, which often leads to discontinuation. Spironolactone does cause hyperkalemia and patients should be monitored for elevated potassium, especially in the setting of chronic kidney disease [60].

Eplerenone. In patients who have LV dysfunction after acute myocardial infarction (MI), eplerenone showed decreased mortality and decreased hospitalization [13]. Eplerenone is a selective mineralocorticoid receptor and does not bind the glucocorticoid, progesterone, or androgen receptors [61]. In contrast with spironolactone, eplerenone does not cause gynecomastia, impotence, or menstrual irregularities.

Antiadrenergic agents
In multiple studies, beta blockers have been shown to reduce mortality [62–66]. The Metoprolol CR/XL Randomized Intervention Trial in Congestive Heart Failure (MERIT-HF) [65] evaluated the effect of metoprolol on mortality in 3991 patients with a mean age of 63 years. Of the patients above age 65, 65% were randomized to metoprolol with standard therapy or standard therapy alone. The study was stopped early because of a 34% decrease in mortality in the metoprolol group. Further analysis of MERIT-HF patients showed improved survival, improved well-being, improved New York Heart Association class, and reduced hospitalization [67].

Studies of beta blockers conducted in elderly patients who have HF have shown benefit regardless of age, gender, or systolic function. Nebivolol, a beta blocker with vasodilating properties related to nitric oxide modulation, was evaluation in 2128 patients with a mean age of 76 years. Nebivolol improved all-cause mortality and cardiovascular hospitalization even though the benefit compared with previous trials was smaller [68]. The

Efficacy of Nebivolol in the Treatment of Elderly Patients with Chronic HF as Add-on Therapy study conducted in 260 patients over the age of 65 years who had an EF of less than 35% documented improvement in LV systolic function with nebivolol [69]. Carvedilol has been shown to improve diastolic function in patients who have diastolic HF [70]. Japanese Diastolic HF is an ongoing trial studying the effects of beta blockers on mortality and hospitalization in patients who have diastolic HF [71].

Beta blockers should be used in HF in the elderly. Benefits might be less than in the younger population, which might be true of all medications in general. Beta blockers should be initiated at a low dose and gradually titrated up over weeks to months. During titration patients should be monitored for hypotension, bradycardia, and worsening heart failure. Reactive airway disease and asymptomatic bradycardia are not absolute contraindications for beta blocker use but beta blockers should not be used with ongoing symptoms [72].

Summary

Summary of the American College of Cardiology/American Heart Association guidelines for treatment of HF in adults as pertaining to the above drugs [73] are as follows:

ACE inhibitors should be used in treatment of elderly patients who have HF. ARBs should be used only if patients are intolerant of ACE inhibitors. Aldosterone antagonists should be used in all patients who have HF and the primary choice should be spironolactone. Beta blockers should be prescribed for all patients who have HF who are already on an ACE inhibitor or ARB.

All patients who have symptoms of fluid overload should be treated with diuretics. ACE inhibitors should be started in all patients who have HF attributable to systolic dysfunction. ACE inhibitors should be started in low doses and titrated slowly. Renal function should be monitored in 1 to 2 weeks. Neither the use of aspirin nor prior kidney disease is a contraindication for treatment with ACE inhibitors. The specific ACE inhibitor does not matter. If hypotension or renal dysfunction occurs reduce the dose of ACE inhibitors or reduce the dose of diuretics or both.

Beta blocker should be used in all patients who have stable HF attributable to reduced systolic function. Beta blockers can be started while the ACE inhibitor dose is being titrated up. Reactive airway disease and asymptomatic bradycardia are not contraindications for beta blocker therapy.

The routine combined use of ARBs and ACE inhibitors is not recommended but can be used in patients who have persistent symptoms.

Aldosterone antagonists should be used in patients who have moderately severe or severe HF symptoms or LV dysfunction early after MI.

Digitalis may be considered in patients who have persistent symptoms of HF during therapy with diuretics, ACE inhibitor, and beta blockers. If the patient is on digoxin and has not been on an ACE inhibitor or beta blocker, digoxin should not be withdrawn.

Positive inotropic agents other than digitalis should not be used for the management of chronic HF unless they are palliative or being used as a bridge to cardiac transplant. In patients who have acute decompensated HF and life-threatening situations, these agents may be used.

References

[1] Thom T, Haase N, Rosamond W, et al. Heart disease and stroke statistics—2006 update: A report from the American Heart Association Statistics Committee and Stroke Statistics Subcommittee. Circulation 2006;113:e85–151.

[2] Adams KF Jr. Pathophysiologic role of the renin-angiotensin-aldosterone and sympathetic nervous systems in heart failure. Am J Health Syst Pharm 2004;61(Suppl 2):S4–13.

[3] Mihata S, Yasutomi N, Mori S, et al. [Effects of dobutamine on hemodynamics, myocardial metabolism and mechanical efficiency in patients with old myocardial infarctions]. Kokyu To Junkan 1987;35(5):541–7.

[4] Grose R, Strain J, Greenberg M, et al. Systemic and coronary effects of intravenous milrinone and dobutamine in congestive heart failure. J Am Coll Cardiol 1986;7(5):1107–13.

[5] Perry GG. The effect of digoxin on mortality and morbidity in patients with heart failure. N Engl J Med 1997;336(8):525–33.

[6] Ahmed A, Rich MW, Love TE, et al. Digoxin and reduction in mortality and hospitalization in heart failure: a comprehensive post hoc analysis of the DIG trial. Eur Heart J 2006;27(2): 178–86.

[7] Rathore SS, Curtis JP, Wang Y, et al. Association of serum digoxin concentration and outcomes in patients with heart failure. JAMA 2003;289(7):871–8.

[8] Uretsky BF, Young JB, Shahidi FE, et al. Randomized study assessing the effect of digoxin withdrawal in patients with mild to moderate chronic congestive heart failure: results of the PROVED trial. PROVED Investigative Group. J Am Coll Cardiol 1993; 22(4):955–62.

[9] Packer M, Gheorghiade M, Young JB, et al. Withdrawal of digoxin from patients with chronic HF treated with angiotensin-converting-enzyme inhibitors. RADIANCE Study. N Engl J Med 1993;329(1):1–7.

[10] Levine TB, Levine AB, Elliott WG, et al. Dobutamine as bridge to angiotensin-converting enzyme inhibitor-nitrate therapy in endstage heart failure. Clin Cardiol 2001;24(3):231–6.

[11] Oliva F, Gronda E, Frigerio M, et al. [Outpatient intermittent dobutamine therapy in congestive heart failure]. Z Kardiol 1999;88(Suppl 3):S28–32.

[12] Applefeld MM, Newman KA, Sutton FJ, et al. Outpatient dobutamine and dopamine infusions in the management of chronic heart failure: clinical experience in 21 patients. Am Heart J 1987;114(3):589–95.

[13] Krell MJ, Kline EM, Bates ER, et al. Intermittent, ambulatory dobutamine infusions in patients with severe congestive heart failure. Am Heart J 1986;112(4):787–91.

[14] Roffman DS, Applefeld MM, Grove WR, et al. Intermittent dobutamine hydrochloride infusions in outpatients with chronic congestive heart failure. Clin Pharm 1985;4(2):195–9.

[15] Oliva F, Latini R, Politi A, et al. Intermittent 6-month low-dose dobutamine infusion in severe heart failure: DICE multicenter trial. Am Heart J 1999;138(2 Pt 1):247–53.

[16] O'Connor CM, Gattis WA, Uretsky BF, et al. Continuous intravenous dobutamine is associated with an increased risk of death in patients with advanced heart failure: Insights from the Flolan International Randomized Survival Trial (FIRST). Am Heart J 1999;138(1): 78–86.

[17] Vandenbrande PP. Intermittent dobutamine infusion in severe chronic heart-failure in elderly patients. Gerontology 1990;36(1):49–54.

[18] Lopez-Candales A, Vora T, Gibbons W, et al. Symptomatic improvement in patients treated with intermittent infusion of inotropes: a double-blind placebo controlled pilot study. J Med 2002;33(1–4):129–46.

[19] Metra M, Nodari S, D'Aloia A, et al. Beta-blocker therapy influences the hemodynamic response to inotropic agents in patients with heart failure: A randomized comparison of dobutamine and enoximone before and after chronic treatment with metoprolol or carvedilol. J Am Coll Cardiol 2002;40(7):1248–58.

[20] Shakar SF, Abraham FWT, Gilbert FEM, et al. Combined oral positive inotropic and beta-blocker therapy for treatment of refractory class IV heart failure. J Am Coll Cardiol 1998; 31(6):1336–40.

[21] Rich MM. A randomized comparison of intravenous amrinone versus dobutamine in older patients with decompensated congestive-heart-failure. J Am Geriatr Soc 1995;43(3): 271–4.

[22] Shipley JJ. Milrinone: basic and clinical pharmacology and acute and chronic management. Am J Med Sci 1996;311(6):286–91.

[23] Cuffe MM. Short-term intravenous milrinone for acute exacerbation of chronic heart failure—A randomized controlled trial. JAMA 2002;287(12):1541–7.

[24] Abraham WT, Adams KF, Fonarow GC, et al. In-hospital mortality in patients with acute decompensated HF requiring intravenous vasoactive medications: an analysis from the Acute Decompensated HF National Registry (ADHERE). J Am Coll Cardiol 2005;46(1): 57–64.

[25] Packer M, Carver JR, Rodeheffer RJ, et al. Effect of oral milrinone on mortality in severe chronic heart failure. The PROMISE Study Research Group. N Engl J Med 1991;325(21): 1468–75.

[26] Lowes BD, Shakar SF, Metra M, et al. Rationale and design of the enoximone clinical trials program. J Card Fail 2005;11(9):659–69.

[27] Uretsky BF, Jessup M, Konstam MA, et al. Multicenter trial of oral enoximone in patients with moderate to moderately severe congestive heart failure. Lack of benefit compared with placebo. Enoximone Multicenter Trial Group. Circulation 1990;82(3):774–80.

[28] Lowes BD, Higginbotham M, Petrovich L, et al. Low-dose enoximone improves exercise capacity in chronic heart failure. J Am Coll Cardiol 2000;36(2):501–8.

[29] Sorsa T, Pollesello P, Permi P, et al. Interaction of levosimendan with cardiac troponin C in the presence of cardiac troponin I peptides. J Mol Cell Cardiol 2003;35(9):1055–61.

[30] Heyndrickx GG. Effect of pimobendan on exercise capacity in patients with heart failure: main results from the Pimobendan in Congestive HF (PICO) trial. Heart 1996;76(3):223–31.

[31] Cleland JG, Freemantle N, Coletta AP, et al. Clinical trials update from the American Heart Association: REPAIR-AMI, ASTAMI, JELIS, MEGA, REVIVE-II, SURVIVE, and PROACTIVE. Eur J Heart Fail 2006;8(1):105–10.

[32] Packer M, Medina N, Yushak M. Hemodynamic and clinical limitations of long-term inotropic therapy with amrinone in patients with severe chronic heart failure. Circulation 1984; 70(6):1038–47.

[33] Pfeffer MA, Braunwald E, Moye LA, et al. Effect of captopril on mortality and morbidity in patients with left ventricular dysfunction after myocardial infarction. Results of the survival and ventricular enlargement trial. The SAVE Investigators. N Engl J Med 1992;327(10): 669–77.

[34] Narang R, Swedberg K, Cleland JGF. What is the ideal study design for evaluation of treatment for heart failure?: insights from trials assessing the effect of ACE inhibitors on exercise capacity. Eur Heart J 1996;17(1):120–34.

[35] Swedberg K, Kjekshus J. Effects of enalapril on mortality in severe congestive heart failure. Results of the Cooperative North Scandinavian Enalapril Survival Study (CONSENSUS). The CONSENSUS Trial Study Group. N Engl J Med 1987;316(23):1429–35.

[36] Garg R, Yusuf S. Overview of randomized trials of angiotensin-converting enzyme inhibitors on mortality and morbidity in patients with heart failure. Collaborative Group on ACE Inhibitor Trials. JAMA 1995;273(18):1450–6.

[37] Heiat A, Gross CP, Krumholz HM. Representation of the elderly, women, and minorities in HF clinical trials. Arch Intern Med 2002;162(15):1682–8.

[38] Flather MD, Yusuf S, Kober L, et al. Long-term ACE-inhibitor therapy in patients with HF or left-ventricular dysfunction: a systematic overview of data from individual patients. Lancet 2000;355(9215):1575–81.

[39] Pernenkil MDR, Vinson MDJM, Shah MDAS, et al. Course and prognosis in patients ≥ 70 years of age with congestive HF and normal versus abnormal left ventricular ejection fraction. Am J Cardiol 1997;79(2):216–9.

[40] Sueta CA, Russo A, Schenck A, et al. Effect of angiotensin-converting inhibitor or angiotensin receptor blocker on one-year survival in patients ≥ 65 years hospitalized with a left ventricular ejection fraction ≥ 50%. Am J Cardiol 2003;91(3):363–5.

[41] Aronow WS, Ahn C, Kronzon I. Comparison of incidences of congestive HF in older African-Americans, Hispanics, and Whites. Am J Cardiol 1999;84(5):611–2.

[42] Bungard TJ, McAlister FA, Johnson JA, et al. Underutilisation of ACE inhibitors in patients with congestive heart failure. Drugs 2001;61(14):2021–33.

[43] Havranek EP, Abrams F, Stevens E, et al. Determinants of mortality in elderly patients with heart failure: the role of angiotensin-converting enzyme inhibitors. Arch Intern Med 1998;158(18):2024–8.

[44] Masoudi FA, Rathore SS, Wang Y, et al. National patterns of use and effectiveness of angiotensin-converting enzyme inhibitors in older patients with HF and left ventricular systolic dysfunction. Circulation 2004;110(6):724–31.

[45] Lewis EJ, Hunsicker LG, Bain RP, et al. The effect of angiotensin-converting-enzyme inhibition on diabetic nephropathy. The Collaborative Study Group. N Engl J Med 1993;329(20):1456–62.

[46] Ravid M, Savin H, Jutrin I, et al. Long-term effect of ACE inhibition on development of nephropathy in diabetes mellitus type II. Kidney Int Suppl 1994;45:S161–4.

[47] Maschio G, Alberti D, Janin G, et al. Effect of the angiotensin-converting-enzyme inhibitor benazepril on the progression of chronic renal insufficiency. The Angiotensin-Converting-Enzyme Inhibition in Progressive Renal Insufficiency Study Group. N Engl J Med 1996;334(15):939–45.

[48] Giatras I, Lau J, Levey AS. Effect of angiotensin-converting enzyme inhibitors on the progression of nondiabetic renal disease: a meta-analysis of randomized trials. Ann Intern Med 1997;127(5):337–45.

[49] Hall D, Zeitler H, Rudolph W. Counteraction of the vasodilator effects of enalapril by aspirin in severe heart failure. J Am Coll Cardiol 1992;20(7):1549–55.

[50] Nguyen MDKN, Aursnes MDPI, Kjekshus MDPJ. Interaction between enalapril and aspirin on mortality after acute myocardial infarction: subgroup analysis of the Cooperative New Scandinavian Enalapril Survival Study II (CONSENSUS II). Am J Cardiol 1997;79(2):115–9.

[51] Kawamura M, Imanashi M, Matsushima Y, et al. Circulating angiotensin II levels under repeated administration of lisinopril in normal subjects. Clin Exp Pharmacol Physiol 1992;19(8):547–53.

[52] Riegger GAJ, Bouzo H, Petr P, et al. Improvement in exercise tolerance and symptoms of congestive HF during treatment with candesartan cilexetil. Circulation 1999;100(22):2224–30.

[53] Cohn JN, Goldstein SO, Greenberg BH, et al. A dose-dependent increase in mortality with vesnarinone among patients with severe heart failure. Vesnarinone Trial Investigators. N Engl J Med 1998;339(25):1810–6.

[54] Granger CB, McMurray JJV, Yusuf S, et al. Effects of candesartan in patients with chronic HF and reduced left-ventricular systolic function intolerant to angiotensin-converting-enzyme inhibitors: the CHARM-Alternative trial. Lancet 2003;362(9386):772–6.

[55] McMurray JJV, Ostergren J, Swedberg K, et al. Effects of candesartan in patients with chronic HF and reduced left-ventricular systolic function taking angiotensin-converting-enzyme inhibitors: the CHARM-Added trial. Lancet 2003;362(9386):767–71.

[56] Yusuf S, Pfeffer MA, Swedberg K, et al. Effects of candesartan in patients with chronic HF and preserved left-ventricular ejection fraction: the CHARM-Preserved Trial. Lancet 2003; 362(9386):777–81.

[57] Granger CB, Ertl G, Kuch J, et al. Randomized trial of candesartan cilexetil in the treatment of patients with congestive HF and a history of intolerance to angiotensin-converting enzyme inhibitors. Am Heart J 2000;139(4):609–17.

[58] Mottram PM, Haluska B, Leano R, et al. Effect of aldosterone antagonism on myocardial dysfunction in hypertensive patients with diastolic heart failure. Circulation 2004;110(5): 558–65.

[59] Roongsritong C, Sutthiwan P, Bradley J, et al. Spironolactone improves diastolic function in the elderly. Clin Cardiol 2005;28(10):484–7.

[60] Juurlink DN, Mamdani MM, Lee DS, et al. Rates of hyperkalemia after publication of the randomized Aldactone evaluation study. N Engl J Med 2004;351(6):543–51.

[61] de Gasparo M, Joss U, Ramjoue HP, et al. Three new epoxy-spirolactone derivatives: characterization in vivo and in vitro. J Pharmacol Exp Ther 1987;240(2):650–6.

[62] Packer M, Coats AJS, Fowler MB, et al. Effect of carvedilol on survival in severe chronic heart failure. N Engl J Med 2001;344(22):1651–8.

[63] Eichhorn EJ, Domanski MJ, Krause-Steinrauf H, et al. The beta-blocker evaluation of survival trial I. A trial of the beta-blocker bucindolol in patients with advanced chronic heart failure. N Engl J Med 2001;344(22):1659–67.

[64] Dargie HJ. Effect of carvedilol on outcome after myocardial infarction in patients with left-ventricular dysfunction: the CAPRICORN randomised trial. Lancet 2001;357(9266): 1385–90.

[65] MERIT-HF Study G. Effect of metoprolol CR/XL in chronic heart failure: Metoprolol CR/XL Randomised Intervention Trial in-Congestive HF (MERIT-HF). Lancet 1999; 353(9169):2001–7.

[66] Cibis-Ii Investigators and C. The Cardiac Insufficiency Bisoprolol Study II (CIBIS-II). A randomised trial. Lancet 1999;353(9146):9–13.

[67] Hjalmarson A, Goldstein S, Fagerberg B, et al. Effects of controlled-release metoprolol on total mortality, hospitalizations, and well-being in patients with heart failure: the Metoprolol CR/XL Randomized Intervention Trial in Congestive HF (MERIT-HF). JAMA 2000; 283(10):1295–302.

[68] Flather MD, Shibata MC, Coats AJS, et al. FASTTRACK Randomized trial to determine the effect of nebivolol on mortality and cardiovascular hospital admission in elderly patients with HF (SENIORS). Eur Heart J 2005;26(3):215–25.

[69] Edes I, Gasior Z, Wita K. Effects of nebivolol on left ventricular function in elderly patients with chronic heart failure: results of the ENECA study. Eur J Heart Fail 2005;7(4): 631–9.

[70] Bergstrom A, Andersson B, Edner M, et al. Effect of carvedilol on diastolic function in patients with diastolic HF and preserved systolic function. Results of the Swedish Doppler-echocardiographic study (SWEDIC). Eur J Heart Fail 2004;6(4):453–61.

[71] Hori M, Kitabatake A, Tsutsui H, et al. The J-DHF Program C. Rationale and design of a randomized trial to assess the effects of [beta]-blocker in diastolic heart failure; Japanese Diastolic HF Study (J-DHF). J Card Fail 2005;11(7):542–7.

[72] Hunt SA, Abraham WT, Chin MH, et al. ACC/AHA 2005 Guideline Update for the Diagnosis and Management of Chronic HF in the Adult—Summary Article: A report of the American College of Cardiology/American Heart Association Task Force on Practice Guidelines (writing committee to update the 2001 guidelines for the evaluation and management of heart failure): developed in collaboration with the American College of Chest

Physicians and the International Society for Heart and Lung Transplantation: Endorsed by the Heart Rhythm Society. Circulation 2005;112(12):1825–52.

[73] Hunt SA, Abraham WT, Chin MH, et al. ACC/AHA 2005 Guideline Update for the Diagnosis and Management of Chronic HF in the Adult: A report of the American College of Cardiology/American Heart Association Task Force on Practice Guidelines (writing committee to update the 2001 guidelines for the evaluation and management of heart failure): developed in collaboration with the American College of Chest Physicians and the International Society for Heart and Lung Transplantation: Endorsed by the Heart Rhythm Society. Circulation 2005;112(12):e154–235.

ELSEVIER
SAUNDERS

Clin Geriatr Med 23 (2007) 155–178

CLINICS IN
GERIATRIC
MEDICINE

Interventional Therapies for Heart Failure in the Elderly

Srihari S. Naidu, MD[a,b], S. Chiu Wong, MD[a,c],
Richard M. Steingart, MD[a,d,e],*

[a]Weill Medical College of Cornell University, 130 York Avenue, New York, NY 10021, USA
[b]Interventional Cardiology, Division of Cardiology, New York Presbyterian Hospital,
520 E. 70th Street, Starr 4, New York, NY 10021, USA
[c]Cardiac Catheterization Laboratory, New York Presbyterian Hospital,
520 E. 70th Street, Starr 4, New York, NY 10021, USA
[d]Cardiology Department, Memorial Sloan Kettering Cancer Center,
1275 York Avenue, New York, NY 10021, USA
[e]Society of Geriatric Cardiology, 2400 N. Street NW, 2nd Floor,
Washington, DC 20037, USA

Hospital discharges for heart failure (HF) rose from 399,000 in 1979 to 1,093,000 in 2003, an increase of 174%. Data from ambulatory care visits to physician offices, hospital outpatient departments, and emergency departments in the United States from 1999 to 2000 showed the number of visits for HF was 3.4 million [1]. The aging of a population replete with risk factors for HF (coronary heart disease, diabetes, and hypertension) coupled with a declining age-adjusted mortality rate for coronary artery and hypertensive heart diseases has created, and will continue to create, a literal explosion in the prevalence of HF in the United States. HF affects more than 5 million Americans, with more than 500,000 new cases diagnosed annually. It is currently the most common diagnosis-related group in adults more than 65 years of age; most hospitalizations occur in patients more than 75 years of age [1]. Despite advances in maximal medical therapy, however, most patients who have symptomatic HF can expect functional impairment, interludes of worsening symptomatology, and a shortened lifespan. Since this question was last addressed in the *Clinics in Geriatric Medicine* it is still appropriate to ask whether the interventional revolution in the management of ischemic cardiovascular disease should be applied to the management of

* Corresponding author. Cardiology Department, Memorial Sloan Kettering Cancer Center, 1275 York Avenue, New York, NY 10021.
  E-mail address: steingar@mskcc.org (R.M. Steingart).

0749-0690/07/$ - see front matter © 2006 Elsevier Inc. All rights reserved.
doi:10.1016/j.cger.2006.09.003   *geriatric.theclinics.com*

HF. This article updates the use of interventional therapies for the treatment of elderly patients who have HF caused by coronary artery disease, valvular heart disease, congential heart disease, myocardial disease, and renal vascular disease.

Heart failure in patients who have coronary artery disease

The greatest survival benefit from revascularization relative to medical therapy is seen among patients who have left ventricular (LV) dysfunction and extensive coronary artery disease, particularly when angina is the primary clinical manifestation [2]. A survival benefit has been more difficult to demonstrate for unselected patients presenting with multivessel disease and LV dysfunction but who do not have important angina. In fact, The Heart Failure Guidelines of the Agency for Health Care Policy and Research state that in the treatment of patients who have moderate to severe LV dysfunction "it is not clear whether patients whose predominant symptom is HF rather than angina would benefit from bypass surgery, or how much ischemia is required to justify surgical intervention" [3]. Yusuf and colleagues [4] in an overview of trials comparing coronary artery bypass grafting (CABG) with medical therapy suggest that CABG provides a survival benefit in high-risk patients (three vessel disease, LV dysfunction, or both). This analysis has been criticized because of the heavy weighting of one trial on these conclusions, a trial that had an unusually high mortality in the medically treated group [5]. Optimal management strategies for these patients are the subject of intense debate and opinion, relying on studies using what are now considered antiquated medical and interventional approaches to the problem. It is important, therefore, to reexamine this vexing issue.

Because ischemia is often silent, it stands to reason that some patients who have HF and multivessel coronary disease without limiting angina would benefit from revascularization. But even in the modern era, the risk of revascularization, and in particular percutaneous coronary intervention (PCI), increases with increasing age, LV dysfunction, HF, and multivessel coronary artery disease. In the most recent New York State Coronary Angioplasty Report, hospital deaths following angioplasty were strongly related to patient age, recent HF, reduced ejection fraction, female sex, and hemodynamic instability at the time of the procedure [6]. In the coronary stent era, older age and more comorbidity, declining ejection fraction, and incomplete revascularization were associated with an adverse impact on long-term mortality [7]. The essential factors associated with HF and coronary disease in the elderly remain to date inextricably tied to worsening outcomes. Recommendations for PCI in the presence of HF and LV function are conspicuously scant in the most recent American College of Cardiology and American Heart Association (ACC/AHA) guidelines [8].

Myocardial viability

For the purposes of this discussion myocardial viability is defined as myocardial dysfunction that is reversible after revascularization [9]. LV dysfunction in patients who have coronary artery disease may be attributable to three disease states: (1) myocardial necrosis, (2) myocardial stunning, and (3) myocardial hibernation.

ACC/AHA guidelines on radionuclide imaging state that there exists an important subpopulation of patients who have obstructive coronary artery disease in which revascularization *may* significantly improve regional or global LV function, symptoms, and potentially natural history [10]. Stunned and hibernating myocardium may coexist in the same patient. These states have in common preserved membrane integrity in the absence of normal contraction attributable to either sustained resting ischemia (hibernation) or transient, usually repetitive, ischemia (stunning). Traditionally, the success of revascularization in the presence of stunned or hibernating myocardium has focused on recovery of regional or global LV function. It is conceivable, however, that revascularization can improve outcome through other mechanisms, including improved diastolic performance, stabilization of the arrhythmic milieu, prevention of myocardial infarction, and attenuation of progressive remodeling [10]. Conversely, it is also conceivable that disruption of the homeostasis established in stunned or hibernating myocardium by opening a chronically stenosed or totally occluded vessel can predispose to an acute catastrophic insult were the target vessel to close abruptly. In a meta-analysis of studies involving more than 3000 patients, patients who had HF and evidence of viability who underwent revascularization had a significant reduction in mortality [11]. On the other hand, perioperative mortality is high when patients who have LV dysfunction undergo surgical revascularization in the absence of viable myocardium. The relationship between viability and outcome is not always straightforward, however. In the presence of viable myocardium, outcome is poor when extensive adverse remodeling has already taken place [12]. Ultimately, controlled prospective clinical trials will be required to answer these questions.

Recently an entity of reversible stress cardiomyopathy has been recognized and described in women, usually older women. In one series women ranged in age from 32 to 89 years with all but one woman over the age of 50 [13]. The initial presentation mimics an acute myocardial infarction with ballooning of the LV apex and sparing of the base of the heart. Extreme emotional or physical stress in the absence of significant coronary disease was the common thread linking the cases, with an acute catecholamine cardiomyopathy postulated as the pathophysiologic mechanism, related to a form of myocardial stunning. In some cases, coronary spasm may have been a contributing factor. The entity, when first recognized in Japan, was named "tako-tsubo" after the LV angiogram resembling an octopus trap. We alert the clinician to this entity because it can mimic closely the acute reversible HF more usually caused by obstructive coronary disease. Interventional techniques have no role in the treatment of this disorder.

The relatively new methodologies of cardiac magnetic resonance imaging (MRI) have proven particularly useful in characterizing the nature of the myocardial insult in these cases of stress stunning. Other widely established techniques for assessing myocardial viability with or without coronary disease include positron emission tomography (PET), myocardial perfusion imaging (MPI), and dobutamine stress echocardiography (DSE).

Positron emission tomography imaging

PET imaging of myocardial blood flow and glucose metabolism is considered to be a gold standard for viability detection. It can predict prognosis, improvement in regional and global ventricular function, and improvement of symptoms of HF. Uptake of [18]fluorodeoxyglucose ([18]FDG) reflects the distribution of glucose use. In fasting patients, normal myocardium uses fatty acids for energy production, whereas ischemic myocardium uses glucose. In the postprandial state, normal myocardium shifts from fatty acid to glucose use. Hibernating myocardium is characterized by an increased [18]FDG uptake compared with normal myocardium in the fasting state. The most commonly used PET protocol involves myocardial glucose metabolism with [18]FDG in conjunction with examination of myocardial blood flow with 13N-ammonia. Meta-analysis of the published data on predicting recovery of regional function after revascularization has suggested that this approach has slightly better overall accuracy than that of single-photon techniques [14]. The magnitude of improvement in HF symptoms after revascularization in patients who have LV dysfunction correlates with the preoperative extent of [18]FDG mismatch pattern (ie, preserved or diminished myocardial blood flow with enhanced or normal glucose metabolism). Moreover, long-term follow-up studies have suggested that the finding of PET mismatch in patients who have coronary artery disease (CAD) and LV dysfunction portends a high risk for cardiac death during medical therapy, whereas that risk is substantially lower after revascularization [15].

Stress-redistribution thallium-201 myocardial perfusion imaging

Normal thallium uptake has a good predictive value for the presence of viable myocardium [16]. The uptake of thallium-201 (Tl-201) is an energy-dependent process requiring intact cell membrane integrity and the presence of Tl-201 implies preserved myocyte cellular viability.

The redistribution properties of Tl-201 have been used as an important marker of myocardial viability in stress imaging followed by a 3- to 4-hour redistribution image. The presence of a reversible perfusion defect or preserved Tl-201 uptake on the 3- to 4-hour redistribution images is an important sign of regional viability. The absence of an important degree of redistribution or Tl-201 uptake on the redistribution images, however, is not a sufficient sign of the absence of regional viability, and iterations of Tl-201 protocols have been investigated to optimize the assessment of regional viability with this tracer. These involve Tl-201 reinjection and late redistribution imaging. In the former protocol, a second dose of Tl-201 is reinjected into the patient after the redistribution images are complete, and a third set of images is obtained 15 to 20 minutes later. It has been demonstrated that approximately 50% of regions with fixed defects on stress/redistribution imaging show significant enhancement of Tl-201 uptake after reinjection [16], and this finding is predictive of future improvement in regional LV function after revascularization. The presence of a severe Tl-201 defect after reinjection identifies areas with a low probability of improvement in function. Late redistribution imaging involves obtaining a third set of images 24 to 48 hours after the initial stress Tl-201 injection, essentially allowing more time for redistribution to occur.

Areas showing redistribution are likely viable, but the negative predictive value is suboptimal because of low Tl-201 blood levels, such that redistribution does not take place even after a prolonged time period. The late redistribution image also may be limited by suboptimal image quality because of continued washout and decay of the tracer. Rest-redistribution Tl-201 protocols also have been studied extensively. After tracer injection at rest, images are obtained 15 to 20 minutes later, which reflect regional blood flow at rest, and images obtained 3 to 4 hours later after redistribution generally reflect preserved viability. The finding of a reversible resting defect may identify areas of myocardial hibernation. Although insensitive for detection of viable myocardium, this is a specific sign of potential improvement in regional function [17].

Technetium 99m

Because the technetium 99m tracers do not redistribute, these agents were not believed well suited to assess myocardial viability. Sestamibi perfusion scans, however, may predict improvement in regional function after revascularization. Sestamibi is relatively overextracted at low blood flows, becoming more a tracer of cell membrane integrity than myocardial blood flow. Quantitative analysis of sestamibi uptake after resting injection provides similar information about myocardial viability as Tl-201. Assessment of sestamibi activity after injection with the administration of nitrates to improve resting blood flow further improves the ability of this tracer to detect myocardial viability. Assessment of wall motion using technetium 99m tracers may further enhance its usefulness as a viability marker [18].

Echocardiography

Contractile reserve is present in hibernating myocardium. Of the echocardiographic techniques, dobutamine stress echo has the largest evidence base supporting its usefulness in the decision to perform revascularization in HF. In patients who have multivessel CAD and depressed LV function, improvement in regional LV function during dobutamine stress echocardiography indicates contractile reserve and is predictive of improved ventricular function after revascularization [19]. The lack of contractile reserve during low-dose dobutamine infusion denotes a low likelihood of improvement after revascularization.

Magnetic resonance imaging

MRI techniques have been used to assess myocardial scar, coronary perfusion, and contractile reserve and are thus well suited to the determination of viability. After the administration of gadolinium-chelate, nonviable tissue appears bright (hyperenhancement). Lack of hyperenhancement in a region with a segmental wall motion abnormality is predictive of recovery after revascularization. Conversely, regional wall motion abnormalities associated with greater than 75% transmural hyperenhancement would not be expected to recover after revascularization. The expected response of segments with intermediate ranges of hyperenhancement (25% to 75%) is less clear, however [20]. The predictive value of dobutamine MRI and echocardiography for functional recovery after revascularization has been shown to be similar [21]. Diastolic wall thickness is a complementary MRI method of determining viability. There are limited prognostic data in patients who have myocardial viability assessed by MRI.

Summary and conclusions: interventional therapies for HF in patients who have coronary artery disease

To quote a recent editorial on the subject, "...there is an astonishing lack of convincing evidence" on whether revascularization improves long-term survival compared with medical therapy in patients who have HF [3]. Randomized controlled trials demonstrating a survival advantage from revascularization in the presence of LV dysfunction have included patients who have angina, not HF, as the dominant complaint. When such trials have been conducted, LV ejection fraction is usually only modestly depressed (eg, ejection fraction 30% to 40%). The Simplified Therapeutic Intervention to Control Hypertension (STITCH) trial is the first randomized controlled trial in more than 10 years to address this issue. Further, there are no randomized controlled trials assessing the role of viability testing in patients who have contractile dysfunction. The studies cited above demonstrating the usefulness of viability assessment for the prediction of outcomes have significant methodological limitations. The STITCH trialists point to selection bias for patients sent for revascularization as the major limitation of all these reports. This bias currently is interfering with the STITCH trial investigators' recruitment of patients into strata in which randomization into the medical treatment arm is possible [3].

Clearly, interventional techniques to maintain sustained vessel patency have greatly improved. Diseased vein grafts and totally occluded vessels are now targets for stent therapy in patients who have LV dysfunction [22]. Medical therapy also has evolved greatly in recent years with demonstrated benefit from beta blockade, angiotensin converting enzyme inhibitor, angiotensin receptor blocker, and Aldactone blockade [23]. Biventricular pacemakers improve LV performance, functional capacity and survival [24]. Implantable defibrillators significantly improve survival [25]. Elderly patients who have coronary disease have access to a wealth of new and effective treatments for HF or systolic LV. Whether interventional therapies will prove superior to medical therapy, biventricular pacing, or implantable defibrillator techniques remains to be determined.

Heart failure in patients who have valvular disease

Valvular heart disease is a common cause of HF in the elderly. Interventional therapies have been developed for the mechanical relief of aortic and mitral valvular obstruction, whereas surgery remains the mainstay for severe valvular regurgitation. Although balloon aortic valvuloplasty (BAV) has limited application in the management of aortic stenosis in the elderly because of frequent restenosis in the first year after successful dilatation, balloon mitral valvuloplasty increasingly has been considered the therapy of choice for patients who have severely symptomatic mitral stenosis. More recently, percutaneous interventional approaches to treat mitral regurgitation and aortic valve disease have been developed and are under investigation as alternatives to surgery.

Aortic stenosis and aortic valve replacement in the elderly

Calcific degenerative aortic stenosis is the most common valvular lesion requiring surgery among elderly patients, accounting for more than 90% of aortic valve replacements (AVR) in patients over age 75. Although the classic symptoms of aortic stenosis are angina, HF, and syncope, the most common initial symptom in the elderly is impaired exercise tolerance [26]. The elderly patient who has symptoms of HF or exercise intolerance and a systolic murmur requires a careful clinical assessment to exclude significant aortic stenosis. A two-dimensional echocardiogram and Doppler are valuable for confirming the presence of calcific stenosis with diminished leaflet excursion, assessing the LV response to pressure overload, and determining the severity as assessed by transvalvular pressure gradient. A well-performed echocardiogram also should exclude other causes of a pressure gradient, including hypertrophic obstructive cardiomyopathy and hypertension-related hypertrophic heart disease. Cardiac catheterization is indicated to confirm or clarify the severity of aortic stenosis, document that the pressure gradient is indeed valvular and not subvalvular, and assess the coronary circulation in patients being considered for surgical intervention.

Because there is no effective medical treatment for severe aortic stenosis, valve replacement must be considered in all symptomatic elderly patients. Advanced age constitutes a surgical risk likely attributable to a greater prevalence of comorbid conditions. The morbid effects of age are extremely variable, however, and an individualized evaluation of each patient is required. The decision to intervene surgically on an elderly patient must take into account three factors:

- Whether the valvular lesion has important hemodynamic consequences
- Whether the symptoms are a product of the lesion and not of concomitant disease
- Whether there are comorbid conditions whose symptoms and prognosis are worse than the valve lesion itself.

The psychologic state of patients and family members is also a factor to be considered. Once a decision is made to proceed with AVR, bioprosthetic valves are most often favored to decrease bleeding risk associated with prolonged Coumadin therapy in this high-risk population. Severe valve calcification may necessitate a mechanical valve, however. Importantly, among elderly patients, freedom from reoperation seems similar for mechanical and biologic valves at 12 to 15 years [27].

Operating on octogenarians has become increasingly commonplace, and for patients who have no other concomitant medical problems the decision to offer surgery is usually straightforward. Published series suggest a surgical mortality in octogenarians of approximately 5% to 10% for isolated AVR and of approximately 10% to 20% for AVR combined with CABG [28–30]. It is likely that there is some selection bias toward more healthy patients in these published series. In addition to death, major morbidity, such as stroke and prolonged ventilatory support, occurs in approximately 5% to 10% of octogenarians undergoing these procedures [29,30]. Long-term survival after AVR for aortic stenosis is excellent with 1-, 3-, and 5-year survival rates of 91%, 84%, and 76%, respectively, in selected patients over age 80 [28]. In fact, the long-term survival following successful AVR in one surgical series compared favorably with unselected healthy 80-year-old people [31]. In a more recent series, survival was similar to the age- and sex-matched population [32]. Moreover, almost all survivors after AVR had improved functional class and relief of HF symptoms [33,34].

Alternatives to aortic valve replacement

Percutaneous BAV has been proposed as a therapeutic option in adults who have severe symptomatic aortic stenosis, especially those who have a high surgical risk because of comorbid conditions or advanced age. BAV is a procedure in which one or more balloons are placed across a stenotic aortic valve and inflated under high pressure to decrease the severity of aortic stenosis [35–40]. The mechanism underlying relief of the stenotic

lesion in older patients is fracture of calcific deposits within the valve leaflets, and to some degree stretching of the annulus and separation of the
fused or calcified commissures [41]. Immediate hemodynamic effects include
a 30% to 50% reduction in the transvalvular aortic pressure gradient, but
the postprocedure aortic valve area frequently ranges from 0.7 to 1 cm^2,
representing substantial residual outflow obstruction [42]. Somewhat higher
efficacy is seen with an antegrade Inoue balloon approach, with postprocedure aortic valve areas of 1.2 to 1.4 cm^2, but the technique is more challenging, requiring puncture of the interatrial septum [43]. Although the absolute
increases in aortic valve areas are generally only 0.2 to 0.4 cm^2, most patients report symptomatic improvement, because a small increase in valve
area may be sufficient to alter the loading conditions of the LV, improve cardiac output, and alleviate symptoms. Most patients report clinical improvement for 12 to 18 months. The in-hospital complication rate of BAV is 30%
with a procedural mortality rate of 3% and in-hospital mortality as high as
8% [44]. The 30-day mortality is substantial at 14% [45,46]. Restenosis with
clinical deterioration occurs within several months in most patients, such
that long-term survival after successful BAV is poor, with 1- and 3-year survival rates of only 55% and 23% (Fig. 1) [46]. This observed mortality rate
is similar to that reported for unoperated patients who have symptomatic
severe aortic stenosis, demonstrating a lack of survival benefit for the procedure [47–49]. In contrast, a subgroup of patients referred for AVR after
a recurrence of symptoms following BAV had a 1-year survival of about
80% [45]. Although statin therapy has shown some usefulness in slowing
the progression of calcific aortic stenosis, any effect on restenosis after
BAV remains to be seen [50].

    Despite the procedural morbidity, mortality, and limited long-term effi-
cacy, BAV can have a temporary role in the management of some elderly

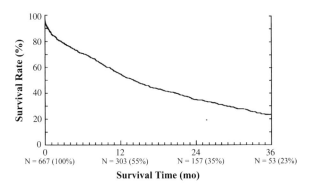

Fig. 1. Survival after balloon aortic valvuloplasty in the entire study population (n = 674), cen-
sored at the time of aortic valve surgery. (*Adapted from* Otto CM, Mickel MC, Kennedy JW,
et al. Three year outcome after balloon aortic valvuloplasty. Circulation 1994;89:642–50;
with permission.)

patients who have symptomatic aortic stenosis who are not candidates for AVR. BAV may be considered as a bridge to AVR in patients who have cardiogenic shock and medically refractory pulmonary edema caused by critical aortic stenosis who are felt to be too ill to undergo surgery [51,52]. A typical patient is someone in the coronary care unit, intubated, with refractory HF from critical outflow obstruction, a low systemic arterial pressure despite vasopressors, and low urine output with elevated filling pressures on pulmonary capillary wedge pressure monitoring. Emergent AVR in this setting has prohibitive risks. The transient improvement in hemodynamics provided by BAV may improve the patient's clinical condition sufficiently to allow urgent AVR to be undertaken with less risk. Although probably the most common use of BAV in clinical practice, there are few indications for palliative BAV in nonoperable symptomatic patients; most patients can expect a temporary relief of symptoms with a limited life expectancy. Because of the high procedural risks and short-lived results, medical therapy should be optimized first for relief of symptoms. If HF symptoms remain refractory, palliative BAV may be considered. In such patients, repeat aortic valvuloplasty is sometimes feasible and may improve short-term survival [53]. BAV also may be considered in patients before urgent noncardiac surgery, to reduce perioperative risk [54]. A final group that may benefit from BAV is HF patients who have low gradient and low cardiac output aortic stenosis. Although no studies have validated this approach, BAV may be used as a diagnostic test to determine whether ventricular function and hemodynamics improve after AVR, which can be undertaken thereafter at lower risk [44].

Recently, a percutaneous approach to aortic valve replacement has been described [55]. In contrast to BAV, replacement addresses aortic insufficiency in addition to aortic stenosis. The percutaneous valve is crimped over a balloon and inflated after careful positioning across the aortic valve by way of a transseptal antegrade approach. Although fewer than a dozen patients have undergone the procedure to date, early results show feasibility with an increase in aortic valve area from 0.5 to 1.7 cm^2 and a decrease in pressure gradient from 44 to 5 mm Hg [56]. Significant improvements in systolic function also have been shown [57]. Early complications in this high-risk, inoperable group have included death, aortic insufficiency, and mitral regurgitation, but the technique shows promise as an alternative to AVR in severely symptomatic patients [56].

Percutaneous balloon mitral valvuloplasty for mitral stenosis

Rheumatic heart disease, the predominant cause of mitral stenosis, usually is acquired before the age of 20 and becomes clinically apparent in most cases in the third, fourth, and fifth decades of life. Inasmuch as rheumatic disease frequently permits survival to old age, mitral stenosis should be considered in the elderly patient who has HF symptoms. Once a patient who has mitral stenosis develops limiting HF symptoms, clinical deterioration is frequently rapid. Percutaneous balloon mitral valvuloplasty (PBMV) has been developed for the mechanical relief of mitral valve obstruction caused by mitral stenosis [58,59]. Compared with BAV, PBMV is associated with less frequent restenosis during the first year and better long-term outcomes. In fact, PBMV is considered the treatment of choice for many patients who have mitral stenosis [60]. PBMV usually is accomplished by interatrial transseptal puncture to gain access to the mitral valve from the left atrium. A balloon catheter is inserted into the femoral vein, passed from the right into the left atrium, and guided across the mitral valve. The balloon is then rapidly inflated and deflated to cause an increase in the area of the mitral valve orifice. The mechanisms involved appear to be commissural splitting, fracture of calcified leaflets, and partial valve disruption, similar to surgical commissurotomy. Both procedures provide excellent results and are associated with low risk in patients who have mobile, pliable, minimally thickened, and only mildly calcified valves. A randomized comparison of PBMV and surgical commissurotomy demonstrated equivalent acute and long-term results [60,61]. Within several minutes of final balloon deflation the immediate hemodynamic results are apparent (Fig. 2). The left atrial pressure falls; the transmitral pressure gradient is decreased; cardiac output increases; and the valve area increases substantially, typically from approximately 1 cm^2 to 1.8 to 2 cm^2 [62]. If blood loss during the procedure is substantial, cardiac output may fall until blood volume is restored. Patients often note a sense of relief of shortness of breath while still on the catheterization table. The major complications of PBMV include death, systemic embolization, severe mitral regurgitation, and cardiac tamponade [63]. Hospital mortality generally is reported as 1% to 3%. Stroke and cardiac tamponade occur in 1% to 2% of cases. The long-term results after PBMV have been excellent in younger patients who have mitral stenosis, who typically have very pliable mitral valve leaflets and mainly commissural fusion. The overall 5-year event-free survival is greater than 70%. Restenosis following successful PBMV occurs in approximately 30% of patients

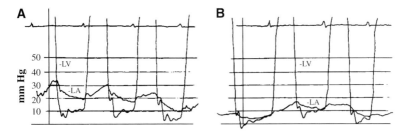

Fig. 2. Left ventricular (LV) and left atrial (LA) pressure tracings before (A) and after (B) percutaneous mitral valvuloplasty. Mitral valve gradient (mm Hg): before, 9; after, 2. Mitral valve area (cm^2): before, 0.7; after, 1.4. Cardiac output (Fick, liter/min): before, 2.9; after, 2.4. Pulmonary artery pressure (mm Hg): before, 38/22 (27); after, 30/15 (22). Left atrial pressure (mm Hg): before, 20; after, 10.

during the first 10 years following the procedure. Patients who have very deformed valves, including the elderly, who in the past would have undergone mitral valve replacement instead of commissurotomy, have displayed more variable acute and chronic results following PBMV [64].

Before consideration of PBMV, two-dimensional echocardiography with Doppler is essential for patient screening. The degree of mitral stenosis, the presence of associated valvular lesions, and the extent of mitral regurgitation are assessed. Anatomic evaluation of the mitral valve, including the extent of commissural fusion, leaflet deformity, leaflet calcification, and involvement of the subvalvular apparatus, allows prediction of the likelihood of a successful and durable result from commissurotomy with PBMV. One semiquantitative system of describing the rheumatic mitral valve assigns a value of 0 to 4 for the degree of leaflet rigidity, thickening, calcification, and subvalvular thickening. High scores indicate more severe rheumatic valvular disease, with a maximum score of 16 [65]. In general, echocardiographic valve scores less than 8 indicate that the patient will have a good response to PBMV, whereas scores greater than 8 indicate less likelihood of success (defined as a postprocedural valve area greater than 1.5 cm^2 or significant worsening of mitral regurgitation). Transesophageal echocardiography (TEE) is also imperative before PBMV to screen for left atrial thrombus, often seen in patients who have severe left atrial dilation or atrial fibrillation. Thrombus in the left atrium is a contraindication to PBMV because of the risk for dislodgement and stroke with catheter manipulation in the left atrium. If present in a patient not chronically anticoagulated, a several-months course of anticoagulation may be tried. If thrombus has resolved on a repeat TEE, PBMV may be performed safely. The presence of significant mitral regurgitation contraindicates PBMV because of the likelihood of deterioration following commissural splitting.

Initial multicenter registries for the evaluation of PBMV generally did not include patients who had severely diseased mitral valves [66]. As operator experience with this technique increased, patient selection for PBMV broadened to include those who had less ideal valves (ie, higher echocardiography scores). Increasingly, older patients who had severe symptomatic mitral stenosis and more advanced rheumatic valvular changes underwent PBMV as an alternative to surgical valve replacement. In one series, patients older than 65 had a success rate of approximately 50% with PBMV compared with the well-reported 90% to 95% success rates in younger patients [67]. More recent series have duplicated this finding, with procedural success of only 53% in those over age 75 [68]. Moreover, increasing age was a risk factor for long-term events. Seventy-five percent of these older patients, however, still had at least a 50% absolute increase in mitral valve area following balloon dilatation. Intermediate follow-up has been favorable with a 3-year survival rate of 80% and 60% of patients in New York Heart Association (NYHA) functional classes I and II following PBMV [67]. Even among patients who have severely diseased valves in which PBMV does not result in mitral valve areas greater than or equal to 1.5 cm^2, many patients still experience clinical improvement (Fig. 3). It must be noted, however, that no randomized comparisons have been made between valve replacement surgery and PBMV in patients who are not well suited by traditional echocardiography criteria for balloon commissurotomy.

Elderly patients who have severe mitral stenosis and who are not suitable candidates for PBMV based on valvular morphology (ie, very high echocardiogram scores, left atrial thrombus, significant mitral regurgitation) or other factors (eg, coexistent severe coronary disease) are usually referred for surgical mitral valve replacement (MVR). Unlike the results following AVR for severe aortic stenosis in the elderly, however, which has an acceptably low mortality rate, surgical mortality for MVR is much higher. Operative mortality rates in selected elderly patients have been reported as approximately 10% to 15%, but the risk increases significantly with LV dysfunction, advanced age, pulmonary hypertension, and other comorbidities [69]. PBMV may be offered to some symptomatic elderly patients as a palliative measure when the risk of MVR is prohibitively high. A clinical profile of such a patient is a frail but functional 80-year-old woman who has NYHA class III symptoms from isolated mitral stenosis, a mitral valve area of 0.8 cm^2, moderate to severe pulmonary hypertension, minimal mitral regurgitation, a very diseased valve evidenced by an echocardiography score of 11, and the absence of left atrial clot on TEE. The surgical mortality risk may be 15% to 20% or higher. PBMV usually increases the mitral valve

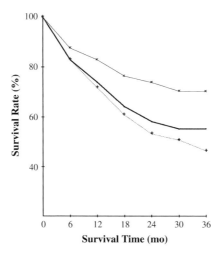

Fig. 3. Acuarial survival (*narrow solid line*), survival with freedom from mitral valve replacement (*heavy solid line*), and survival with freedom from mitral valve replacement and New York Heart Association functional class III or IV (*dotted line*) in 99 patients 65 years of age or more undergoing percutaneous balloon mitral valvuloplasty. (*Adapted from* Tuzcu EM, Block PC, Griffin BP, et al. Immediate and long-term outcome of percutaneous mitral valvulotomy in patients 65 years and older. Circulation 1992;85:963–71; with permission.)

area by at least 50% with an acceptably low procedural risk in such elderly patients, supporting this approach.

In summary, the management strategy for an older patient who has symptomatic mitral stenosis and class III to IV HF is best made on an individual basis. Patients who have symptomatic mitral stenosis, favorable valve morphology, and no contraindications are best served with PBMV. Surgical treatment is a better option for symptomatic patients who have advanced rheumatic disease. If the surgical risk is prohibitively high because of other comorbidities, PBMV may be a form of palliation with acceptable early and intermediate-term results.

Percutaneous mitral valve repair for mitral regurgitation

Among elderly patients, mitral regurgitation is most commonly attributable to myxomatous degeneration with resultant prolapse, severe mitral annular calcification, or papillary muscle dysfunction from myocardial ischemia or infarction [70,71]. Surgery is recommended for those who have moderate to severe (3+) or severe (4+) regurgitation. In addition, surgery is recommended when secondary effects of chronic mitral regurgitation are seen, such as LV dysfunction and dilation, atrial fibrillation, or pulmonary hypertension, regardless of symptom status [72].

Whenever possible, the favored surgical technique for mitral regurgitation is a repair procedure [73,74]. In a series of elderly patients, in-hospital and 5-year mortality were significantly reduced with mitral repair versus replacement [75]. Recently, a percutaneous approach to mitral repair has been devised, based on the edge-to-edge repair technique of Alfieri [76]. The Alfieri approach apposes the middle scallops of the anterior and posterior leaflets to create a "double-orifice" mitral valve. This approach typically reduces the degree of regurgitation without producing significant stenosis [76,77]. Using a transseptal approach to gain access to the mitral valve, the percutaneous approach involves precise positioning and deployment of a clip to hold together the anterior and posterior leaflets. Results of the Phase I safety and feasibility study were reported recently. Successful edge-to-edge coaptation could be performed in all 27 patients, with full deployment in 24. In 67%, mitral regurgitation was reduced to 2+ or less [78]. Although still experimental, this approach may ultimately prove beneficial in elderly patients who have multiple comorbidities, in whom surgery carries prohibitive risk.

Heart failure in patients who have renal artery stenosis

HF has been reported as a complication of renal artery stenosis [79]. In a study of elderly patients who had HF in the United Kingdom, 86 patients (mean age 77.5 years) were screened for renovascular disease. Magnetic resonance angiography showed severe renovascular disease (> 50% renal artery stenosis) in 34% of patients; one quarter of these had bilateral disease. Predictors of renal artery stenosis were advanced age, peripheral vascular disease, and impaired renal function. Complications of renal artery stenosis, such as HF and hypertension, appear most often with bilateral involvement. Indeed, among 90 consecutive patients who had renovascular disease who were treated with percutaneous renal artery stent placement, 41% of patients who had bilateral renal artery stenosis had a history of HF before stent placement, compared with only 12% of subjects who had unilateral stenosis [80]. In patients who had prior HF, 77% of those who had bilateral stenosis were free of HF after stent placement, compared with only 33% of patients who had unilateral stenosis after a mean follow-up of 18.4 months. The subjects who had bilateral stenosis who had recurrent HF had evidence of stent restenosis. The authors concluded that bilateral but not unilateral renal artery stenosis is associated with HF, and that stent placement can lower the risk. Another study randomized 55 patients who had refractory hypertension to continued medical therapy or renal artery stenting. Blood pressure was reduced only in stented patients who had bilateral renal artery stenosis [81]. Major outcome events, including HF, were similar in the medical and angioplasty groups, however, raising concern over the benefits of renal artery stenting even in bilateral disease. In this limited series, intervention was accompanied by a significant complication rate, without clear clinical benefit. Khosla and colleagues [82] studied 120 elderly patients who underwent renal artery stenting for refractory hypertension. At baseline, 28 patients had HF (mean age 67 years) and 43% of patients who had HF also had unstable angina. Six patients who had HF underwent coronary intervention in addition to renal artery stenting. Most patients who had HF had bilateral renal artery stenosis. Five of 28 patients who had HF died during follow-up, but most surviving patients were reported to have sustained clinical improvement in functional status. Most recently, Gray and coworkers [83] reported on 39 patients undergoing renal artery stenting for the control of recurrent or refractory HF. All patients had evidence of bilateral disease or disease to a solitary functioning kidney. After renal artery stenting, the mean NYHA functional class decreased from 2.9 to 1.6, and the mean number of HF hospitalizations was reduced from 2.4 in the year preceding intervention to 0.3 in the year following intervention. Thirty of 39 patients (77%) had no HF hospitalizations for a mean follow-up period of 21 months. Although select patients who have bilateral renal artery stenosis and HF benefit from bilateral renal artery stenting, the data remain too preliminary and varied to recommend widespread screening for renal artery stenosis in the elderly patient who has HF.

Heart failure in patients who have hypertrophic cardiomyopathy

Hypertrophic cardiomyopathy occurs in approximately 1 of 500 individuals, making it the most common genetic cardiac disorder [84]. It is relatively unique in that the disease may manifest clinically at any age, or not at all. The most severe symptoms often are found in those who have the ob-structive form of the disease, representing up to 25% of cases [85]. The com-bination of subaortic obstruction, mitral regurgitation attributable to systolic anterior motion of the mitral valve, and severe hypertrophy, results in the typical symptoms of dyspnea on exertion, chest pain, or syncope. If left untreated, patients may present later in life with classic signs of HF.

Treatment of hypertrophic obstructive cardiomyopathy involves negative inotropic medications that improve ventricular relaxation and increase pre-load, thereby reducing the propensity to intracavitary obstruction. These most typically include nondihydropyridine calcium channel blockers and beta-blockers. When medication fails to relieve symptoms, proven alterna-tives include surgical myectomy and percutaneous alcohol septal ablation.

Surgical myectomy has been the gold standard invasive treatment since the 1960s with good long-term success. Elderly patients, those with concom-itant medical conditions, and those who have undergone prior cardiac sur-gery might not be considered favorable candidates, however [86]. In these patients, alcohol septal ablation may be considered. The technique uses standard angioplasty equipment to selectively infuse a small amount of ab-solute alcohol into the septal perforator that perfuses the area of the septum where obstruction to outflow occurs. This area may be localized by trans-thoracic echocardiographic guidance during the procedure with improved outcome [87]. Approximately 5% to 10% of the myocardium is necrosed, resulting in an immediate fall in outflow tract gradient in 90% of selected patients [88]. Acute reduction in the gradient is attributable to an immediate decrease in septal contraction that reduces subaortic narrowing during systole [89]. Over the ensuing 1 to 2 years, gradients typically reduce further because of scar contraction of the necrosed area, regression of global ventricular hypertrophy, a decrease in interstitial collagen, and improved di-astolic function (Fig. 4) [90,91].

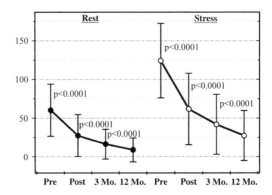

Fig. 4. Acute and chronic effects of alcohol septal ablation on resting and provocable gradients (*Adapted from* Seggewiss H. Medical therapy versus interventional therapy in hypertrophic ob-structive cardiomyopathy. Curr Control Trials Cardiovasc Med 2000;1:115; with permission.)

Although no randomized trials exist to date, it seems that surgical myec-tomy and alcohol septal ablation produce similar results, at least over the intermediate term [92,93]. Although younger patients may be better treated with septal myectomy, older patients and those who have comorbidities may be better candidates for alcohol septal ablation. In addition, patients who have recurrence of symptoms after surgical myectomy may still benefit from the percutaneous approach [94].

Heart failure in patients who have atrial septal defect

Large atrial septal defects, defined by a pulmonary to systemic flow ratio of greater than 1.5:1, typically manifest in the second decade of life. If un-diagnosed or left untreated, patients develop progressive symptoms, includ-ing a decline in exercise tolerance or overt HF, in the later decades. Symptoms of orthodeoxia and platypnea can occur in the late stage, culmi-nating in true Eisenmenger physiology in extreme cases.

Because of the propensity to progressive clinical deterioration, closure of an atrial septal defect is recommended when the flow ratio exceeds 1.5:1, re-gardless of symptom status [95]. Corroborating evidence for hemodynamic significance includes right ventricular and right atrial volume overload or the presence of pulmonary hypertension. In such patients, closure is recom-mended at any age. Severe pulmonary hypertension with pulmonary vas-cular resistance greater than 7 Woods Units, or the development of Eisenmenger physiology with reversal of flow across the atrial septal defect, are generally considered contraindications to closure, but fortunately occur only in the minority of cases [96].

Currently, percutaneous closure of atrial septal defects is possible only for ostium secundum defects. Other defects, such as ostium primum or sinus ve-nosus defects, generally require surgical correction because of their proximity to important structures or the presence of other anomalies that warrant sur-gical correction. The device consists of a tightly woven nitinol mesh that is shaped into two flat disks with an intervening waist that traverses the septum. Various sizes are available, from 4 to 40 mm, depending on the size of the de-fect [97]. Transesophageal echocardiogram is necessary before the procedure to delineate the anatomy and confirm the absence of atrial thrombus. The procedure involves a delivery system that crosses the septum from the right atrial side, using a femoral venous approach. Intracardiac echocardiographic guidance is used to position the device properly before its release.

Results using the Amplatzer closure device have been excellent, with 96% procedural success and significantly less morbidity than traditional surgical closure. In one study comparing percutaneous versus surgical closure in 442 patients, the complication rate was significantly less (7.2% versus 24.0%), and mean length of hospital stay significantly lower (1.0 versus 3.4 days) in patients undergoing a percutaneous approach, with no mortality in either group [98]. Particularly relevant to the elderly who have advanced disease,

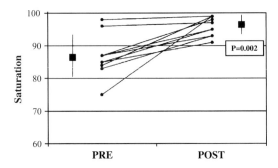

Fig. 5. Improvement in arterial oxygen saturation before and after percutaneous atrial septal defect closure in patients who have systemic hypoxemia. (*Adapted from* Ilkhanoff, L, Naidu SS, Rohatgi S, et al. Transcatheter device closure of interatrial septal defects in patients who have hypoxia. J Interven Cardiol 2005;18:227; with permission.)

a recent study evaluated percutaneous closure in late-stage patients who had HF, platypnea–orthodeoxia syndrome, and resultant systemic hypoxemia. Percutaneous closure was safe and improved systemic arterial saturation from a mean preprocedure value of 86.7% to postprocedure value of 95.9% (Fig. 5) [99]. Patients tolerated the procedure well without clinical deterioration.

Summary

Coronary artery bypass surgery is the treatment of choice for elderly patients who have HF who have predominant angina and multivessel or left main coronary disease. In patients who do not have angina, aggressive medical therapy remains the preferred treatment. Revascularization probably improves outcomes when a sufficient mass of viable myocardium is supplied by stenosed coronary arteries that are suitable for revascularization. The likelihood for recovery of ventricular function and improvement of symptoms increases when there is substantial dysfunctional myocardium caused by ischemia (eg, >15% to 20% of the left ventricle), particularly if the left anterior descending coronary artery territory is involved. Both PCI and surgical risk increase with increasing age, worsening LV dysfunction, and the presence of clinical HF. Until direct comparative data are available for PCI and CABG, the technique that produces the most complete, enduring revascularization should be the procedure of choice when medical therapy has failed; however, some patients may be better suited for PCI based on comorbidities. Consideration also must be given to the implications of ventricular resynchronization or defibrillation therapy when deciding on the merits of medical therapy versus catheter or surgical revascularization for HF in patients who have ischemic cardiomyopathy.

For elderly patients who have HF caused by valvular stenosis, BAV can be used as a bridge to valve replacement surgery, whereas PBMV can stand alone as definitive therapy in select patients. Newer techniques, including percutaneous aortic valve replacement and mitral valve repair, may prove beneficial in select patients. In elderly patients who have HF, especially those who have refractory hypertension, renal insufficiency, or repeated bouts of flash pulmonary edema, consideration should be given to the possibility of bilateral renal artery stenosis. Renal artery stenting is a promising interventional technique, but further investigation is required before its routine application can be recommended. Hypertrophic cardiomyopathy and untreated atrial septal defects are rare causes of HF in elderly patients that can now be treated percutaneously, particularly when medical therapy fails to relieve symptoms.

References

[1] Thom T, Haase N, Rosamond W, et al. Heart disease and stroke statistics—2006 update: a report from the American Heart Association Statistics Committee and Stroke Statistics Subcommittee. Circulation 2006;113:e85–151.
[2] Alderman EL, Fisher LD, Litwin P, et al. Results of coronary artery surgery in patients with poor left ventricular function (CASS). Circulation 1983;68:785.
[3] Doenst T, Velazquez EJ, Beversdorf F, et al. To STICH or not to STICH: we know the answer, but do we understand the question? J Thorac Cardiovasc Surg 2005;129:246–9.
[4] Yusuf S, Zucker D, Peduzzi P, et al. Effect of coronary artery bypass graft surgery on survival: overview of 10-year results from randomized trials by the Coronary Artery Bypass Surgery Trialists Collaboration. Lancet 1994;344:563–70.
[5] Hampton JR. Coronary artery bypass grafting for the reduction of mortality: an analysis of the trials. BMJ 1984;289:1166–70.
[6] New York State Department of Health. Percutaneous coronary interventions in New York State 2001–2003. New York State Department of Health. 2005.
[7] Hannan EL, Racz M, Holmes DR, et al. Impact of completeness of percutaneous coronary intervention revascularization on long-term outcomes in the stent era. Circulation 2006;113: 2406–12.
[8] Smith Sc, Jr, Feldman TE, Hirshfield JW, Jr, et al. ACC/AHA/SCAI 2005 guideline update for percutaneous coronary intervention: a report of the American College of Cardiology/ American Heart Association Task Force on Practice Guidelines (ACC/AHA/SCAI Writing committee to update the 2001 guidelines for percutaneous intervention). American College of Cardiology. Available at: http://www.acc.org/clinical/guidelines/percutaneous/update/index.pdf.
[9] Rahimtoola S. Importance of diagnosing hibernating myocardium: how and in whom. J Am Coll Cardiol 1997;30:1701.
[10] Klocke FJ, Gaird MG, Bateman TM, et al. ACC/AHA/ASNC guidelines for the clinical use of cardiac radionuclide imaging. Available at: http://www.acc.org/clinical/guidelines/radio/rni/fultext.pdf.
[11] Allman KC, Shaw LJ, Hachamovitch R, Udelson JE. Myocardial viability testing and impact of revascularization on prognosis in patients with coronary artery disease and left ventricular dysfunction: a meta-analysis. J Am Coll Cardiol 2002;39:1151–8.
[12] Di Carli MF, Asgarzadie F, Schelbert HR, et al. Quantitative relation between myocardial viability and improvement in heart failure symptoms after revascularization in patients with ischemic cardiomyopathy. Circulation 1995;92:3436–44.
[13] Sharkey SW, Lesser JR, Zenovich AG, et al. Acute and reversible cardiomyopathy provoked by stress in women from the United States. Circulation 2005;111:472–9.
[14] Bax JJ, Wijns W, Cornel JH, et al. Accuracy of currently available techniques for prediction of functional recovery after revascularization in patients with left ventricular dysfunction

due to chronic coronary artery disease: comparison of pooled data. J Am Coll Cardiol 1997;
30:1451–60.

[15] Di Carli MF, Davidson M, Little R, et al. Value of metabolic imaging with positron emission tomography for evaluating prognosis in patients with coronary artery disease and left ventricular dysfunction. Am J Cardiol 1994;73:527–33.

[16] Dilsizian V, Rocco TP, Freedman NM, et al. Enhanced detection of ischemic but viable myocardium by the reinjection of thallium after stress-redistribution imaging. N Engl J Med 1990;323:141–6.

[17] Mori T, Minamiji K, Kurogane H, et al. Rest-injected thallium-201 imaging for assessing viability of severe asynergic regions. J Nucl Med 1991;32:1718–24.

[18] Maurea S, Cuocolo A, Soricelli A, et al. Enhanced detection of viable myocardium by technetium-99m-MIBI imaging after nitrate administration in chronic coronary artery disease. J Nucl Med 1995;36:1945–52.

[19] Cheitlin MD, Armstrong WF, Aurigemma GP, et al. ACC/AHA/ASE 2003 guideline update for the clinical application of echocardiography: a report of the American College of Cardiology/American Heart Association Task Force on Practice Guidelines (ACC/AHA/ASE Committee to Update the 1997 Guidelines for the Clinical Application of Echocardiography). 2003. American College of Cardiology Web Site. Available at: www.acc.org/clinical/guidelines/echo/index.pdf.

[20] Shan K, Godwin C, Sivananthan M, et al. Role of cardiac magnetic resonance imaging in the assessment of myocardial viability. Circulation 2004;109:1328–34.

[21] Baer FM, Theissen P, Crnac J, et al. Head to head comparison of dobutamine-transoesophageal echocardiography and dobutaminemagnetic resonance imaging for the prediction of left ventricular functional recovery in patients with chronic coronary artery disease. Eur Heart J 2000;21:981–91.

[22] Serruys PW, Kutryk MJB, Ong ATL. Drug therapy. Coronary artery stents. N Engl J Med 2006;354:483–95.

[23] Jessup M, Brozena S. Medical progress: heart failure. N Engl J Med 2003;348:2007–18.

[24] Turer AT, Rao SV. Device therapy in the management of congestive heart failure. Cardiol Rev 2005;13:130–8.

[25] Goldberger Z, Lampert R. Implantable cardioverter-defibrillators. expanding indications and technologies. JAMA 2006;295:809–81.

[26] Otto CM, Bunwash IG, Legget ME, et al. A prospective study of asymptomatic valvular AS: clinical, echocardiographic and exercise predictors of outcome. Circulation 1997;95:2262.

[27] Prasongsukarn K, Jamieson WR, Lichtenstein SV. Performance of bioprostheses and mechanical prostheses in age group 61–70 years. J Heart Valve Dis 2005;14(4):501–8.

[28] Elayda MA, Hall RJ, Reul RM, et al. Aortic valve replacement in patients 80 years and older: operative risk and long term results. Circulation 1993;88:II11.

[29] Zaidi AM, Fitzpatrick AP, Keenan DJ, et al. Good outcomes from cardiac surgery in patients over the age of 70. Heart 1999;82:134.

[30] Collart F, Feier H, Kerbaul F, et al. Primary valvular surgery in octogenarians: perioperative outcome. J Heart Valve Dis 2005;14(2):238–42.

[31] Levinson JR, Akins CW, Buckley MJ, et al. Octogenarians with aortic stenosis: outcome after aortic valve replacement. Circulation 1989;80(suppl 1):I-49.

[32] Wasywich CA, Ruygrok PN, West TM, et al. Extended follow up after isolated aortic valve replacement in the elderly. Heart Lung Circ 2003;12(2):103–7.

[33] Gehlot A, Mullany CJ, Ilstrup D, et al. Aortic valve replacement in patients aged eighty years and older: early and long-term results. J Thorac Cardiovasc Surg 1996;111(5):1026–36.

[34] Salazar E, Torres J, Barragan R, et al. Aortic valve replacement in patients 70 years and older. Clin Cardiol 2004;27(10):565–70.

[35] Block PC, Palacios IF. Clinical and hemodynamic follow-up after percutaneous aortic valvuloplasty in the elderly. Am J Cardiol 1988;62:760.

[36] Letac B, Cribier A, Koning R, et al. Results of percutaneous transluminal valvuloplasty in 218 patients with valvular aortic stenosis. Am J Cardiol 1988;6:598.
[37] McKay RG. The Mansfield Scientific Aortic Registry. Overview of acute hemodynamic results and procedural complications. J Am Coll Cardiol 1991;17:485.
[38] Balloon Valvuloplasty Participants NHLBI. Percutaneous balloon aortic valvuloplasty: Acute and 30 day follow-up in 674 patients from the NHLBI Balloon Valvuloplasty Registry. Circulation 1991;84:2383.
[39] Nishimura RA, Holmes DR, Reeder GS, et al. Doppler evaluation of results of percutaneous aortic balloon valvuloplasty in calcific aortic stenosis. Circulation 1988;78:791.
[40] Rahimtoola SH. Catheter balloon valvuloplasty for severe calcific aortic stenosis: A limited role. J Am Coll Cardiol 1994;23:1076.
[41] Safian RD, Mandell VS, Thuren RE, et al. Postmortem intra-operative balloon valvuloplasty of calcific aortic stenosis in older patients: mechanisms of successful dilation. J Am Coll Cardiol 1987;9:655.
[42] Cribier A, Savin T, Rocha P, et al. Percutaneous transluminal valvuloplasty of acquired aortic stenosis in elderly pateitnes: An alternative to valve replacement? Lancet 1986; 11:63.
[43] Sakata Y, Syed Z, Salinger MH, et al. Percutaneous balloon aortic valvuloplasty: antegrade transseptal vs. conventional retrograde transarterial approach. Catheter Cardiovasc Interv 2005;64(3):314–21.
[44] Feldman TE, Sanborn TA, O'Neill WW. Balloon aortic and pulmonic valvuloplasty. In: Herrmann HC, editor. Interventional cardiology: percutaneous non-coronary intervention. Totowa (NJ): Human Press; 2005.
[45] Davidson CJ, Harrison JK, Leithe MB, et al. Failure of balloon aortic valvuloplasty to result in sustained clinical improvement in pateitns with depressed LV function. Am J Cardiol 1990;65:72.
[46] Otto CM, Mickel MC, Kennedy JW, et al. Three-year outcome after balloon aortic valvuloplasty. Circulation 1994;89:642.
[47] Kastrup J, Wennevold A, Thuesen L, et al. Short- and long-term survival after aortic balloon valvuloplasty for calcified aortic stenosis in 137 elderly patients. Dan Med Bull 1994;41(3): 362–5.
[48] Eltchaninoff H, Cribier A, Tron C, et al. Balloon aortic vavluloplasty in elderly patients at high risk for surgery, or inoperable. Immediate and mid-term results. Eur Heart J 1995;16(8): 1079–84.
[49] Lieberman EB, Bashore TM, Hermiller JB, et al. Balloon aortic valvuloplasty in adults: failure of procedure to improve long-term survival. J Am Coll Cardiol 1995;26(6): 1522–8.
[50] Novaro GM, Tiong IYU, Pearce GL, et al. Effect of hydroxymethylglutaryl coenzyme a reductase inhibitors on the progression of calcific aortic stenosis. Circulation 2001;104(18): 2205–9.
[51] Desnoyers MR, Salem DN, Rosenfeld K, et al. Treatment of cardiogenic shock by emergency aortic balloon valvuloplasty. Ann Intern Med 1988;108:833.
[52] Buchwald AB, Meyer T, Scholz K, et al. Efficacy of balloon valvuloplasty in patients with critical aortic stenosis and cardiogenic shock—the role of shock duration. Clin Cardiol 2001;24(3):214–8.
[53] Agarwal A, Kini AS, Attanti S, et al. Results of repeat balloon valvuloplasty for treatment of aortic stenosis in patients aged 59 to 104 years. Am J Cardiol 2005;95(1):43.
[54] Roth RB, Palacios F, Block PC. Percutaneous aortic valvuloplasty: its role in the management of patients with aortic stenosis requiring major non cardiac surgery. J Am Coll Cardiol 1989;13:1039.
[55] Cribier A, Eltchaninoff H, Bash A, et al. Percutaneous transcatheter implantation of an aortic valve prosthesis for calcific aortic stenosis: first human description. Circulation 2002;106: 3006–8.

[56] Cribier A, Eltchaninoff H, Tron C, et al. Early experience with percutaneous transcatheter implantation of heart valve prosthesis for the treatment of end-stage inoperable patients with calcific aortic stenosis. J Am Coll Cardiol 2004;43(4):698–703.

[57] Bauer F, Eltchaninoff H, Tron C, et al. Acute improvement in global and regional left ventricular systolic function after percutaneous heart valve implantation in patients with symptomatic aortic stenosis. Circulation 2004;110(11):1473–6.

[58] Herrmann HC, Wilkins GT, Block PC. Percutaneous balloon mitral valvulotomy for patients with mitral stenosis: Analysis of factors influencing early results. J Thorac Cardiovasc Surg 1988;96:33.

[59] Reyes VP, Raju BS, Wynne J, et al. Percutaneous balloon valvuloplasty compared with opoen surgical commissurotomy for mitral stenosis. N Engl J Med 1994;331:961.

[60] Ben Farhat M, Ayari M, Maatouk F, et al. Percutaneous balloon versus surgical closed and open mitral commissurotomy: Seven-year follow-up results of a randomized trial. Circulation 1998;97:245.

[61] Bonow RO, Carabello B, de Leon AC Jr, et al. ACC/AHA guidelines for the management of patients with valvular heart disease: American College of Cardiology/American Heart Association Task Force on Practice Guidelines (Committee on Management of Patients with Valvular Heart Disease). J Am Coll Cardiol 1998;32:1448.

[62] Marzo KP, Herrmann H, Mancini DM. Effect of balloon mitral valvuloplasty on exercise capacity, ventilation and skeletal muscle oxygenation. J Am Coll Cardiol 1993;21:856.

[63] Tuzcu EM, Block PC, Palacios IF. Comparison of early versus late experience with percutaneous mitral balloon valvotomy. J Am Coll Cardiol 1991;17:1121.

[64] Post JR, Feldman T, Isner J, et al. Inoue balloon mitral valvotomy in patients with valvular and subvalvular deformity. J Am Coll Cardiol 1995;25:1129.

[65] Wilkins GT, Weyman AE, Abascal VM, et al. Percutaneous balloon dilatation of the mitral valve: An analysis of echocardiographic variables related to outcome and the mechanism of dilatation. Br Heart J 1988;60:299.

[66] Lefevre T, Bonan R, Serra A, et al. Percutaneous mitral valvuloplasty in surgical high risk patients. J Am Coll Cardiol 1991;17:348.

[67] Tuzcu EM, Block PC, Griffin BP, et al. Immediate and long-term outcome of percutaneous mitral valvulotomy in patients 65 years and older. Circulation 1992;85:963.

[68] Sanchez PL, Rodriguez-Alemparte M, Inglessis I, et al. The impact of age in the immediate and long-term outcomes of percutaneous mitral balloon valvuloplasty. J Interv Cardiol 2005;18(4):217.

[69] Fremes SE, Goldman IV BS, Ivanow J, et al. Valvular surgery in the elderly. Circulation 1989;80:177.

[70] Otsufi Y, Handschumacher MD, Liel-Cohen N, et al. Mechanism of ischemic mitral regurgitation with segmental left ventricular dysfunction: three-dimensional echocardiographic studies in models of acute and chronic progressive regurgitation. J Am Coll Cardiol 2001;37(2):641.

[71] Levine RA, Hung J, Otsuji Y, et al. Mechanistic insights into functional mitral regurgitation. Curr Cardiol Rep 2002;4(2):125.

[72] Bonow RO, Carabello B, de Leon AC Jr, et al. Guidelines for management of patients with valvular heart disease: executive summary. Circulation 1998;98:1949.

[73] Miller DC. Ischemic mitral regurgitation redux—to repair or replace? J Thorac Cardiovasc Surg 2001;122(6):1059.

[74] Lawrie GM. Mitral valve repair vs. replacement: current recommendations and long-term results. Cardiol Clin 1998;16(3):437.

[75] Gogbashian A, Sepic J, Soltesz EG, et al. Operative and long-term survival of elderly is significantly improved by mitral valve repair. Am Heart J 2006;151(6):1325.

[76] Alfieri O, Maisano F, DeBonis M, et al. The edge-to-edge technique in mitral valve repair: a simple solution for complex problems. J Thorac Cardiovasc Surg 2001;122:674.

[77] Umana JP, Salehizadeh B, DeRose JJ, et al. "Bow-tie" mitral valve repair: an adjuvant technique for ischemic mitral regurgitation. Ann Thorac Surg 1998;66:1640.

[78] Herrmann HC, Wasserman HS, Whitlow PL, et al. Percutaneous edge-to-edge mitral valve repair; preliminary results of the EVEREST-I Study. Circulation 2004;10:III-438.

[79] MacDowall P, Kalra PA, O'Donoghue DJ, et al. Risk of morbidity from renovascular disease in elderly patients with congestive heart failure. Lancet 1998;35:12.

[80] Bloch MJ, Trost DW, Pickering TG, et al. Prevention of recurrent pulmonary edema in patients with bilateral renovascular disease through renal artery stent placement. Am J Hypertens 1999;12:1.

[81] Webster J, Marshall F, Abdalla M, et al. Randomized comparison of percutaneous angioplasty vs continued medical therapy for hypertensive patients with atheromatous renal artery stenosis. J Hum Hypertens 1998;12:329.

[82] Khosla S, White CJ, Collins TJ, et al. Effects of renal artery stent implantation in patients with renovascular hypertension presenting with unstable angina or congestive heart failure. Am J Cardiol 1997;80:363.

[83] Gray BH, Olin JW, Childs MB, et al. Clinical benefit of renal artery angioplasty with stenting for the control of recurrent and refractory congestive heart failure. Vasc Med 2002;7(4):275.

[84] Maron BJ. Hypertrophic cardiomyopathy. Circulation 2002;106:2419.

[85] Maron BJ, Olivotto I, Spirito P, et al. Epidemiology of hypertrohic cardiomyopathy-related death: revisited in a large non-referral-based patient population. Circulation 2000; 102:858.

[86] Maron BJ. Hypertrophic cardiomyopathy: a systematic review. JAMA 2001;287:1308.

[87] Nagueh SF, Lakkis NM, He ZX, et al. Role of myocardial contrast echocardiography during nonsurgical septal reduction therapy for hypertrophic obstructive cardiomyopathy. J Am Coll Cardiol 1998;32:225.

[88] Kuhn H, Gietzen FH, Schafers M, et al. Changes in the left ventricular outflow tract after transcoronary ablation of septal hypertrophy (TASH) for hypertrophic obstructive cardiomyopathy as assessed by transesophageal echocardiography and by measuring myocardial glucose utilization and perfusion. Eur Heart J 1999;20:1808.

[89] Flores-Ramirez R, Lakkis NM, Middleton KJ, et al. Echocardiographic insights into the mechanisms of relief of left ventricular outflow tract obstruction after nonsurgical septal reduction therapy in patients with hypertrophic obstructive cardiomyopathy. J Am Coll Cardiol 2001;37:208.

[90] Nagueh SF, Lakkis NM, Middleton KJ, et al. Changes in left ventricular diastolic function 6 months after nonsurgical septal reduction therapy for hypertrophic obstructive cardiomyopathy. Circulation 1999;99:344.

[91] Mazur W, Nagueh SF, Lakkis NM, et al. Regression of left ventricular hypertrophy after nonsurgical septal reduction therapy for hypertrophic obstructive cardiomyopathy. Circulation 2001;103:1492.

[92] Firoozi S, Elliott PM, Sharma S, et al. Septal myotomy-myectomy and transcoronary septal alcohol ablation in hypertrophic obstructive cardiomyopathy. A comparison of clinical, hemodynamic and exercise outcomes. Eur Heart J 2001;23:1617.

[93] Nagueh SF, Ommen SR, Lakkis NM, et al. Comparison of ethanol septal reduction therapy with surgical myectomy for the treatment of hypertrophic obstructive cardiomyopathy. J Am Coll Cardiol 2001;38:1701.

[94] Juliano N, Wong SC, Naidu SS. Alcohol septal ablation for failed surgical myectomy. J Invasive Cardiol 2005;17(10):569.

[95] Porter CJ, Feldt RH, Edwards WD, et al. Atrial septal defects. In: Allen HD, Gutgesell HP, Clark EB, et al, editors. Moss and Adams' heart disease in infants, children, and adolescents: including the fetus and young adult. 6th edition. Baltimore, MD: Williams and Wilkins; 2001. p. 603–17.

[96] Steele PM, Fuster V, Cohen M, et al. Isolated atrial septal defect with pulmonary vascular obstructive disease—long term follow-up and prediction of outcome after surgical correction. Circulation 1987;76(5):1037.
[97] Masura J, Gavora P, Formanek A, et al. Trans-catheter closure of secundum atrial septal defects using the new self-centering Amplatzer septal occluder: initial human experience. Cathet Cardiovasc Diagn 1997;42:388.
[98] Du ZD, Hijazi ZM, Kleinman CS, et al. Comparison between transcatheter and surgical closure of secundum atrial septal defect in children and adults: results of a multi-center non-randomized trial. J Am Coll Cardiol 2001;39:1836.
[99] Ilkhanoff L, Naidu SS, Rohatgi S, et al. Transcatheter device closure of interatrial septal defects in patients with hypoxia. J Interv Cardiol 2005;18(4):227–32.

ELSEVIER
SAUNDERS

CLINICS IN
GERIATRIC
MEDICINE

Clin Geriatr Med 23 (2007) 179–192

Surgical Treatment of Heart Failure in the Elderly

Ramin Malekan, MD, Steven L. Lansman, MD, PhD*

*New York Medical College, Westchester Medical Center,
Macy Pavilion 114 West, Valhalla, NY 10595, USA*

Because the number of elderly people who have heart disease will increase during the next few decades, heart failure (HF) will likely remain a great challenge for the practitioner [1]. HF in elderly patients who may benefit from surgical therapy is usually secondary to ischemic or valvular heart disease. When referring such patients for surgery, life expectancy, along with the expectations of the patient and family with regard to the surgical treatment, must be considered. The goals of cardiac surgery in this patient population are to maintain or improve cardiac function, decrease HF episodes, reduce hospital admissions, and improve functional class. Safer surgical techniques developed during the last two decades have allowed high-risk patients well into their 80s to undergo complex cardiac operations with decreasing morbidity and mortality. Successful surgical intervention often leads to a more productive and independent life for elderly patients who have HF. This article discusses myocardial revascularization procedures, valve repair or replacement, myocardial remodeling procedure, and the limited option of ventricular assist devices (VADs) in the elderly who have HF.

Preoperative evaluation of patients who have heart failure

The cardiac surgeon usually is consulted to see a patient who has been admitted with HF and subsequently found to have ischemic or valvular heart disease. Elderly patients who present with HF can be divided into two categories. The first group presents in severe, refractory HF with severely depressed ventricular function secondary to chronic ischemia or valvular heart disease with ejection fractions (EFs) well below 20%. In some

---

* Corresponding author.
E-mail address: lansmans@wcmc.com (S.L. Lansman).

0749-0690/07/$ - see front matter © 2006 Elsevier Inc. All rights reserved.
doi:10.1016/j.cger.2006.08.007
geriatric.theclinics.com

patients the coronary disease is so severe and extensive that grafting may not be feasible. Most patients describe chronic shortness of breath with severe decrease in exercise capacity. These patients may exhibit pulmonary hypertension as a manifestation of their chronic condition, and they may also suffer from cardiac cachexia. Many have refused surgery in the past, yet others may have had previous open heart surgery making reoperation difficult, high risk, and without clear benefit. Comorbidities, such as severe peripheral vascular disease, chronic obstructive pulmonary disease, renal insufficiency, or renal failure, add significantly to the risk for operation and the chance of a successful outcome with long-term benefits. These patients have limited life expectancy and surgical intervention is unlikely to alter their prognosis. Cardiac transplantation is the best chance for long-term survival in patients who have end-stage heart disease; however, given the limited number of donor hearts, cardiac transplantation usually is not an option for most patients who have end-stage HF [2]. Clinical trials show improved survival and better quality of life in patients who have end-stage HF receiving left ventricular assist devices [3], although these devices have not gained widespread clinical use as destination therapy. For this group of patients, medical therapy with the goal of palliation of symptoms is the preferred treatment. As technology continues to improve, ventricular assist devices will have a greater role in treatment of these patients.

The second group that presents with HF has a broad range of ventricular dysfunction, from a relatively normal ventricle to one with moderate to severe dysfunction. Most of these patients benefit from revascularization or valve repair or replacement procedures. A detailed history and physical examination is essential to determine the duration of symptoms, presence of angina, and limitations in function, and to fully investigate the cause in these patients. Although angina indicates ongoing ischemia and myocardium at risk, which could potentially benefit from revascularization, silent ischemia is an increasingly recognized entity, especially in patients who have longstanding diabetes. HF can also be the initial presenting symptom for many. Patients often describe having symptoms dating back weeks or months. They often limit their activity with the onset of angina or shortness of breath, and learn to "live around their disease."

If an acute myocardial infarction (MI) is the presenting symptom and the patient has presented within a few hours, immediate revascularization of the culprit vessel, whether biochemical or mechanical, is desirable. In such situations communication between the interventional cardiologist and cardiac surgeon is paramount. For patients presenting within a few hours of the evolving MI, often the culprit vessel can undergo angioplasty and stenting. This procedure salvages myocardium and allows the patient to be stabilized for future surgical therapy. For patients who have left main coronary or severe three-vessel disease who are not amenable to coronary angioplasty and stenting and present in severe HF, the surgical intervention may become necessary during the same hospital admission. The intra-aortic balloon pump (IABP) is useful in providing mechanical assist for the failing heart and augmenting coronary blood flow in patients who await coronary revascularization [4]. Its contraindications for use are moderate to severe aortic insufficiency and aortic pathology that precludes percutaneous placement. The IABP reduces myocardial oxygen consumption [5] and may reduce infarct size in post-MI patients. In patients who have decreased ventricular function, it reduces the need for cardiac inotropic therapy and hence may lower the risk for ventricular arrhythmias.

Patients presenting in cardiogenic shock have a high rate of mortality and require close monitoring, inotropic therapy, and frequent assessment of cardiac output and end-organ perfusion (acidosis and urine output). These patients should have a pulmonary artery catheter placed either during cardiac catheterization or at the bedside. Frequent monitoring of cardiac output along with arterial and mixed venous blood gas determinations dictate the course of inotropic treatment. This treatment is continued until acidosis is resolved and mixed venous saturation and end-organ perfusion is adequate. Most patients have severely elevated pulmonary and central venous pressures. They usually present in severe fluid overload, which manifests as pulmonary, lower extremity, or generalized edema, and benefit from aggressive diuresis. Although therapy with nesiritide has gained popularity in HF therapy in recent years, most patients who respond do well with conventional diuretic therapy. Furosemide as a continuous infusion is more effective than bolus therapy [6]. Zaroxolyn usually is added to augment the response of the continuous infusion of furosemide. Evidence no longer supports the use of renal dose dopamine to augment renal function [7]. Patients in HF usually respond with brisk diuresis and require frequent monitoring of their electrolytes and renal function. Patients in cardiogenic shock on high-dose inotropic treatment should undergo elective intubation and mechanical ventilation. This intervention decreases the work of breathing and stress on the cardiopulmonary system. In patients who have right ventricular infarct, mechanical ventilation allows lower levels of P_{CO_2}, which dilates the pulmonary arteries and lowers pulmonary artery pressures. Cardiac arrhythmias are treated aggressively with the correction of electrolyte abnormalities and with anti-arrhythmic agents.

Most patients presenting with HF symptoms recover in response to the treatment and then undergo definitive surgical intervention. Performing serial echocardiograms is an excellent diagnostic modality in such patients. Specifically, wall motion abnormalities, global heart function, chamber sizes, and presence of valvular disease can be assessed. Echocardiograms also serve as an excellent tool in assessing the degree and the mechanism of valvular regurgitation (ie, ischemic versus degenerative) and the need for valvular repair in conjunction with the revascularization procedure. Changes in ventricular function during the perioperative period can be documented by way of echocardiogram and are compared with the postoperative function.

Once HF has been treated adequately, a coronary angiogram, if not performed initially, is done to rule out coronary artery disease. Coronary disease is common in this population and the authors believe that this is the preferred, definitive test, rather than an additional screening test before angiography. If the patient does not have significant elevations of his BUN and creatinine, multiple views of coronary arteries and a ventriculogram are performed to assess wall motion and ventricular function. In patients found to have pulmonary hypertension or elevated right-sided pressures (by way of pulmonary artery catheter or echocardiography), right heart catheterization should also be performed.

Patients presenting with a non–Q-wave MI can undergo revascularization once stabilized [8]. Patients who have a Q-wave MI show decreased mortality if the revascularization is delayed for at least 3 days [9], provided that the patient remains stable, the cardiac enzymes levels are trending downward, and there is no evidence of ongoing ischemia (angina) or further myocardial injury. An IABP can be left in place in these patients until revascularization has been performed. The authors have had few complications from IABPs in these patients, especially with the smaller IAPB catheters, and the complications that do arise are manageable.

Patients who have preserved heart function or mild to moderate decrease in EF can undergo revascularization with excellent early and long-term results. In most of these patients revascularization preserves EF, prevents further myocardial ischemia or infarction, and decreases congestive HF (CHF) episodes. In patients who have decreased EF, revascularization often drastically improves wall motion abnormality and ventricular function [10]. This change usually is evident on intraoperative transesophageal echocardiogram (TEE). In the latter group of patients, revascularization also drastically improves survival compared with the medically treated group [11].

In patients who have severe decrease in ventricular function, dilated cardiomyopathy, and severe HF, the benefit of revascularization may be less clear. These patients should undergo viability studies to document areas with reversible ischemia in territories to be grafted. If areas of reversible ischemia are small and unlikely to change based on coronary angiography, surgical revascularization should be questioned. In these patients intractable HF with severe decrease in EF is likely attributable to the combination of coronary artery disease and a nonischemic cardiomyopathy. Nonetheless, most patients who have EFs between 15% and 25% and evidence of reversible ischemia benefit from revascularization. It is important, therefore, to reevaluate patients who have a low EF who have been treated in the hospital for HF because their treatment may result in significant improvement in EF, which will in turn make them possible candidates for surgical intervention.

Many elderly patients undergoing open heart surgery have other comorbidities that may complicate their perioperative course. Patients who have left main coronary disease, severe peripheral vascular disease, or history of a prior cerebrovascular accident (CVA) should have carotid artery studies with Doppler echocardiogram to rule out significant carotid lesions. Patients who have significant carotid lesions need to have higher systemic pressures during cardiopulmonary bypass to decrease the chance of cerebral ischemia secondary to decreased flow through narrowed arteries. The benefit from carotid endarterectomy (CEA) in asymptomatic patients is substantially less than in patients who are symptomatic from their carotid lesions [12,13]. These patients can be followed postoperatively for possible surgical intervention in the future. Although some groups advocate combined CEA and coronary artery bypass graft (CABG) [14], others suggest that the symptomatic lesion (in this case heart disease) should be addressed first [15]. Patients who have had a prior CVA should have a computed tomography of the brain to document the extent of the infarct before cardiac surgery.

Valvular heart disease in elderly patients

A significant number of patients who present in HF with decreased EF have mitral regurgitation (MR) as a result of an inferior wall MI (IWMI) or a dilated left ventricle (LV). The mechanism of MR is different in each scenario. Patients who have an IWMI have shortened posterior papillary muscle and asymmetric dilatation of the posterior annulus as a result of previous MI in the circumflex coronary artery distribution; patients who have a dilated LV generally have a dilated posterior annulus. Patients also can present with a combination of the above lesions, such as a patient who has ischemic MR (IMR) with a tethered posterior leaflet and chronic HF with cardiac enlargement and a grossly dilated annulus. Although the leaflets in both types of MR may appear normal during valve repair analysis, the valve apparatus is dysfunctional resulting in various degrees of MR. In IMR valvular dysfunction is secondary to ventricular disease rather than leaflet disease, and in dilated cardiomyopathy MR is from a dilated annulus. The MR jet in the former group is directed toward the anterior leaflet, whereas in the latter group the jet is central. These characteristics are used in preoperative echocardiogram to examine the mechanism of valvular insufficiency and to formulate an operative plan for correction of the defect. Because the intraoperative TEE is done under general anesthesia, which decreases peripheral vascular resistance, MR is usually downgraded by 1 to 2+ [16]. Patients suspected of having mitral valve disease, either from the presentation, history, or during angiography, therefore should undergo transthoracic echocardiography (TTE) before the operation to assess their MR and degree of pulmonary hypertension. Patients who have moderate to severe MR on preoperative TTE should have mitral valve repair or replacement during the revascularization procedure. The same rationale is used for patients who have not had a preoperative TTE and whose intraoperative TEE shows at lease moderate (2+) MR. Patients who present with functional MR (ie, MR during ischemic episodes) may respond to revascularization without a need for mitral valve intervention, although predicting which patients would respond to revascularization alone may not always be possible.

Elevated pulmonary artery pressures, dilated left atrium, and atrial fibrillation (AF) often hint at the chronicity of MR and point toward a more aggressive approach to mitral valve repair or replacement. There are a few exceptions to the generalized approach outlined above. Mitral valve replacement or repair in a very old patient who has a heavily calcified annulus may require removal of annular calcifications, which carries the risk for atrioventricular disruption, a complication that is usually fatal. It is safer to leave the mitral valve alone in these patients. In those who have severe aortic stenosis and moderate MR, reduction in left ventricular outflow track obstruction by aortic valve replacement reduces MR in most of these patients. Aortic valve replacement may be all that is needed to reduce mitral insufficiency in the presence of severe aortic stenosis.

In elderly patients the aortic valve is the most common valvular pathology. In patients presenting with HF, aortic stenosis, aortic insufficiency, or mixed lesions must be ruled out. Aortic stenosis (AS) causes ventricular hypertrophy, which increases myocardial oxygen demand and exaggerates ischemia in patients who have coronary artery disease who already have a fixed cardiac output secondary to the stenotic valve. Aortic insufficiency, although well tolerated, also can cause ventricular hypertrophy and enlargement and HF symptoms. Patients who have aortic valve pathology respond well to valve replacement. Even patients who have moderate to severe decrease in EF and severe AS should undergo aortic valve replacement. The new advances in tissue valve engineering make bioprosthetic valves an attractive option because anticoagulation is not required, and the actuarial freedom from valve replacement in elderly patients is high [17]. In patients who have AF who are already on Coumadin, tissue valve is again a reasonable option because anticoagulation for AF can be stopped if the patient has a bleeding episode, but the current mechanical valves require lifelong anticoagulation. The question arises in patients undergoing CABG who have moderate AS. Because AS is a progressive lesion, it is reasonable to replace the aortic valve in these patients and accept a small increase in operative risk rather than have the patient return with symptoms from aortic valve pathology requiring reoperation in a patient who is older and generally has more risk factors. Reoperation in this setting carries a greater risk for complications and death.

General considerations for open heart surgery in the elderly

Most revascularization procedures and essentially all valve repair or replacement procedures require cardiopulmonary bypass (CPB) with cardiac arrest. Improvement in survival in patients who undergo open heart surgery is directly related to advancements in surgical techniques and improvements in myocardial protection. Myocardial protection is paramount in patients who have low EF who require prolonged cross-clamping for complex operations. Patients who have severe AS and hypertrophic ventricle are at increased risk for myocardial ischemia during CPB. During cardiopulmonary bypass the heart is arrested and isolated from systemic circulation by clamping of the ascending aorta. Myocardial oxygen consumption is directly related to cardiac activity and temperature. The heart undergoes diastolic arrest with electrical silence using antegrade (given to the ascending aorta or directly down to coronary ostia) and retrograde (given through a catheter placed in the coronary sinus by way of the right atrium) cold blood cardioplegia at least every 20 minutes. Addition of topical ice slush to the heart surface helps keep myocardial temperature low and decreases myocardial oxygen demand to very low levels. Given this approach, prolonged cross-clamp times are well tolerated even in patients who have low EFs. This tolerance allows complex procedures requiring cross-clamp times in excess of 3 hours to be performed with a low risk for postcardiotomy HF. The authors' intraoperative IABP use is generally less than 5% even in patients who have a moderately low EF.

Although traditionally the ascending aorta is used for inflow cannulation there are circumstances that prevent the use of the aorta as a suitable access site. Patients who have a thin, aneurysmal ascending aorta and severe aortic atherosclerosis and calcification present a risk for aortic dissection and embolization. The authors' policy is to scan the ascending aorta in all patients using a hand-held transthoracic echo probe inserted into a sterile sheath to rule out significant atheromatous plaques. These plaques can be a source of cerebral and peripheral embolization during arterial inflow cannulation, decannulation, aortic cross-clamping, and unclamping maneuvers [18]. Patients found to have significant atheromatous plaques in the ascending aorta undergo direct inflow cannulation of their axillary artery. The risk for complications from axillary artery cannulation (brachial plexus injury or vascular injury) should be less than 1%. Using this approach the authors' stroke rate is only about 1%.

Revascularization procedures

CABG remains the gold standard for coronary revascularization. It is the preferred approach for patients who have three-vessel coronary disease, patients who have diabetes, and patients who require additional open-heart surgery for other indications, such as valve repair or replacement. It is also the preferred approach in patients who have stent stenosis. The authors' approach is to bypass all areas involved with coronary disease (total revascularization) and use arterial grafts when feasible. Most patients require two to five bypass grafts. The left internal mammary artery (LIMA) has excellent long-term patency and almost always is anastomosed to the anterior descending artery. Its use is directly associated with improvement in the hospital and long-term survival. Traditionally, poor LV function contraindicated the use of the IMA. This is no longer the case. The authors harvest the LIMA as a skeletonized pedicle graft, in which there is no disruption of the internal mammary veins and endothoracic fascia. Although technically more challenging, the LIMA harvested with this technique has more usable length and improved flow and can be used in sequential grafting. In elderly patients who lack adequate saphenous vein for conduit, either secondary to its previous harvest, varicosities, or other disease processes, the radial artery is usually the second conduit of choice. It is sensitive to competitive flow from the native coronary artery, which means that it should be used to bypass lesions with greater than 70% stenosis [19]. Although there is concern regarding spasm with the use of this conduit in patients who have a low EF who require cardiac pressors postoperatively, with the use of the no-touch technique of conduit harvest the authors have not encountered this problem in more than 500 cases involving the use of this artery, including patients who have severe decrease in LV function. Antegrade and retrograde cardioplegia are given after the construction of each anastomosis as described above.

Transmyocardial laser revascularization

The idea of providing blood to the ischemic myocardium directly from the left ventricular cavity dates back to the 1960s when Sen used transmyocardial acupuncture to provide channels to feed the ischemic myocardium [20]. Mirhoseini attempted the same concept in the 1980s using laser energy [21]. Although transmyocardial laser revascularization (TMR) gained considerable attention during the 1990s, it has been used infrequently in patients who have nongraftable coronary arteries. Controversy exists regarding patency of transmyocardial channels and whether blood can flow into the myocardium during the cardiac cycle if the intramyocardial pressure exceeds the ventricular pressure at any point in the cardiac cycle [22]. Moreover, proposed angiogenesis induced by TMR is likely secondary to a nonspecific response to injury rather than the effect of laser on the ischemic myocardium [23]. TMR has been shown to improve angina class and decrease the need for antianginal medications [24]. Positron emission tomography studies of myocardial perfusion, however, do not consistently demonstrate improved perfusion in the lasered areas [25]. Although most TMR used today is in conjunction with CABG in territories not amenable to bypass grafting, TMR should not be used as a revascularization procedure. The authors currently do not use TMR in the authors' practice.

Valve repair or replacement

Following revascularization the valvular pathology is addressed. Aortic valve pathology in elderly patients almost always is managed with valve replacement. The new generations of bioprosthetic aortic valves (tissue valves) have good long-term durability and do not require lifelong anti-coagulation. The actuarial freedom from reoperation for aortic valve bio-prostheses in elderly patients (greater than age 70) is greater than 95%, whereas the complication rates are much lower than for mechanical valves in this age group [17]. Aortic bioprosthesis is therefore a good choice in the elderly patient. Bioprostheses in the mitral position gener-ally lack the long-term durability seen in aortic prostheses. In addition, mechanical valves need life-long anticoagulation with inherent risk for bleeding and thromboembolism, especially in the elderly. Mitral valve re-pair is therefore the preferred approach to mitral valve pathology when feasible. With new techniques of valve repair, greater than 95% of mitral valves not involved with rheumatic heart disease can be repaired successfully.

Most mitral valve disease seen in elderly patients who have HF in the United States is secondary to ischemic mitral regurgitation (IMR) from a previous MI of the circumflex artery territory or from annular dilatation attributable to the cardiac enlargement of chronic HF. In patients who have IMR or MR secondary to dilated cardiomyopathy, the repair is fairly straightforward. These types of valvular insufficiency can be repaired with the placement of a simple annuloplasty ring that reduces the anterior–pos-terior (AP) dimension of the mitral valve annulus and hence coapts the leaf-lets. Because the leaflets are usually structurally normal, the increased coaptation surface eliminates MR. Annular dilatation alone is repaired with the placement of a "true size" annuloplasty ring, one that approxi-mates the size of the anterior leaflet of the mitral valve and restores annular AP dimensions. In IMR, the annuloplasty exaggerates the reduction in AP diameter by "undersizing" the annuloplasty ring. This undersizing brings the tethered posterior leaflet toward the anterior annulus to coapt with the anterior leaflet. In occasional patients who have degenerative mitral valve pathology and flail leaflet, limited resection of the prolapsed segment (usually P2 scallop of the posterior leaflet) and the addition of annuloplasty eliminate the MR.

Mitral valve stenosis is an infrequent cause of HF in the United States. It is often the result of rheumatic heart disease. If the leaflets are not involved excessively with fibrosis and calcification and mitral regurgitation is not se-vere, a commissurotomy may be all that is needed to reduce the stenosis without the need for valve replacement. In cases in which some but not all of the chordae tendineae are fused and thickened, fenestration of the fused cords may elongate the shortened cords. The addition of commissur-otomy alleviates stenosis. In cases in which the valve is severely damaged from rheumatic heart disease or in the presence of significant MR in addition to stenosis, valve replacement often is necessary.

Modified maze procedure or pulmonary vein isolation

AF frequently occurs in elderly patients who have longstanding valvular or ischemic heart disease. Elderly patients in HF who present in AF require anticoagulation and attempts at rhythm or rate control. AF increases hospital length of stay and is an independent risk factor for postoperative morbidity and mortality [26]. Most foci responsible for AF generation and propagation are near the orifices of the pulmonary veins [27]. Although the Cox-Maze is considered the gold standard operation for treatment of AF, its complexity has prevented its widespread use in treatment of AF in elderly patients who have HF. Also known as the cut and sew Maze, the operation requires cutting and then suturing of the left atrium from a cuff of pulmonary veins and lesions in the right atrium [28,29]. The cut areas healed with fibrosis electrically isolate the atria from signals that induce and maintain AF. The operation is technically demanding, requiring prolonged cross-clamp times, and imposes a significant risk for morbidity. Over the past few years simpler operations requiring fewer lesion sets using various energy sources have been devised, although general agreement regarding the energy source and the number and location of these lesions is lacking.

The most commonly used energy sources are radiofrequency (RF) and liquid nitrogen. The simplest form of the modified maze procedure is pulmonary vein isolation using a liquid nitrogen probe that creates transmural lesions in the left atrium around the orifices of the pulmonary veins. The left atrial appendage also can be ligated as part of electrical isolation and to reduce the risk for embolization of clot from the atrial appendage if the patient does not remain in sinus rhythm. In patients requiring mitral valve repair who have a history of AF, the addition of the pulmonary vein isolation procedure may prevent recurrent AF. It entails creating transmural lesions encircling the orifices of the pulmonary veins from inside the left atrium during mitral valve procedures so the foci responsible for AF are isolated from entering the atria. The left atrial appendage also can be oversewn during this procedure. Whether the last maneuver reduces the risk for embolic events in patients who have recurrent AF has not been evaluated clinically. The pulmonary vein isolation procedure reportedly is successful in 90% of patients who have a history of paroxysmal AF alone. In patients who have ischemic or valvular heart disease, chronic AF, and grossly dilated atria, the success rate is probably close to 50%. The pulmonary vein isolation procedure also can be performed during a CABG procedure by using a liquid nitrogen probe or an RF clamp to create transmural lesions from outside the left atrium. The authors reserve this approach for patients who present with paroxysmal AF with near normal size atria.

Ventricular remodeling procedure

Because of widespread use of fibrinolytic compounds and increased sophistication of catheter-based intervention in reestablishing coronary flow after an acute MI, the incidence of large ventricular aneurysms has been declining [30]. In patients who present with a completed infarction of a large anterior wall MI the ventricle undergoes a complex remodeling process. This change is secondary to fibrosis of the infarcted region and mechanical stretch of the area surrounding the infarct. This remodeling leads to ventricular aneurysm formation and cardiac enlargement. The thin aneurysmal region, by definition, paradoxes with the cardiac cycle, bulging during systole. This phenomenon causes some of the mechanical work to be lost in the aneurysmal sac, leading to ineffective cardiac work, LV dilatation, and symptoms of HF. The Dor procedure [31] or ventricular remodeling procedure aims at eliminating the aneurysmal region of the heart and restoring a more normal geometry to the infarcted ventricle. It is known from clinical and animal studies that the process of aneurysm formation takes about 6 to 8 weeks to develop [32]. In addition, freshly infarcted tissue is difficult to manipulate. If the HF symptoms can be managed medically it is therefore optimal to wait a few weeks in these patients so the aneurysm wall becomes demarcated from the rest of the LV.

The Dor procedure is performed through a median sternotomy under cardiopulmonary bypass. If another procedure is contemplated it is performed before the remodeling procedure. Some patients require CABG in other regions of myocardium, and mitral valve repair is often necessary if significant MR is present. The infarcted area usually involves a substantial portion of the LV anterior wall that has become fibrotic and thin over time. Grafting the LAD that is chronically occluded usually is not indicated, because reestablishing flow to this region is unlikely to change the infarcted area or lead to improvement in ventricular function.

The aneurysm sac is opened and thrombus, which is often adherent to the infarcted area, is evacuated. A circular patch of Dacron graft is sewn over the neck of the aneurysm. It usually is necessary to place the patch near the base of the papillary muscles. After placement of the patch, the fibrotic LV wall that was previously opened is closed in layers over the patch to ensure a secure closure. The patient then is weaned off CPB.

Ventricular assist devices

For patients who present with severe refractory HF cardiac transplantation offers the best chance of long-term survival and improved quality of life. Given the limited number of donors each year, cardiac transplantation is a limited option for most HF patients. Moreover, many elderly patients have other chronic diseases that make them less suitable candidates for heart transplant. The REMATCH trial, which was completed in 2001, showed a 48% reduction in risk for death in a group of patients who received a VAD as destination therapy, compared with a similarly matched group of patients who had end-stage HF who were only treated medically [33]. The patients receiving a VAD reported better quality of life despite being twice as likely to suffer an adverse event and required more frequent hospitalizations. Ventricular assist devices, therefore, have become an option not necessarily as a bridge to transplant but as destination therapy. As the technology improves, these devices will assume a greater role in elderly patients who have end-stage HF.

Postoperative care

Ventricular function is the most important factor in predicting postoperative recovery following open heart surgery. The postoperative care of elderly patients who have HF should start with briefing of the ICU staff. This report should include important medical and surgical history, intraoperative events, significant comorbidities, and anticipated postoperative course. The staff also is made aware of possible complications the patient may face during the recovery period. To ensure adequate cardiac function, the authors follow the mixed venous blood gases in addition to serial cardiac output measurements in all patients. This approach also helps guide patient treatment and weaning of cardiac pressors postoperatively. Patients who have severe decrease in EF may show further reduction in EF after CPB and in the early postoperative period, requiring significant inotropic support in addition to IABP placement. Patients who have mild to moderate reduction in LV function can be weaned off the inotropes and extubated when awake and stable. For patients who have severe decrease in EF and pulmonary hypertension, the process of weaning from inotropes should be slower. These patients should remain intubated until their hemodynamics are stabilized, cardiac function is adequate, and there is minimal or no acidosis present. Extubating an elderly, frail patient who has a low EF and pulmonary hypertension in the presence of significant inotropic support can be disastrous. Older patients who undergo TEE and endotracheal intubation have a high incidence of oropharyngeal dysfunction. In addition, postoperative sedation exaggerates the risk for aspiration in these patients. To minimize the risk for postoperative aspiration and pneumonia in elderly patients who require prolonged intubation, the authors obtain a speech and swallow evaluation before the start of any diet.

Weaning of inotropes is continued in small increments as long as mixed venous saturation remains satisfactory and end-organ perfusion is adequate. The authors tend to keep the IABP in place until most of the inotropes have been weaned off. Most patients have significant weight gain as a result of CPB and preoperative CHF. Once stable, diuresis usually begins and is continued until weight returns close to baseline. For patients admitted in CHF the baseline weight maybe a few kilograms less than the admission weight.

Patients who have a low EF may need daily diuretics continued after discharge. Milrinone is used in patients who require long-term inotropic support but are otherwise stable enough to be transferred to a step-down unit. β-receptor blockers can be started when the patient is on a milrinone tapering dosage. The patients also are started on angiotensin-converting enzyme inhibitors. Patients are encouraged to ambulate once transferred to the step-down ward, where they then receive physical therapy. When the patient is off all cardiac pressors, a follow-up echocardiogram is performed to assess ventricular function. All patients who have mitral valve repair also need documentation of valvular and ventricular function before discharge.

References

[1] Levy D, Kenchaiah S, Larson MG, et al. Long-term trends in the incidence of and survival with heart failure. N Engl J Med 2002;347:1397–402.
[2] Hosenpud JD, Bennett LE, Keck BM, et al. The registry of the International Society for Heart and Lung Transplantation: seventeenth official report — 2000. J Heart Lung Transplant 2000;19:909–31.
[3] Rose EA, Gelijns AC, Moskowitz AJ, et al. Long-term use of a left ventricular assist device for end-stage heart failure: the randomized evaluation of mechanical assistance for the treatment of congestive heart failure (REMATCH) study group. N Engl J Med 2001;345:1435–43.
[4] Ohman EM, George BS, White CJ, et al. Use of aortic counterpulsation to improve sustained coronary artery patency during acute myocardial infarction. Circulation 1994;90:792–9.
[5] Bolooki H. The effects of counterpulsation with an intra-aortic balloon on cardiovascular dynamics and metabolism. In: Bolooki H, editor. Clinical application of intra-aortic balloon pump. New York: Futura; 1977. p. 13–8.
[6] Makhoul N, Riad T, Friedstorm S, et al. Frusemide in pulmonary oedema: continuous versus intermittent. Clin Intensive Care 1997;8(6):273–6.
[7] Korkeila M, Ruokonen E, Takala J. Low-dose dopamine in patients with early renal dysfunction: a placebo-controlled randomised trial. Lancet 2001;356:2139–43.
[8] Lee DC, Oz MC, Weinberg AD, et al. Optimal timing of revascularization: transmural versus nontransmural acute myocardial infarction. Ann Thorac Surg 2001;71:1198–204.
[9] Lee DC, Oz MC, Weinberg AD, et al. Appropriate timing of surgical intervention after transmural acute myocardial infarction. J Thorac Cardiovasc Surg 2003;125:115–20.
[10] Ross J Jr. Myocardial perfusion-contraction matching. Implications for coronary heart disease and hibernation. Circulation 1991;83:1076–83.
[11] Allman KC, Shaw LJ, Hachamovitch R, et al. Myocardial viability testing and impact of revascularization on prognosis in patients with coronary artery disease and left ventricular dysfunction: a meta-analysis. J Am Coll Cardiol 2002;39:1151–8.
[12] Barnett HJM, Taylor DW, Eliasziw M, et al. Benefit of carotid endarterectomy in patients with symptomatic moderate or severe stenosis: the North American symptomatic carotid endarterectomy trial collaborators. N Engl J Med 1998;39:1415–25.
[13] The Executive Committee for the Asymptomatic Carotid Atherosclerosis Study. Endarterectomy for asymptomatic carotid artery stenosis. JAMA 1995;273:1421–8.
[14] Hertzer NR, Loop FD, Beven EG, et al. Surgical staging for simultaneous coronary and carotid disease: a study including prospective randomization. J Vasc Surg 1989;9:455–63.
[15] Borger MA, Tremes SE, Weisel RD, et al. Coronary bypass and carotid endarterectomy: does a combined approach increase risk? A meta-analysis. Ann Thorac Surg 1999;68:14.
[16] Aklog L, Filsoufi F, Flores QK, et al. Does coronary artery bypass grafting alone correct moderate ischemic mitral regurgitation? Circulation 2001;104:68–75.

[17] Chan V, Jamieson WRE, Germann E, et al. Performance of bioprostheses and mechanical prostheses assessed by composites of valve-related complications to 15 years after aortic valve replacement. J Thorac Cardiovasc Surg 2006;131(6):1267–73.

[18] Van der Linden J, Hadjinikolaou L, Bergman P, et al. Postoperative stroke in cardiac surgery is related to the location and extent of atherosclerotic disease in the ascending aorta. J Am Coll Cardiol 2001;38:131–5.

[19] Desai ND, Cohen EA, Naylor CD, et al. The radial artery patency study investigators. A randomized comparison of radial-artery and saphenous-vein coronary bypass grafts. N Engl J Med 2004;351:2302–9.

[20] Sen PK, Udwadia TE, Kinare SG, et al. Transmyocardial acupuncture: a new approach to myocardial revascularization. J Thorac Cardiovasc Surg 1965;50:181–9.

[21] Mirhoseini M, Fisher JC, Cayton M. Myocardial revascularization by laser: a clinical report. Lasers Surg Med 1983;3:241–5.

[22] Pifarre R, Jasuja ML, Lynch RD, et al. Myocardial revascularization by transmyocardial acupuncture: a physiologic impossibility. J Thorac Cardiovasc Surg 1969;58:424–31.

[23] Malekan R, Reynolds C, Narula N, et al. Angiogenesis in transmyocardial laser revascularization: a nonspecific response to injury. Circulation 1998;98:II62–5.

[24] Cooley DA, Frazier OH, Kadipasaoglu KA, et al. Transmyocardial laser revascularization: clinical experience with twelve-month follow-up. J Thorac Cardiovasc Surg 1996;111:791–9.

[25] Horvath KA, Cohn LH, Cooley DA, et al. Transmyocardial laser revascularization: results of a multicenter trial with transmyocardial laser revascularization used as sole therapy for end-stage coronary artery disease. J Thorac Cardiovasc Surg 1997;113:645–54.

[26] Creswell LL, Schessler RB, Rosenbloom M, et al. Hazards of post operative atrial arrhythmias. Ann Thorac Surg 1993;56:539–49.

[27] Haïssaguerre M, Jaïs P, Shah DC, et al. Spontaneous initiation of atrial fibrillation by ectopic beats originating in the pulmonary veins. N Engl J Med 1998;339:659–66.

[28] Cox JL, Ad N, Palazzo T, et al. Current status of the maze procedure for the treatment of atrial fibrillation. Semin Thorac Cardiovasc Surg 2000;12:15–9.

[29] Gaynor SL, Diodato MD, Prasad SM, et al. A prospective, single center clinical trial of a modified Cox maze procedure with bipolar radiofrequency ablation. J Thorac Cardiovasc Surg 2004;124:535–42.

[30] Coltharp WH, Hoff SJ, Stoney WS, et al. Ventricular aneurysmectomy: a 25-year experience. Ann Surg 1994;219:707–13.

[31] Dor V, Saab M, Coste P, et al. Left ventricular aneurysm: a new surgical approach. Thorac Cardiovasc Surg 1989;37:11–9.

[32] Markovitz LJ, Savage EB, Ratcliffe MB, et al. Large animal model of left ventricular aneurysm. Ann Thorac Surg 1989;48:838–45.

[33] Rose EA, Gelijns AC, Moskowitz AJ. long-term use of a left ventricular assist device for end-stage heart failure: the randomized evaluation of mechanical assistance for the treatment of congestive heart failure (REMATCH) study group. N Engl J Med 2001;345:1435–43.

ELSEVIER
SAUNDERS

CLINICS IN
GERIATRIC
MEDICINE

Clin Geriatr Med 23 (2007) 193–203

Cardiac Resynchronization Therapy for Treatment of Heart Failure in the Elderly

Jordana Kron, MD[a], Jamie B. Conti, MD[a,b],*

[a]Division of Cardiovascular Medicine, Department of Medicine, University of Florida,
Box 100277, Gainesville, FL 32610-0277, USA
[b]Clinical Cardiac Electrophysiology, University of Florida,
Box 100277, 1600 SW Archer Road, Gainesville, FL 32610, USA

Case presentation

A 92-year-old man presents to the Heart Failure Clinic because of shortness of breath on exertion. He has a history of coronary artery disease and ischemic cardiomyopathy with a recent echocardiogram demonstrating a left ventricular ejection fraction of 20% to 25%. Despite being on stable doses of lisinopril, carvedilol, atorvastatin, spironolactone, digoxin, and aspirin, he fatigues easily and cannot walk more than one block without stopping to rest. An electrocardiogram shows normal sinus rhythm with a left bundle branch block and a QRS duration of 160 milliseconds. He asks if there are any additional therapies available to treat his heart failure (HF).

Introduction

HF affects 5 million patients each year [1]. Both the prevalence and incidence of HF increase with age. Specifically, the incidence per 1000 population of new and recurrent HF events for white American men is 21.5 for ages 65 to 74, 43.3 for ages 75 to 84, and 73.1 for ages 85 and older. The rates for women (black or nonblack) and black men similarly increase with age. In fact, in patients older than 65 at least 20% of hospital admissions are attributable to HF [2].

Despite advances in pharmacologic therapy, the prognosis of patients who have New York Heart Association (NYHA) functional class III and

---

* Corresponding author. Division of Cardiovascular Medicine, Department of Medicine, University of Florida, Box 100277, Gainesville, FL 32610-0277.
E-mail address: jamie.conti@medicine.ufl.edu (J.B. Conti).

0749-0690/07/$ - see front matter © 2006 Elsevier Inc. All rights reserved.
doi:10.1016/j.cger.2006.08.008
geriatric.theclinics.com

IV HF remains poor and thus has led to the development of innovative strategies for better management of this common clinical problem. Cardiac resynchronization therapy (CRT), known alternatively as biventricular pacing, is the simultaneous pacing of the right and left ventricles, an approach that can improve symptoms and outcomes in some patients who have HF. The use of devices—implantable cardioverter defibrillators (ICDs) with biventricular pacing capabilities and biventricular pacemakers—in addition to aggressive medical therapy has become a mainstay of HF treatment. Clinical trial data indicate a decrease in mortality and considerable improvement in symptoms with both types of devices [3–5]. In this article the authors review the role of CRT in the treatment of elderly patients who have HF.

Background

Ventricular dysfunction is a hallmark of HF and frequently is associated with ventricular conduction delays. Stevenson and colleagues [6] reported that 30% of patients who have HF have intraventricular conduction disturbances severe enough to cause dyssynchronous ventricular contractions resulting in abnormal decreased ventricular filling and decreased cardiac output. Intraventricular conduction delays, usually left bundle branch blocks, may cause segments of the heart to contract at different times resulting in worsening mitral regurgitation, increased systolic ejection time, and a subsequent decrease in diastolic filling time (Box 1). CRT is a relatively new therapy for patients who have HF and mechanical dyssynchrony. Its therapeutic intent is to activate both ventricles simultaneously, thus improving the mechanical efficiency of the heart by "resynchronizing" ventricular contraction.

CRT has two components. First, atrioventricular synchrony should be established with traditional atrioventricular pacing. The increase in cardiac output with an appropriate atrial contribution to diastolic filling is well established [7]. In addition to coordinating atrial and ventricular contraction, biventricular cardiac pacemakers stimulate the right and left ventricles almost simultaneously as a means to resynchronize ventricular contraction.

Box 1. Adverse consequences of intraventricular conduction delays

- Worsening mitral regurgitation
- Increase in systolic ejection time
- Decrease in diastolic filling time
- Decreased cardiac output
- Decreased ventricular filling

This therapy for HF significantly improves outcomes in patients who have left ventricular dysfunction and concomitant intraventricular conduction delays (Table 1) [3,8–10]. Specifically, CRT has been shown to improve distance walked in 6 minutes, NYHA functional class, quality of life, ejection fraction, mortality, and time to first hospitalization.

Current implantation techniques

Standard atrial and ventricular pacing leads are placed in the right atrium and the right ventricle, respectively. To achieve ventricular resynchronization, a specially designed lead is advanced into a lateral or posterolateral branch of the coronary sinus to pace the left ventricle. To achieve accurate lead placement, retrograde venography is performed by inserting commercially available balloon-tipped catheters into the coronary sinus through a separate access from that used for standard right ventricular pacemaker implantation. The balloon is inflated temporarily to occlude flow in the coronary sinus, and nonionized contrast is injected to opacify the left ventricular venous system. Images are captured as a "roadmap" in multiple views, generally 30 degrees right anterior oblique, 30 degrees left anterior oblique, and anteroposterior, to best define the major venous structures and their branches (Fig. 1). The balloon catheter is removed, and a guide catheter is inserted into the coronary sinus os. Next, the coronary sinus pacing lead is advanced into an anterior or lateral venous branch of the coronary sinus, and threshold testing is performed (Fig. 2). All leads are then connected to the pulse generator—either a pacemaker or an ICD.

Pacing the left ventricle by way of the coronary sinus is accepted practice, although other means of pacing the left ventricle when the coronary sinus cannot be entered successfully have been described. Epicardial placement of the left ventricular lead is accomplished easily by a cardiothoracic surgeon if access to the coronary sinus is impossible or if pacing from the coronary sinus is impractical. Interestingly, Jais and coworkers [11] published

Table 1
Outcomes in major randomized CRT trials

Trial	Patients	Results
MIRACLE	453	• Improvement in 6-minute walk test
		• Improvement in NYHA functional class
		• Improvement in quality of life
		• Improvement in ejection fraction
MIRACLE-ICD	369	• Improvement in NYHA functional class
		• Improvement in quality of life
COMPANION	1520	• Reduced all-cause mortality or hospitalization
CARE-HF	813	• Reduced mortality or hospitalization
		• Improvement in NYHA functional class
		• Improvement in quality of life
		• Increased ejection fraction

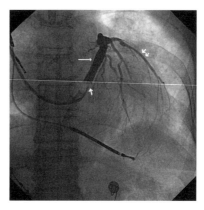

Fig. 1. Venogram of the coronary sinus in an anteroposterior (AP) view. The single short arrow indicates the inflated balloon occluding flow in the coronary sinus. The long arrow identifies the trunk of the coronary sinus. The two short arrows identify one of the lateral cardiac veins.

a case in which left ventricular pacing was accomplished transseptally. In this case report, the patient had an improvement in NYHA class. This method cannot be recommended routinely, though, because of the risk for thromboembolic complications.

Efficacy of cardiac resynchronization therapy in the geriatric population

To date, no prospective randomized trial has addressed CRT specifically in an elderly population. Many of the patients included in the major CRT trials were aged 70 and older, however. In the Cardiac Resynchronization–Heart Failure (CARE-HF) trial, 813 patients who had NYHA class III or IV HF attributable to left ventricular systolic dysfunction and cardiac

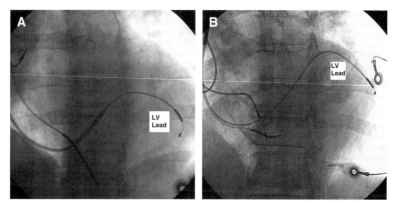

Fig. 2. The left ventricular pacing lead is advanced into the lateral coronary sinus. (A) An AP projection shows the LV lead in a midlateral venous branch of the coronary sinus. (B) Another LV lead is positioned in a more superior lateral venous branch of the coronary sinus.

dyssynchrony who were receiving optimal medical therapy were randomized to medical therapy versus CRT [3]. Included in the trial were patients who had a left ventricular ejection fraction of less than or equal to 35%, a left ventricular end-diastolic dimension of at least 30 mm, and a QRS duration of 120 milliseconds or greater. The primary endpoint was time to death from any cause or hospitalization for a major cardiovascular event. The secondary endpoint was death from any cause.

In CARE-HF, 404 patients were randomized to receive medical therapy alone and 409 were randomized to receive medical therapy and CRT. The mean age of the patients was 66 in the medical therapy alone group and 67 in the medical therapy plus CRT group. The primary endpoint was reached in 224 patients in the medical therapy group compared with 159 patients in the medical therapy plus CRT group (55% versus 39%, $P < .0001$). Eighty-two patients who received CRT died compared with 120 patients who received medical therapy only (20% versus 30%, $P < .002$). Prespecified subgroup analyses were performed to detect heterogeneity in the response of patients to CRT. These analyses compared patients less than 66.4 years old to patients greater than or equal to 66.4 years old and showed no difference in the primary endpoint.

Another landmark CRT trial, the Comparison of Medical Therapy, Pacing, and Defibrillation in Heart Failure (COMPANION) study, also included many elderly patients [10]. A total of 1520 patients with NYHA class III or IV HF and a QRS duration of at least 120 milliseconds were randomized to medical therapy alone, medical therapy plus CRT, or medical therapy plus CRT with an ICD in a 1:2:2 ratio. Patients who had both ischemic and nonischemic cardiomyopathies were included. All patients were on optimal medical therapy as tolerated, including diuretics, angiotensin-converting enzyme inhibitors (or angiotensin-receptor blockers if not tolerated), beta-blockers, and spironolactone. The primary endpoint was a composite of the time to death or hospitalization attributable to any cause.

Of the patients randomized, 308 received optimal medical therapy, 617 received biventricular pacemakers, and 595 received biventricular ICDs. The mean ages of the groups were 68, 67, and 66, respectively. The composite endpoint analyzed at 12 months was reached in 68% of the pharmacologic therapy only group compared with 56% in the biventricular pacemaker group ($P = .014$, adjusted $P = .015$ with log-rank test) and 56% in the biventricular ICD group ($P = .010$, adjusted $P = .011$.) Overall, CRT with or without defibrillator reduced the risk for reaching the primary endpoint by approximately 20%. Again, subgroup analysis was performed on patients less than or equal to 65 years old and those greater than 65 years old and showed consistent efficacy for each device equal to that of the younger patients.

One observational trial compared the effectiveness of CRT in patients less than 70 years old versus those greater than or equal to 70 years old [12]. One hundred seventy consecutive patients who had NYHA class III or IV HF who underwent biventricular pacemaker placement were included. All patients had a left ventricular ejection fraction of less than or equal to 35% and a measured QRS interval greater than 120 milliseconds with left bundle branch block morphology. Exclusion criteria included myocardial infarction within 3 months and decompensated HF.

Before pacemaker implantation, each patient underwent clinical evaluation and two-dimensional echocardiography to measure left ventricular volumes and ejection fraction. Clinical evaluation included assessment of NYHA functional class, quality of life assessment using the Minnesota Living with Heart Failure Questionnaire, and a 6-minute walk test. Tissue Doppler imaging was used to evaluate left ventricular dyssynchrony. Tissue Doppler imaging was performed again immediately after pacemaker implantation to assess resynchronization. Clinical status and left ventricular volumes and ejection fraction were reevaluated at 6 months. Patients were classified as responders if they experienced an improvement of greater than or equal to one NYHA functional class after 6 months of follow-up.

The echocardiographic and clinical results were similar in both age groups. Both groups had similar rates of immediate resynchronization based on tissue Doppler imaging. Improvements in NYHA class, quality-of-life score, and 6-minute walk distance were also comparable in the two groups. The rate of responders was 75% in patients less than 70 years old and 78% in those greater than or equal to 70 years old (P not significant). Improvements in left ventricular ejection fraction and the degree of left ventricular remodeling were also similar in the two groups. Survival at 1 year was 90% in those less than 70 years old and 83% in those greater than or equal to 70 years old (P not significant).

Age as a predictor of response to cardiac resynchronization therapy

About 20% to 30% of patients who receive CRT do not respond [13,14]. Although the topic of response versus nonresponse is complex [15], clinical or echocardiographic parameters typically are used in this assessment. Other parameters considered are clinical symptoms, which are subjective, and rates of hospitalization and mortality that can be measured more reliably. Echocardiographic measurements suggesting response include improvement in left ventricular ejection fraction and evidence of reverse left ventricular remodeling (decrease in left ventricular systolic and diastolic diameters and volumes) [16]. The identification of responders is complicated by discrepancies between clinical and echocardiographic responses.

One study evaluated 143 consecutive patients who received CRT to determine predictors of nonresponse to CRT [17]. Twenty-eight patients (20%) who died of HF, underwent cardiac transplantation, or did not have a greater than 10% increase in 6-minute walk distance were identified as nonresponders. Independent predictors of nonresponse, identified by logistic regression analysis, were ischemic heart disease, severe mitral regurgitation, and left ventricular end-diastolic diameter greater than or equal to 75 mm. The mean age was 68 in both nonresponding and responding patients (P not significant). In this study, age was not a predictor of nonresponse.

Complications of implantation

The complications of implantation are similar to those encountered with standard pacemaker implantation. They include pneumothorax, perforation of the great vessels or myocardium, air embolus, infection, bleeding, and arrhythmias. Complications unique to this procedure include coronary sinus dissection (Fig. 3), perforation, and thrombosis. One study reviewed the safety of CRT in 2078 patients from three large clinical trials [18]. The implantation was successful in 1903 patients (91.6%), with 35 patients (1.8%) requiring more than one attempt to achieve successful implantation. There were 333 perioperative complications in 287 patients (15%), with the perioperative period defined as the day of implantation and the 7 subsequent days. There were 243 postoperative complications in 209 patients (11%), with the postoperative period including day 8 through 6 months. Eight patients (0.3%) died as a result of the procedure. Coronary sinus dissection or perforation, cardiac perforation, or cardiac vein dissection or perforation occurred in 45 patients. Overall, transvenous biventricular pacemaker placement was safe with a high rate of successful implantation. Additionally, the safety of CRT implantation improved with operator experience and the introduction of new technologies. No study has evaluated the effect of age on implantation complication rates.

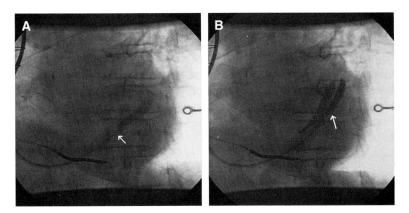

Fig. 3. Coronary sinus dissection is one complication of cardiac resynchronization. (A) Balloon-occluded venogram fails to opacify the lateral branches of the coronary sinus. (B) The arrow identifies a coronary sinus dissection during a balloon-occluded venogram.

Cost effectiveness

In the United States, the estimated direct and indirect cost of HF for 2006 will total $29.6 billion. In 2001, $4 billion was paid on behalf of Medicare beneficiaries for HF [1]. Although CRT devices are expensive, the costs of implantation and complications are partially offset by reductions in hospitalizations for HF. COMPANION trial data were analyzed to estimate incremental cost-effectiveness ratios for CRT alone and CRT with an ICD [19]. Over 2 years, follow-up hospitalization costs were reduced by 29% for CRT with an ICD and 37% for CRT alone. Projecting the analysis over 7 years, the incremental cost-effectiveness ratio was $43,000 per quality-adjusted life-years for CRT with an ICD and $19,600 per quality-adjusted life-years for CRT alone. Although by this analysis CRT is below the $50,000 benchmark generally accepted for medical interventions in the United States, the assumptions chosen in cost-effectiveness analysis can influence the results sharply. One study calculated a cost of $107,800 per quality-adjusted life-years for CRT [20]. Although the COMPANION cost-effectiveness analysis did not make calculations based on patient age, the mean age of patients in this study was 67 years. Given the high rate of hospitalizations for HF in elderly patients, CRT may indeed prove cost-effective by reducing hospitalization expenses [2].

Cardiac resynchronization therapy and arrhythmias

Biventricular pacing alone without an ICD decreases mortality [3]. In addition to the hemodynamic and functional benefits described with biventricular pacing, many believe that CRT decreases ventricular arrhythmias also. This reduction is not specific to elderly patients, but would certainly be of benefit to them. Higgins and colleagues [21] hypothesized that biventricular pacing would decrease the need for appropriate therapy in patients with previously implanted ICDs. They reviewed the frequency of therapy in patients, serving as their own controls, who were enrolled in the Ventak CHF biventricular pacing study. Participants had an epicardial LV lead placed by way of thoracotomy. Of the 54 patients enrolled, 32 could be analyzed, with each completing 3 blinded months programmed to biventricular pacing and a second randomly assigned 3-month period of no pacing. These investigators found that of the 32 patients, 13 (41%) received appropriate therapy for ventricular tachycardia at least once in the 6 months of follow-up. Five (16%) had at least one episode while being paced biventricularly, whereas 11 (34%) had at least one episode while programmed to no pacing. This decrease was significant ($P = .035$). The authors concluded that ICD therapy is less common with biventricular pacing. They speculated that the mechanism might be related to hemodynamic improvement, concluding that ICD therapy may be less common when HF is compensated clinically.

Another study evaluated 18 consecutive ICD patients who underwent an upgrade to CRT with an ICD [22]. The mean age of the patients was 69 years old. Medical therapy for HF was not altered during the study. ICD data were studied to determine whether CRT decreases susceptibility to life-threatening arrhythmias. Before CRT, the frequency of ventricular tachycardia, ventricular fibrillation, and appropriate ICD shocks was 0.31 ± 1.23, 0.047 ± 0.083, and 0.048 ± 0.085 episodes per month per patient, respectively. An average of 14 months after CRT, the frequency of ventricular tachycardia, ventricular fibrillation, and appropriate ICD shocks was 0.13 ± 0.56, 0.001 ± 0.004, and 0.003 ± 0.016 episodes per month per patient, respectively ($P = .59$, $.03$, and $.05$ versus pre-CRT). In this small study, CRT decreased tachyarrhythmias and the frequency of ICD therapy, either shock or antitachycardia pacing. In contrast, one case report described the development of torsades de pointes in a patient whenever biventricular or epicardial pacing was used [23]. There remains concern that reversing the direction of the activation of the left ventricular wall by epicardial pacing by way of the coronary sinus may have a pro-arrhythmic effect [24].

Quality of death

In clinical practice, most patients who receive CRT are also candidates for ICD therapy. Combination devices account for more than 80% of CRT implants [25]. In most cases, combination devices are appropriate. ICD implantation can cause various psychological complications, however, including anxiety, depression, fear of ICD firings, and decreased quality of life [26]. Although the ICD can prevent premature death in patients who have HF, ultimately it does not prevent death itself. The ICD converts an acute life-threatening disease into a chronic illness, which can have significant implications for a patient's quality of death [27]. Achieving quality of death suggests minimizing pain, respecting the patient's desires, and preserving the sanctity of life. Compared with deaths because of HF, progressive lung disease, or cancer, arrhythmic deaths can be viewed as rapid and painless. Some patients, particularly elderly patients, may wish to die naturally of cardiac arrhythmias rather than prevent death with ICD therapy only to succumb to a chronic disease.

One study investigated end-of-life issues in ICD patients [28]. Twenty-seven of 100 ICD patients received a shock in the month preceding their deaths, with one third of those receiving a shock within the last minute of life. As a patient's HF or other disease progresses to a life-threatening illness, doctors may wish to discuss end-of-life issues with the patient, including the possibility of ICD deactivation. To preserve quality of death, ICDs should not be implanted in patients who have severe comorbid diseases that limit life expectancy to less than 6 months. With the high frequency of comorbidities in geriatric patients, comorbid diseases should be factored into the decision of whether or not to implant any HF device. Conversely, a biventricular pacemaker without defibrillator capabilities certainly should be considered for palliation of severe HF symptoms.

Case presentation: decision making

Because our 92-year-old patient has an ejection fraction of less than 30%, he would likely benefit from primary prophylaxis of sudden cardiac death by implantation of an ICD. Additionally, because he has class IV HF and a wide QRS complex suggesting intraventricular dyssynchrony, he would likely benefit also from CRT. The risks and benefits of CRT with and without an ICD were discussed with the patient. He is hopeful that CRT will improve his exercise capacity and enable him to resume activities he has been unable to perform, such as playing golf. Although he is elderly, he is fortunate to have no comorbidities other than hypertension and coronary disease. His quality of life is good and he enjoys spending time with his children and grandchildren. After discussions with his doctors and family, he decided to proceed with implantation of a CRT and ICD combination device.

References

[1] Thomas T, Haase N, Rosamond W, et al. Heart disease and stroke statistics—2006 update: a report from the AHA statistics committee and stroke statistics subcommittee. Circulation 2006;113:e85–151.
[2] Jessup M, Brozena S. Heart failure. N Engl J Med 2003;348:2007–18.
[3] Cleland JGF, Daubert JC, Erdmann E, et al. The effect of cardiac resynchronization on morbidity and mortality in heart failure. N Engl J Med 2005;352:1539–49.
[4] Moss AJ, Hall WJ, Cannom DS, et al. Improved survival with an implantable defibrillator in patients with coronary disease at high risk for ventricular arrhythmia. N Engl J Med 1996; 335:1933–40.
[5] Moss AJ, Wojciech Z, Hall WJ, et al. Prophylactic implantation of a defibrillator in patients with myocardial infarction and reduced ejection fraction. N Engl J Med 2002;346:877–83.
[6] Stevenson W, Stevenson L, Middlekauf H, et al. Improving survival for patients with advanced heart failure: a study of 737 consecutive patients. J Am Coll Cardiol 1995;26:1417–23.
[7] Rediker DE, Eagle KA, Homma S, et al. Clinical and hemodynamic comparison of VVI versus DDD pacing in patients with DDD pacemakers. Am J Cardiol 1988;61:323–9.
[8] Abraham WT, Westby GF, Smith AL, et al. Cardiac resynchronization in chronic heart failure. N Engl J Med 2002;346:1845–53.
[9] Young JB, Abraham WT, Smith AL, et al. Combined cardiac resynchronization and implantable cardioversion defibrillation in advanced chronic heart failure: The MIRACLE ICD trial. JAMA 2003;289:2685–94.
[10] Bristow MR, Saxon LA, Boehmer J, et al. Cardiac-resynchronization therapy with or without an implantable defibrillator in advanced chronic heart failure. N Engl J Med 2004;350: 2140–50.
[11] Jais P, Douard H, Shah DC, et al. Endocardial biventricular pacing. Pacing Clin Electrophysiol 1998;21:2128–31.
[12] Bleeker GB, Schalij MJ, Molhoek SG, et al. Comparison of effectiveness of cardiac resynchronization therapy in patients < 70 versus ≥ 70 years of age. Am J Cardiol 2005;96(3): 420–2.

[13] Abraham WT, Fisher WG, Smith AL, et al. Cardiac resynchronization in chronic heart failure. N Engl J Med 2002;346:1845–53.

[14] Bax JJ, Van der Wall EE, Schalij MJ. Correspondence: Cardiac resynchronization therapy for heart failure. N Engl J Med 2002;347:1803.

[15] Aranda JM Jr, Woo GW, Schofield RS, et al. Management of heart failure after cardiac resynchronization therapy: integrating advanced heart failure therapy with optimal device function. J Am Coll Cardiol 2005;46:2193–8.

[16] Bax JJ, Abraham T, Barold SS, et al. Cardiac resynchronization therapy. Part 1—issues before device implantation. J Am Coll Cardiol 2005;46:2153–67.

[17] Díaz-Infante E, Mont L, Leal J, et al. Predictors of lack of response to resynchronization therapy. Am J Cardiol 2005;95:1436–40.

[18] León AR, Abraham WT, Curtis AB, et al. Safety of transvenous cardiac resynchronization system implantation in patients with chronic heart failure: combined results of over 2,000 patients from a multicenter study program. J Am Coll Cardiol 2005;46:2348–56.

[19] Feldman AM, de Lissovoy G, Bristow MR, et al. Cost effectiveness of cardiac resynchronization therapy in the Comparison of Medical Therapy, Pacing, and Defibrillation in Heart Failure (COMPANION) trial. J Am Coll Cardiol 2005;45:2311–21.

[20] Nichol G, Kaul P, Huszti E, et al. Cost-effectiveness of cardiac resynchronization therapy in patients with symptomatic heart failure. Ann Intern Med 2004;141:343–51.

[21] Higgins SL, Yong P, Sheck D, et al. Biventricular pacing diminishes the need for implantable cardioverter defibrillator therapy. Ventak CHF Investigator. J Am Coll Cardiol 2000;36:824–7.

[22] Ermis C, Seutter R, Ahu AX, et al. Impact of upgrade to cardiac resynchronization therapy on ventricular arrhythmia frequency in patients with implantable cardioverter-defibrillators. J Am Coll Cardiol 2005;46:2258–63.

[23] Medina-Ravell VA, Lankipalli RS, Yan GX, et al. Effect of epicardial or biventricular pacing to prolong QT interval and increase transmural dispersion of repolarization. Does resynchronization therapy pose a risk for patients predisposed to long QT or torsade de pointes? Circulation 2003;107:740–6.

[24] Fish JM, Brugada J, Antzelevitch C. Potential proarrhythmic effects of biventricular pacing. J Am Coll Cardiol 2005;46:2340–7.

[25] Saxon LA, Kumar UN, DeMarco T. Cardiac resynchronization therapy (biventricular pacing) in heart failure. Available at: http://www.uptodate.com. 2006. Accessed June 30, 2006.

[26] Sears S, Lewis TS, Kuhl E, et al. Predictors of quality of life in patients with implantable cardioverter defibrillators. Psychosomatics 2005;46:451–7.

[27] Sears SF, Vasquez Sowell L, Kuhl EA, et al. Quality of death: implantable cardioverter defibrillators and proactive care. Pacing Clin Electrophysiol 2006;29:637–42.

[28] Goldstein NE, Lampert R, Bradley E, et al. Management of implantable cardioverter defibrillators in end-of-life care. Ann Intern Med 2004;141:835–8.

CLINICS IN
GERIATRIC
MEDICINE

ELSEVIER
SAUNDERS

Clin Geriatr Med 23 (2007) 205–219

Treatment of Arrhythmias and Use of Implantable Cardioverter-Defibrillators to Improve Survival in Elderly Patients with Cardiac Disease

Ilan Goldenberg, MD*, Arthur J. Moss, MD

Heart Research Follow-up Program, Cardiology Unit, Department of Medicine, Box 653, University of Rochester Medical Center, Rochester, NY 14642, USA

Introduction

Sudden cardiac death (SCD) is responsible for more than 300,000 deaths annually in the United States, overwhelmingly as a result of ventricular fibrillation. The causes of SCD are numerous and vary depending on the age and ethnicity of the population studied. They include hereditary and acquired disorders, such as the congenital or acquired long QT syndromes, Brugada syndrome, arrhythmogenic right ventricular dysplasia, hypertrophic or dilated cardiomyopathies, and most commonly coronary heart disease. The latter condition accounts for more than 80% of cases of SCD, especially in patients 65 years or older [1]. Heart failure (HF) represents an important substrate for malignant ventricular arrhythmias in patients who have coronary artery disease, with both hospitalizations and deaths related to HF having doubled in the past 20 years [2]. The risk for SCD varies between 20% and 30% among patients who have depressed left ventricular (LV) systolic function. Furthermore, the risk for SCD increases in a nearly exponential manner as ejection fraction (EF) decreases to less than 30% [3]. In addition to the severity of LV dysfunction, the degree of functional impairment as evaluated by New York Heart Association (NYHA) functional classification also has been shown to be a powerful independent predictor of SCD [4,5]. Although the absolute SCD number is greatest for patients who have NYHA functional class IV symptoms, this mode of death accounts for

Dr. Arthur J. Moss is a research grant recipient from Guidant Corp.
* Corresponding author.
E-mail address: ilan.goldenberg@heart.rochester.edu (I. Goldenberg).

only 35% of all-cause mortality in this group of patients. Conversely, SCD accounts for 64% of deaths among patients who have compensated NYHA functional class II HF symptoms [5–7]. Patients who have mildly symptomatic (ie, well-compensated) HF thus should not be viewed as being at low risk for SCD.

Currently, HF is the leading admission diagnosis for people older than 65 years of age. It is important therefore to recognize the effectiveness and limitations of current therapies for the management of malignant arrhythmias in the older age group.

Ventricular arrhythmias in elderly patients have traditionally been managed with various pharmacologic agents. Drug absorption, distribution, metabolism, and efficacy are often altered in elderly patients, however, resulting in a substantially narrowed therapeutic window. Moreover, emerging data from recent studies have demonstrated consistently that most antiarrhythmic drugs do not reduce the risk for SCD in adult patients who have acquired heart disease [8–12], whereas several recent studies have shown that device-based therapy with an implantable cardioverter defibrillator (ICD) provides superior protection from malignant arrhythmias for primary and secondary prevention of SCD [13–18]. Most of these studies suggest that the benefits of device-based therapy are conferred to patients independent of age. Furthermore, recent technological advances in transvenous lead design and improved programming flexibility and reduction in device size have increased the usage of device-based therapy for the management of malignant ventricular arrhythmias and prevention of SCD in elderly patients.

In this article we (1) provide a summary of current data regarding pharmacologic management of ventricular arrhythmias, and (2) focus on device therapy for the management of ventricular arrhythmias and prevention of SCD in elderly patients who have HF.

Pharmacologic therapy

Medical therapy with antiarrhythmic drugs has several important limitations in elderly patients. Pharmacokinetic and pharmacodynamic data concerning commonly used cardioactive drugs are limited for patients older than 65 years of age and mostly nonexistent for octogenarians. Available data are often extrapolated from studies performed in younger people who are usually free of multisystem disease. Reduction in gastric motility, renal function, and hepatic blood flow coupled with changes in lean body mass affect volume of distribution and elimination half-life in older patients. In addition, alterations in autonomic balance, receptor density, and baroreceptor response can influence the pharmacodynamics of drugs in the elderly [19]. These factors contribute to a narrowing of the therapeutic–toxic window and can increase the likelihood of adverse drug reactions in older patients. Multisystem disease and the concomitant use of multiple medications can contribute to drug–drug interactions that may limit therapeutic efficacy and increase toxicity of pharmacologic agents for this population. Pharmacologic therapy of cardiac arrhythmias thus can be particularly difficult in elderly individuals.

Data on the effectiveness of antiarrhythmic drugs for the prevention of arrhythmic mortality have shown limited success. The Vaughn-Williams class Ic agents (encainide, flecainide, and moricizine) were tested in the Cardiac Arrhythmia Suppression Trial (CAST). The study was designed to test the hypothesis that suppression of ventricular ectopy after a myocardial infarction (MI) reduces the incidence of SCD. Patients in whom ventricular ectopy could be suppressed with encainide, flecainide, or moricizine were randomly assigned to receive either active drug or placebo. The use of encainide and flecainide was discontinued because of excess mortality. There was an excess of deaths (2.4-fold) attributable to arrhythmia and deaths attributable to shock in patients treated with encainide or flecainide [8]. d-sotalol, a Vaughn-Williams class III pure potassium-channel blocker without clinically significant beta-blocking activity, was tested in a similar population of patients who had EF less than or equal to 40% (mean age 66 years; 99% men) and either a recent (6–42 days) MI or symptomatic HF with a remote (>42 days) MI. The trial was stopped because of excess deaths in the treatment arm. A nearly twofold increase in the risk for arrhythmic death accounted for the increased mortality [9].

Several studies have evaluated the efficacy of another class III agent, amiodarone, with complex pharmacology, including sodium, potassium, calcium, and beta-blocking properties. In the Congestive Heart Failure: Survival Trial of Antiarrhythmic Therapy (CHF-STAT), amiodarone had no effect on survival or SCD despite a significantly better suppression of ventricular arrhythmias compared with placebo [10]. Treatment with amiodarone was associated with a trend to a reduction in mortality risk among nonischemic HF patients enrolled in this trial, and in the Grupo de Estudio de la Sobrevida en la Insuficiencia Cardiaca en Argentina (GESICA) trial [11] that enrolled a substantial proportion of patients who had nonischemic cardiomyopathy. The neutral effect of amiodarone on all-cause mortality and cardiac mortality in survivors of MI who had depressed LV function was further supported by the results of the European and Canadian trials of amiodarone [12,13]. Side effects of amiodarone include thyroid abnormalities, pulmonary toxicity, hepatotoxicity, neuropathy, insomnia, and numerous other reactions. Amiodarone therefore should not be considered as part of the routine treatment of patients who have HF, with or without frequent premature ventricular depolarizations or asymptomatic nonsustained ventricular tachycardia (VT); however, it remains the agent most likely to be safe and effective when antiarrhythmic therapy is necessary to prevent recurrent symptomatic ventricular arrhythmias. The other pharmacologic antiarrhythmic therapies described above rarely are indicated in HF, but may be used occasionally to suppress recurrent ICD shocks when amiodarone has been ineffective or discontinued because of toxicity.

β-blockers have been shown to be effective in reducing the risk for all-cause mortality and arrhythmic death in patients who have chronic HF [20–23]. β-blockers act principally to inhibit the adverse effects of the sympathetic nervous system in patients who have HF, and these effects far outweigh their well-known negative inotropic effects. Three beta-blockers have been shown to be effective in patients who have HF: bisoprolol [20] and sustained-release metoprolol (succinate) [21] that selectively block beta-1 receptors, and carvedilol [22,23] that blocks alpha-1, beta-1, and beta-2 receptors. Patients who have Stage C HF (eg, patients who have structural heart disease with prior or current symptoms of HF) should be treated with one of these three β-blockers [24]. Cardiovascular side effects of β-blockers, including symptomatic bradyarrhythmias, hypotension, lethargy, and weakness, may be more common in elderly patients. Treatment with a β-blocker should be initiated at low doses, followed by gradual increments in dose if lower doses have been well tolerated.

Device therapy in high-risk subsets

The results of prospective controlled trials of ICD therapy for the primary and secondary prevention of SCD are presented in Table 1. The patient populations studied in these studies mostly consisted of relatively young (mean age 55–65 years) white men with NYHA class II and III HF symptoms. Data on the benefit of ICD therapy among older patients, in whom HF may be more severe and comorbidities are more common, are limited and are provided in the following sections.

Secondary prevention

The American College of Cardiology/American Heart Association/North American Society for Pacing and Electrophysiology 2002 guidelines for implantation of cardiac pacemakers and antiarrhythmia devices [25] consider ICD therapy as a Class I indication for patients who experienced the following conditions: (1) cardiac arrest attributable to VT or ventricular fibrillation, not attributable to a transient reversible cause; and (2) spontaneous sustained VT in association with structural heart disease. This indication is mainly based on three prospective controlled secondary-prevention trials [18,26,27].

The Antiarrhythmics Versus Implantable Defibrillators (AVID) trial enrolled 1016 patients who were resuscitated from either ventricular fibrillation, sustained ventricular tachycardia with syncope, or sustained ventricular tachycardia with EF of less than or equal to 40%, and symptoms suggesting severe hemodynamic compromise [18]. Eligible patients were randomized to receive an ICD or treatment with a class III antiarrhythmic drug, primarily amiodarone, at empirically determined doses. The primary end point of this trial was all-cause mortality. The study showed that ICD therapy was superior to antiarrhythmic-drug therapy at 1, 2, and 3 years

Table 1
Randomized trials of implantable cardioverter-defibrillator therapy

Trial	N	Mean age ± SD (years)	Setting	Mortality ICD (%)	Mortality non-ICD (%)	P value
AVID	1016	64 ± 9	Secondary prevention	24	16	.02
CIDS	659	64 ± 10	Secondary prevention, ischemic	30	25	.14
CASH	288	58 ± 11	Secondary prevention, ischemic	44	36	.08
MADIT-I	196	63 ± 9	Primary prevention, ischemic	39	16	.009
MADIT-II	1,232	64 ± 10	Primary prevention, ischemic	20	14	.007
DINAMIT	674	62 ± 11	Primary prevention, ischemic (recent acute MI)	7.5	6.9	.66
CABG-Patch	900	64 ± 9	Primary prevention, ischemic (elective CABG)	21	22	.64
CAT	104	52 ± 10	Primary prevention, nonischemic	31	26	.55
AMIOVERT	103	58 ± 11	Primary prevention, nonischemic	13	12	.80
DEFINITE	450	58	Primary prevention, nonischemic	14	6	.06
SCD-HeFT	2,521	60 (52, 68)*	Primary prevention, nonischemic	29	22	.007

Abbreviations: AMIOVERT, Amiodarone Versus Implantable Cardioverter Defibrillator Randomized Trial; AVID, Antiarrhythmics Versus Implantable Defibrillators; CABG Patch, Coronary Artery Bypass Graft Patch; CASH, Cardiac Arrest Study Hamburg; CAT, Cardiomyopathy Trial; CIDS, Canadian Implantable Defibrillator Study; DEFINITE, DEFibrillator Implantation in Non-Ischemic cardiomyopathy Treatment Evaluation; DiNAMIT, Defibrillator in Acute Myocardial Infarction Trial; ICD, implantable cardioverter-defibrillator; MADIT, Multicenter Automatic Defibrillator Implantation Trial; SCD-HeFT, Sudden Cardiac Death-Heart Failure Trial.

* Age was provided in this study as median (interquartile range).

of follow-up. The mean age of patients enrolled in this trial was 63 ± 9 in the ICD group and 64 ± 9 in the control group. Separate Cox regression analyses were performed for each of the 10 prespecified covariates, including age, NYHA functional class, EF, and presence or absence of diabetes mellitus, and no significant interaction with implanted defibrillator therapy was found (ie, the hazard ratios for patients randomized to ICD therapy versus nondevice therapy were similar among subgroups defined according to the covariates). Treatment with an ICD in this secondary prevention trial therefore seemed to be beneficial regardless of age or additional comorbidities. Similar results have been reported in two small, randomized trials—the Canadian Implantable Defibrillator Study (CIDS) (mean age 64 ± 10 years) [28] and the Cardiac Arrest Study Hamburg (CASH) [17]. In a subanalysis of the CIDS trial, only three variables were significant predictors of all-cause mortality in the amiodarone-treated patients. These included age greater than 70 years (*P* = .0005), decreasing EF (*P* = .0001), and NYHA functional class III or IV (*P* = .0009). When study patients were stratified into four risk quartiles by the three risk factors, the benefit of ICD therapy was significant only in the highest risk quartile (relative risk reduction 50% [95% CI, 21% to 68%]. These results suggest that secondary prevention with ICD is highly effective in patients who have multiple risk factors, including advancing age. Patients included in the CASH trial were relatively younger (mean age 58 ± 11 years); no interaction was shown among subgroups analyzed in the trial, including age, suggesting similar ICD efficacy in older patients [27].

Pooled data from these three secondary prevention trials [29] indicate that the benefit of ICD versus amiodarone therapy was consistent, with an overall 28% reduction in the relative risk for death with the ICD that is attributable almost entirely to a 50% reduction in arrhythmic mortality.

A recent large retrospective observational study of more than 6900 patients admitted to Veteran's Administration hospitals that evaluated the efficacy of ICD therapy (n = 1442) versus medical management alone among patients who had new-onset ventricular arrhythmias (ventricular tachycardia, fibrillation, or cardiac arrest) and known ischemic heart disease [30] showed that ICD treatment significantly lowered all-cause mortality (odds ratio 0.52 [95% CI, 0.45–0.60]) at 3-year follow-up. When the entire cohort was stratified on age (≥ 70 years, <70 years), multivariate regression analysis for 3-year all-cause mortality gave an odds ratio of 0.54 (95% CI, 0.44 to 0.67) for age greater than or equal to 70 years and 0.46 (95% CI, 0.38–0.55) for age less than 70 years. Because the mortality risk was higher in the 70 years or older group (58.1% versus 44.2%), patients in the older age group derived a relatively greater benefit.

In all secondary prevention studies little advantage for ICD therapy over drug therapy was observed in patients who had EF greater than 35% [29]. Electrophysiologic studies (EP), performed after resuscitation, are insensitive predictors of risk for recurrent life-threatening arrhythmias during long-term follow-up.

Primary prevention

Several randomized clinical trials have evaluated ICD treatment for primary prevention of SCD among patients who had impaired LV systolic function because of underlying ischemic heart disease. The first Multicenter Automatic Defibrillator Implantation Trial (MADIT-I) randomized 196 patients who had coronary artery disease, spontaneous nonsustained ventricular tachycardia during EP testing, EF less than or equal to 35%, and inducible ventricular tachycardia that was not suppressed during intravenous procainamide administration to an ICD or conventional medical therapy [17]. The ICD resulted in a significant reduction in overall mortality (Table 1). The mean age of study patients in the first MADIT study was 63 ± 9 years. Separate Cox regression analyses revealed no evidence that any of the 11 preselected baseline variables, including age, had a meaningful influence on the hazard ratio ($P > .2$ for all interactions).

The Multicenter Unsustained Tachycardia Trial (MUSTT) enrolled a patient population similar to that of the MADIT I trial and evaluated the efficacy of EP-guided antiarrhythmic therapy. Patients who had inducible ventricular tachycardia on EP testing (n = 704) were assigned to receive either conventional medical therapy or antiarrhythmic therapy as guided by serial EP testing [16]. Individuals could receive an ICD without randomization (n = 161) if one or more drug trials showed inadequate arrhythmia suppression. At 5-year follow-up, all-cause mortality was 24% in the ICD group, 55% for patients who received EP-guided antiarrhythmic therapy, and 48% in patients who did not receive any antiarrhythmic treatment (P <.001) [16]. The median age of patients allocated to EP-guided therapy was 66 (interquartile range: 60–72) years. After adjustment for baseline clinical risk factors, including age, ICD therapy was associated with a significant 55% reduction in the risk for death compared with non-ICD therapy.

The Multicenter Automatic Defibrillator Implantation Trial-II (MADIT-II) enrolled 1232 patients (mean age 64 ± 10 years) with ischemic cardiomyopathy and an EF less than or equal to 30%. No documentation of spontaneous or inducible arrhythmias was required for enrollment [15]. Antiarrhythmic therapy was prescribed in less than 20% of both groups. During an average follow-up of 20 months, all-cause mortality was 20% in the control group versus 14% in the defibrillator group [15]. The hazard ratio for death in the ICD group was 0.69 (95% CI, 0.51–0.93, P = .016). There were no significant differences in the effect of defibrillator therapy on survival in subgroup analyses stratified according to age, sex, EF, NYHA class, or the QRS interval.

A recent meta-analysis of all major primary prevention SCD trials showed a significant benefit in favor of ICD placement with a risk reduction for all-cause mortality of 34% (P = .03), which was independent of age [31]. Current practice guidelines support ICD implantation as a primary prevention strategy in patients who have a prior MI and an EF less than 30% [25].

Several recent trials have studied the role of ICDs for the primary prevention of SCD in patients who have nonischemic cardiomyopathy [32–35]. The Cardiomyopathy Trial (CAT) enrolled 104 relatively young patients (mean age 52 ± 10) who had recent onset of nonischemic dilated cardiomyopathy (<9 months) and an EF less than or equal to 30% [32]. Patients were assigned to either ICD implantation or conventional therapy. The primary endpoint was all-cause mortality at 1 year of follow-up. No significant difference in survival was noted among patients undergoing ICD implantation compared with control patients. The study was underpowered, however, because of a low event rate in the control group [32]. Similarly, the Amiodarone Versus Implantable Cardioverter Defibrillator Trial (AMIOVIRT) showed no improvement in survival or arrhythmia-free survival with ICD therapy compared with amiodarone treatment in 103 patients (mean age 58 ± 11) who had nonischemic dilated cardiomyopathy, EF less than or equal to 35%, and asymptomatic nonsustained ventricular tachycardia

[33]. The Defibrillators in Non-Ischemic Cardiomyopathy Treatment Evaluation (DEFINITE) trial randomized 458 subjects (mean age 58 years, 71% men) who had nonischemic dilated cardiomyopathy, EF less than 36%, and more than 10 premature ventricular complexes per hour or nonsustained ventricular tachycardia on 24-hour ambulatory monitoring, to receive standard medical therapy alone or in combination with a single-chamber ICD [34]. All patients had NYHA functional class II or higher HF symptoms within 6 months of randomization. Both arms of the study received optimal medical therapy, including β-blockers, angiotensin-converting enzyme inhibitors, and angiotensin-II receptor blockers, with little use of antiarrhythmic medications. Defibrillator therapy resulted in a significant reduction in SCD from arrhythmia, but the beneficial impact of device therapy on all-cause mortality did not reach statistical significance [34]. Although the study was not powered for subgroup analysis, patients older than 65 years ($n = 157$) derived a mortality benefit.

The recently completed Sudden Cardiac Death in Heart Failure Trial (SCD-HeFT) was a three-armed study that randomized 2521 patients who had left ventricular ejection fractions less than 35% (median age 60.4 years, interquartile range 51.7–68.3 years), ischemic (52%) or nonischemic (48%) cardiomyopathy, and NYHA functional class II (70%) or III (30%) HF symptoms, to conventional pharmacologic therapy alone or in combination with either amiodarone or a single-lead ICD [35]. Median follow-up averaged 45.5 months. The SCD-HeFT trial showed a significant 33% reduction in total mortality in the ICD group. Amiodarone therapy failed to improve survival. The survival benefit was similar in magnitude between ischemic and nonischemic patients. No interaction between age and ICD benefit was shown in this study: the hazard ratio for ICD versus placebo among patients 65 years or older was 0.86 (95% CI, 0.62–1.18) and the hazard ratio among patients younger than 65 years was 0.68 (95% CI, 0.50–0.93). The findings of DEFINITE and SCD-HeFT are likely to result in a change in current recommendation for ICD implantation, favoring more widespread use of ICDs in the nonischemic HF population who have EF less than 35%.

Primary ICD therapy was not shown to be effective in patients who had LV dysfunction scheduled for elective coronary bypass surgery [36] or in patients who had recently suffered an MI (6–40 days after MI) [37]. In addition, ICD therapy is not recommended for patients who have advanced HF symptoms (NYHA functional class IV) who remain refractory to optimal medical therapy.

Primary prevention with ICDs in age subsets and by risk groups: analysis of data from MADIT-II

Because of the relative paucity of data regarding ICD efficacy in elderly patients, we performed a retrospective analysis of the MADIT-II trial in which ICD benefit was assessed within prespecified age groups ($<$65 years, 65–74 years, and $\geq$75 years). The Cox proportional-hazards regression model was used to evaluate the independent contribution of baseline clinical factors within age groups to the endpoints of all-cause mortality and SCD; the probability of death by treatment group within each age group was estimated and graphically displayed according to the method of Kaplan and Meier, with comparison of cumulative events by the log-rank test.

Baseline laboratory and clinical characteristics of study patients in the prespecified age categories are shown in Table 2. Increasing age among patients enrolled in MADIT-II was associated with an increasing proportion of abnormal parameters of renal function, including higher serum creatinine and blood urea nitrogen serum levels, and a significantly higher proportion

Table 2
Characteristics of MADIT-II patients by age groups

Characteristic	Age group (years)		
	$<$65 (n = 574)	65–74 (n = 455)	$\geq$75 (n = 204)
Estimated glomerular filtration rate (mL/min/1.73 m^2)	79 ± 25	66 ± 23	59 ± 22*
eGFR$<$30 (%)	3	8	13*
Creatinine (mg/dL)	1.1 ± 0.4	1.3 ± 0.6	1.4 ± 0.5*
Blood urea nitrogen (mg/dL)	20 ± 10	26 ± 13	29 ± 14*
Female gender (%)	16	15	15
New York Heart Association functional class $\geq$2[a] (%)	62	66	63
Angina pectoris functional class $\geq$2[a] (%)	71	72	76
Hypertension (%)	50	60	49*
Diabetes (%)	35	40	25*
Past coronary artery bypass graft surgery (%)	54	61	59*
Left bundle branch block (%)	12	23	26*
QRS duration, msec	11 ± 3	13 ± 3	13 ± 4*
Ejection fraction $<$25 (%)	67	68	68
Systolic blood pressure (mm Hg)	119 ± 18	123 ± 19	125 ± 18*
Heart rate per ECG $\geq$80 beats per minute (%)	26	35	33
Medical therapy			
Angiotensin-converting enzyme inhibitors (%)	81	75	73*
β-blockers (%)	69	60	50*
Amiodarone (%)	6	8	8
Lipid-lowering agents[b] (%)	73	64	52*
Diuretics	70	79	78*

Values are means ± SD or percentages.

[a] New York Heart Association and angina pectoris functional class represent highest class during the 3 months before enrollment.

[b] Statins composed 95% of lipid-lowering agents.

* P value for difference among three groups $<$.05.

Table 3
Adjusted risk for all-cause mortality and sudden cardiac death in the conventional therapy group

| Variable | Age group (years) | | | |
	<65	65–74 HR (95% CI)	≥75 HR (95% CI)	P for trend
All-cause mortality*	1	2.06 (1.29–3.28)	2.94 (1.70–5.14)	<.001
SCD**	1	2.46 (1.21–5.05)	2.61 (1.06–6.47)	.01

Abbreviation: SCD, sudden cardiac death.

* Findings were adjusted for the additional covariates: age, NYHA functional class, smoking, ejection fraction, diabetes mellitus, diastolic blood pressure, heart rate, body mass index, eGFR, and treatment with beta-blockers.

** Findings were adjusted for the additional covariates: age, EF, diastolic blood pressure, eGFR, and heart rate.

of patients who had severe renal failure as defined by estimated glomerular filtration rate (eGFR) less than 30 mL per minute per 1.73 m^2. Medical therapy with angiotensin-converting enzyme inhibitors and β-blockers was administered less frequently to older patients compared with the younger age group.

In multivariate analysis, non-ICD–treated patients in the age groups of 65 to 74 years and 75 years and older had a respective twofold and threefold increase in the risk for all-cause mortality (P <.001) and a respective 2.5-fold and 2.6-fold increase in the risk for SCD (P = .01) compared with patients younger than 65 years (Table 3).

Defibrillator therapy was independently associated with a significant overall 32% reduction in the risk for all-cause mortality and a 68% reduction in the risk for SCD. The analysis of the efficacy of ICD therapy within the prespecified age groups (Table 4) did not demonstrate a significant

Table 4
Efficacy of defibrillator therapy for all–cause mortality and sudden cardiac death within age groups

| | Endpoint: all-cause mortality* | | Endpoint: sudden cardiac death[†] | |
	HR (95% CI)	P value	HR (95% CI)	P value
Total population (n = 1223)	0.68 (0.51–0.90)	.006	0.32 (0.18–0.55)	<.001
Age group (years)				
<65 (n = 574)	0.79 (0.48–1.29)	.35	0.32 (0.12–0.84)	.02
65–74 (n = 455)	0.63 (0.41–0.95)[‡]	.03	0.35 (0.17–0.73)[§]	.005
≥75 (n = 204)	0.70 (0.41–1.20)[‡]	.20	0.32 (0.10–1.00)[§]	.05

* The hazard ratio is the risk of death with ICD versus convention medical therapy after adjustment for age, NYHA functional class, smoking, ejection fraction, diabetes mellitus, diastolic blood pressure, heart rate, body mass index, eGFR, and β-blockers.

[†] Adjusted for age, EF, diastolic blood pressure, eGFR, and heart rate.

[‡] p-value for interaction = 0.75.

[§] p-value for interaction = 0.74.

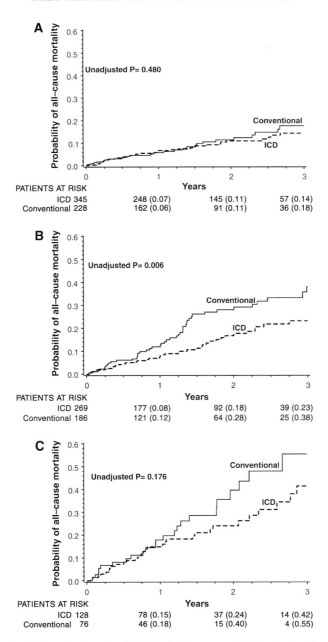

Fig. 1. Kaplan-Meier estimates of probability of all-cause mortality by treatment group within patient age ranges of (*A*) less than 65 years, (*B*) 65 to 74 years, and (*C*) 75 years or older.

interaction effect, suggesting that ICD is effective in all age categories. The reduction in the risk for SCD with ICD therapy was similar in patients 65 to 74 and greater than or equal to 75 years old (65% and 68%, respectively). The benefit of ICD therapy for the endpoint of all-cause mortality, however, was most prominent among patients 65 to 74 years old (37% reduction, $P = .03$), intermediate among older patients (30% reduction, $P = .20$), and lowest in the younger age group (21% reduction, $P = .35$). Accordingly, Kaplan-Meier estimates of the probability of death (Fig. 1, A–C) showed that the cumulative probability of death at 2 years was significantly lower in the ICD group compared with the conventional therapy group among patients in the age range of 65 to 74 years (see Fig. 1B), a trend to lower 2-year mortality rates with ICD therapy was shown in patients greater than or equal to 75 years (see Fig. 1C), and similar mortality rates in the ICD and conventional therapy groups were observed in patients less than 65 years of age (see Fig. 1A).

The overall beneficial effects of primary ICD implantation in the older age groups in the current analysis, however, should be interpreted with caution, because these patients exhibited a higher proportion of comorbidities, including a significantly higher frequency of advanced renal dysfunction. Recent data from MADIT-II show that the efficacy of defibrillator is attenuated with declining renal function and is no longer evident among patients who have advanced renal dysfunction [38]. Notably, the proportion of patients who have severe renal disease as defined by eGFR less than 30 mL per minute per 1.73 m^2 increased more than fourfold in the older age group (Table 2). It is possible that among this subset of elderly patients who have significant renal disease ICD therapy is not associated with a significant survival benefit.

Summary

Medical therapy with antiarrhythmic drugs has not been shown to reduce mortality in patients who have LV dysfunction. Implantation of an ICD is the only mode of therapy that has been shown to be effective for the primary and secondary prevention of arrhythmic mortality in cardiac patients who have compromised LV function. Prospective randomized trials of ICD therapy enrolled mostly younger patients who had a mean age less than 65 years. Nevertheless, subanalyses of these studies did not show a significant interaction between age and ICD efficacy, suggesting that the benefit of defibrillator therapy is maintained in older patients. Moreover, the current analysis of the MADIT-II study suggests that the benefit of ICD therapy may be even more pronounced among patients older than 65 years (mainly in the 65–74 age range) compared with younger patients.

Despite these findings regarding the beneficial effects of defibrillator therapy in older patients, caution should be exhibited when extrapolating data from prospective ICD trials because the number of elderly patients randomized to ICD or medical therapy was limited. Furthermore, advanced comorbidities that are common in the older age groups may attenuate the survival benefit of ICD therapy. The growing number of elderly patients who have LV dysfunction and HF warrants a prospective randomized ICD trial in this population.

References

[1] American Heart Association. Heart disease and stroke statistics—2004 update. Dallas, TX: American Heart Association; 2003.

[2] Schulman SP. Cardiovascular consequences of the aging process. Cardiol Clin 1999;17: 35–49.

[3] Echt DS, Liebson PR, Mitchell LB, et al. Mortality and morbidity in patients receiving encainide, flecainide, or placebo. N Engl J Med 1991;324:781–8.

[4] The Multicentre Postinfarction Research Group. Risk stratification and survival after myocardial infarction. N Engl J Med 1983;309:331–6.

[5] The MERIT-HF Investigators. Effect of metoprolol CR/XL in chronic heart failure Metoprolol CR/XL Randomised Intervention Trial in Congestive Heart Failure (MERIT-HF). Lancet 1999;353:2001–7.

[6] Bigger JT Jr, Fleiss JL, Kleiger R, et al. The relationships among ventricular arrhythmias, left ventricular dysfunction, and mortality in the 2 years after myocardial infarction. Circulation 1984;69:250–8.

[7] Luu M, Stevenson WG, Stevenson LW, et al. Diverse mechanisms of unexpected cardiac arrest in advanced heart failure. Circulation 1989;80:1675–80.

[8] Huikuri HV, Castellanos A, Myerburg RJ. Sudden death due to cardiac arrhythmias. N Engl J Med 2001;345:1473–82.

[9] Waldo AL, Camm AJ, deRuyter H, et al. Effect of d-sotalol on mortality in patients with left ventricular dysfunction after recent and remote myocardial infarction. Lancet 1996;348: 7–12.

[10] Singh SN, Fletcher RD, Fisher SG, et al. Amiodarone in patients with congestive heart failure and asymptomatic ventricular arrhythmia. N Engl J Med 1995;333:77–82.

[11] Doval HC, Nul DR, Grancelli HO, et al. Randomized trial of low-dose amiodarone in severe congestive heart failure. Grupo de Estudio de la Sobrevida en la Insuficiencia Cardiaca en Argentina (GESICA). Lancet 1994;344:493–8.

[12] Julian DG, Camm AJ, Frangin G, et al. Randomised trial of effect of amiodarone on mortality in patients with left-ventricular dysfunction after recent myocardial infarction: EMIAT. Lancet 1997;349:667–74.

[13] Cairns JA, Connolly SJ, Roberts R, et al. Randomised trial of outcome after myocardial infarction in patients with frequent or repetitive premature depolarisations: CAMIAT. Lancet 1997;349:675–82.

[14] Bardy GH, Lee KL, Mark DB, et al. Sudden cardiac Death in Heart Failure Trial (SCD-HeFT) Investigators. Amiodarone or an implantable cardioverter-defibrillator for congestive heart failure. N Engl J Med 2005;352:225–37.

[15] Moss AJ, Zareba W, Hall WJ, et al. Multicenter Automatic Defibrillator Implantation Trial II Investigators. Prophylactic implantation of a defibrillator in patients with myocardial infarction and reduced ejection fraction. N Engl J Med 2002;346:877–83.

[16] Buxton AE, Lee KL, Fisher JD, et al. A randomized study of the prevention of sudden death in patients with coronary artery disease. Multicenter Unsustained Tachycardia Trial Investigators. N Engl J Med 1999;341:1882–90.

[17] Moss AJ, Hall WJ, Cannom DS, et al. Improved survival with an implanted defibrillator in patients with coronary disease at high risk for ventricular arrhythmia. Multicenter Automatic Defibrillator Implantation Trial Investigators. N Engl J Med 1996;335:1933–40.

[18] A comparison of antiarrhythmic-drug therapy with implantable defibrillators in patients resuscitated from near-fatal ventricular arrhythmias. The Antiarrhythmics versus Implantable Defibrillators (AVID) Investigators. N Engl J Med 1997;337:1576–83.

[19] Podrazik PM, Schwartz JB. Cardiovascular pharmacology of aging. Cardiol Clin 1999;17: 17–34.

[20] The Cardiac Insufficiency Bisoprolol Study II (CIBIS-II): a randomised trial. Lancet 1999; 353:9–13.

[21] Hjalmarson A, Goldstein S, Fagerberg B, et al. MERIT-HF Study Group. Effects of controlled-release metoprolol on total mortality, hospitalizations, and well-being in patients with heart failure: the Metoprolol CR/XL Randomized Intervention Trial in congestive heart failure (MERIT-HF). JAMA 2000;283:1295–302.

[22] Dargie HJ. Effect of carvedilol on outcome after myocardial infarction in patients with left-ventricular dysfunction; the CAPRICORN randomised trial. Lancet 2001;357: 1385–90.

[23] Cleland JG, Pennell DJ, Ray SG, et al. Myocardial viability as a determinant of the ejection fraction response to carvedilol in patients with heart failure (CHRISTMAS trial) randomised controlled trial. Lancet 2003;362:14–21.

[24] Abraham WT, Chin MH, Feldman AM, et al. Chronic heart failure in the adult: ACC/AHA 2005 Guideline update for the diagnosis and management of heart failure in the adult. J Am Coll Cardiol 2005;46:1116–43.

[25] Gregoratos G, Abrams J, Epstein AE, et al. ACC/AHA/NASPE 2002 guideline update for implantation of cardiac pacemakers and antiarrhythmia devices: summary article: a report of the American College of Cardiology/American Heart Association Task Force on Practice Guidelines (ACC/AHA/NASPE Committee to Update the 1998 Pacemaker Guidelines). Circulation 2002;106:2145–61.

[26] Connolly SJ, Gent M, Roberts RS, et al. Canadian Implantable Defibrillator Study (CIDS) a randomized trial of the implantable cardioverter defibrillator against amiodarone. Circulation 2000;101:1297–302.

[27] Siebels J, Cappato R, Ruppel R, et al. Investigators CASH. Preliminary results of the Cardiac Arrest Study Hamburg (CASH). Am J Cardiol 1993;72:109F–13F.

[28] Sheldon R, Connolly S, Krahn A, et al. Identification of patients most likely to benefit from implantable cardioverter-defibrillator therapy: the Canadian Implantable Defibrillator Study. Circulation 2000;101:1660–4.

[29] Connolly SJ, Hallstrom AP, Cappato R, et al. Meta-analysis of the implantable cardioverter defibrillator secondary prevention trials. AVID, CASH and CIDS studies. Antiarrhythmics vs Implantable Defibrillator study. Cardiac Arrest Study Hamburg. Canadian Implantable Defibrillator Study. Eur Heart J 2000;21:2071–8.

[30] Chan PS, Hayward RA. Mortality reduction by implantable cardioverter-defibrillators in high-risk patients with heart failure, ischemic heart disease, and new-onset ventricular arrhythmia an effectiveness study. J Am Coll Cardiol 2005;45:1474–81.

[31] Lee DS, Green LD, Liu PP. Effectiveness of implantable defibrillators for preventing arrhythmic events and death a meta-analysis. J Am Coll Cardiol 2003;41:573–82.

[32] Bansch D, Antz M, Boczor S, et al. Primary prevention of sudden cardiac death in idiopathic dilated cardiomyopathy the Cardiomyopathy Trial (CAT). Circulation 2002;105: 1453–8.

[33] Strickberger A, Hummel JD, Bartlett TG, et al. Amiodarone versus implantable cardioverter-defibrillator randomized trial in patients with nonischemic dilated cardiomyopathy and asymptomatic nonsustained ventricular tachycardia—AMIOVIRT. J Am Coll Cardiol 2003;41:1707–12.

[34] Kadish A, Dyer A, Daubert JP, et al. Prophylactic defibrillator implantation in patients with nonischemic dilated cardiomyopathy. N Engl J Med 2004;350:2151–8.

[35] Bardy GH, Lee KL, Mark DB, et al. Amiodarone or an implantable cardioverter-defibrillator for congestive heart failure. N Engl J Med 2005;352:225–37.

[36] Bigger T Jr. Coronary Artery Bypass Graft (CABG) Patch Trial Investigators. Prophylactic use of implanted cardiac defibrillators in patients at high risk for ventricular arrhythmias after coronary-artery bypass graft surgery. N Engl J Med 1997;337:1569–75.

[37] Hohnloser SH, Kuck KH, Dorian P, et al. Prophylactic use of an implantable cardioverter-defibrillator after acute myocardial infarction. N Engl J Med 2004;351:2481–8.

[38] Goldenberg I, Moss AJ, McNitt S, et al. for the Multicenter Automatic Defibrillator Implantation Trial-II Investigators. Relationship between renal function, risk of sudden cardiac death, and benefit of the implanted cardiac defibrillator in post-myocardial infarction patients with left ventricular dysfunction. Am J Cardiol 2006;98:485–90.

ELSEVIER
SAUNDERS

CLINICS IN
GERIATRIC
MEDICINE

Clin Geriatr Med 23 (2007) 221–234

Exercise Therapy for Elderly Heart Failure Patients

Jerome L. Fleg, MD

Division of Cardiovascular Diseases, National Heart, Lung, and Blood Institute,
6701 Rockledge Drive, Room 8126, Bethesda, MD 20892-7936, USA

Low aerobic capacity: hallmark of both normal aging and heart failure

Both the normative aging process and heart failure (HF) are character-ized by a reduced aerobic exercise capacity, best quantified by peak oxygen consumption (VO_2). Multiple cross-sectional studies have shown declines in peak VO_2 of 8% to 10% per decade in apparently healthy populations (Fig. 1) [1–4]. Peak VO_2 typically declines from approximately 45 mL/kg/min in a healthy 25-year-old man to approximately 25 mL/kg/min in a 75-year-old (see Fig. 1). Comparable values in women are approximately 20% lower because of their smaller proportion of muscle mass and lower hemoglo-bin levels. Of note, a healthy 80-year-old woman typically has a peak VO_2 of 15 to 20 mL/kg/min, a range characteristic of mild HF. Furthermore, these cross-sectional studies represent a best-case scenario because healthy older adults are a highly selected group. Elderly individuals often have comorbidities, such as arthritis, orthopedic or neurologic disorders, pulmonary disease, and coronary or peripheral arterial disease, that further impair aerobic capacity. In addition, recent data suggest that longitudinal age-associated declines in peak VO_2 in healthy volunteers accelerate with age, exceeding 20% per decade after age 70 (see Fig. 1) [5].

Peak VO_2 is the product of cardiac output (CO) and arteriovenous oxy-gen (AVO_2) difference. Data from the Baltimore Longitudinal Study of Ag-ing indicate that declines in peak heart rate (HR) and AVO_2 difference make similar contributions to the decline in peak VO_2 with aging [6]. In contrast, exercise stroke volume (SV) is not age related among individuals screened for the absence of coronary heart disease by clinical criteria and exercise thallium scintigraphy; enhanced use of the Frank–Starling mechanism to augment left ventricular end-diastolic volume (LVEDV) compensates for

E-mail address: flegj@nhlbi.nih.gov

0749-0690/07/$ - see front matter. Published by Elsevier Inc.
doi:10.1016/j.cger.2006.08.011   *geriatric.theclinics.com*

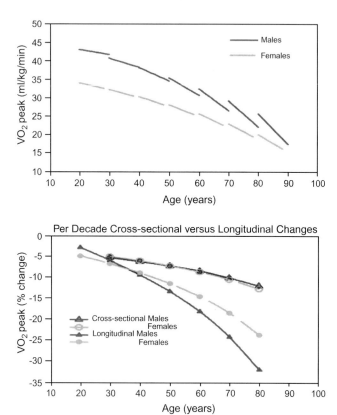

Fig. 1. Cross-sectional and longitudinal changes in peak VO_2 per kg weight in healthy adults by age decade and gender. (*Top panel*) The per-decade longitudinal change in peak VO_2 for age decades from the 20s through the 70s, predicted from a mixed-effects regression model. Peak VO_2 declines more steeply with successive age decades, especially in men. (*Bottom panel*) Per-decade percent cross-sectional and longitudinal changes in peak VO_2 by age decade and gender, derived from the mixed-effects model. From the 50s onward, longitudinal declines in peak VO_2 substantially exceed cross-sectional declines. (*From* Fleg JL, Morrell CH, Bos AG, et al. Accelerated longitudinal decline of aerobic capacity in healthy older adults. Circulation 2005;12:674–82.)

a modest blunting of systolic emptying with age [7]. Plasma catecholamines are increased with age at peak exercise [8]. This exercise hemodynamic profile of normal aging resembles that of beta adrenergic blockade of a young adult [9].

An impaired peak VO_2 is characteristic of patients who have HF and is a strong predictor of survival and the need for cardiac transplantation [10–12]. The impairment in peak VO_2 in these patients is attributable to cardiac and peripheral factors; peak HR and SV are reduced about 20% and 45%, respectively, in patients who have systolic HF compared with normal individuals [13,14]. Peripheral factors contributing to reduced AVO_2 difference, and thence peak VO_2, include reduced muscle mass, decreased mitochondrial density in exercising muscle, and peripheral vasoconstriction because of intrinsic abnormalities of smooth muscle vasodilation and neurohormonal factors [15,16]. A similar constellation of peripheral abnormalities contributes to the age-associated decrease in AVO_2 difference at peak exercise (Table 1) [17]. In patients who have HF and preserved systolic function, so-called "diastolic HF," peak VO_2 is reduced to nearly the same degree as in patients who have systolic HF [18]. The reduction in SV, however, is primarily because of a failure to use the Frank–Starling mechanism to enhance LVEDV rather than a deficiency of systolic emptying [19].

Do older people who do not have heart failure respond to aerobic training like younger adults?

Early studies suggested that aerobic capacity could not be augmented by exercise training in healthy older adults. Multiple subsequent investigations have documented 10% to 25% increases in peak VO_2 in previously sedentary people through the ninth decade—comparable to those seen in young adults [20–23]. These improvements in peak VO_2 are mediated by enhanced AVO_2 difference and augmented SV secondary to a larger LVEDV; maximal HR is unaffected by exercise training in healthy older adults.

Salutary responses to aerobic training also have been shown convincingly in older coronary patients. In nonrandomized clinical studies of patients participating in traditional cardiac rehabilitation programs after a coronary event, men and women older than 70 years of age have derived relative improvements in exercise capacity and reduction of coronary risk factors similar to those in younger patients [24–27]. For example, in 60 patients aged 65 ± 5 years who underwent 3 months of training beginning 8 weeks after myocardial infarction or coronary revascularization, Ades and colleagues [26] noted a 16% increase in peak VO_2. The augmentation in peak VO_2 was entirely attributable to increased AVO_2 difference, similar to the training response in younger coronary patients.

Table 1
Physiologic similarities between normative aging and heart failure

	Aging*	Heart failure
Peak VO_2	↓↓	↓↓↓
Maximal stroke volume	↔ or ↓	↓↓
Maximal heart rate	↓↓	↓
Maximal AV oxygen difference	↓↓	↓↓
Skeletal muscle mass	↓↓	↓↓
Mitochondrial oxidative enzymes	↓	↓↓↓

* Between the third and ninth decades.

From Fleg JL. Can exercise conditioning be effective in older heart failure patients? Heart Failure Rev 2002;7:99–103.

Exercise training in patients who have heart failure: state of the evidence

Before focusing specifically on the role of exercise training in elderly patients who have HF, it may be useful to review the evidence in the general HF population. Although patients who have clinical HF have been excluded systemically from traditional cardiac rehabilitation programs, multiple studies over the past decade have demonstrated that aerobic exercise training is effective and safe in patients with HF. Among such patients who were receiving diuretics, converting enzyme inhibitors, and digitalis at baseline, randomized trials have demonstrated increases in peak VO_2 of 12% to 33% [28,29]. The limited data available in patients on beta blockers suggest similar training-induced improvements in aerobic capacity [30]. Increased AVO_2 difference is the primary contributor to the training-induced augmentation of peak VO_2 in patients who have HF, with modest increases in cardiac output also observed in some studies [31]. Parallel improvement in ventilatory or lactate threshold typically has been observed, along with lower HR and lactate levels at fixed submaximal workloads. These physiologic changes translate into improved exercise tolerance with fewer symptoms—both highly relevant clinical outcomes. Although early concerns were raised that aerobic training might exacerbate adverse LV remodeling, especially in coronary patients who have pre-existing wall motion abnormalities [32], many subsequent investigations have shown no deterioration in LV structure or resting function after training.

Much of the benefit of aerobic exercise training in patients who have HF is mediated by improvement in peripheral blood flow and skeletal muscle morphology and function. Increases in peak leg blood flow and oxygen delivery and reduced leg vascular resistance have been demonstrated [33]. Training also augments the blunted endothelium-mediated flow-dependent vasodilation seen in patients who have HF [34,35]. Several investigations have documented decreases in muscle acidosis and phosphocreatine depletion during localized limb exercise plus accelerated adenosine triphosphate resynthesis after exercise cessation post-training [36–38]. Increases of approximately 20% in mitochondrial volume density and 41% in cytochrome C oxidase–positive mitochondria were observed after 6 months of aerobic training; these increases correlated with improvements in exercise tolerance [39].

Aerobic training also elicits favorable alterations in autonomic function and neurohormonal profile in HF. The increased resting plasma levels of vasopressin, atrial natriuretic peptides, angiotensin, and aldosterone characteristic of HF are reduced after training [40]. Decreases in norepinephrine spillover are accompanied by a parallel reduction in low-frequency heart rate variability and reciprocal increases in high-frequency peaks, consistent with enhanced vagal tone [41].

Although no published studies of exercise training in HF have been adequately powered to detect an effect on clinical events or survival, Belardinelli and colleagues [42] observed reduced rates of hospital admissions and cardiac mortality in patients randomized to 14 months of supervised aerobic training compared with controls. Some of the reduction in events by training in this primarily ischemic sample may have been mediated by improved myocardial perfusion, observed in 75% of trained patients but only 2% of controls.

Aerobic exercise training in elderly patients who have heart failure: clinical trial evidence

Although multiple clinical trials have demonstrated favorable effects of aerobic exercise training in HF, most such trials have enrolled predominantly younger patients. A similar age bias has been observed in non-exercise HF trials [43]. Nevertheless, the advanced age typical of patients who have HF in the general community makes it imperative to extract data specific to the elderly from the literature of HF training studies. In a 1998 review of randomized exercise training trials in HF, only 2 of 14 trials had a mean patient age greater than 65 years [44]. A more recent review of 29 such trials in 2004 revealed only 4 with a mean age greater than 65 years [45]. Furthermore, 11 of these 29 trials included only men and another 11 enrolled less than 25% women. Clearly, more data for elderly HF patients are needed.

In the few exercise training trials that have included meaningful numbers of older patients who have HF, results have been generally favorable (Table 2). Willenheimer and coworkers [46] randomized 54 patients of mean age 64 years to 4 months of supervised cycle ergometry or a control group; an improved quality of life but no significant changes in peak VO_2 or the dyspnea–fatigue index were found in those who trained. In 67 men with New York Heart Association (NYHA) class 2 or 3 HF and LVEF less than 40% who underwent 12 weeks of aerobic training, Wielenga and colleagues [47] observed similar increases in peak VO_2 and exercise duration in patients younger versus those older than 65 years; however, the change in peak VO_2 was not statistically significant in either group. In a study of 33 older HF patients, Gottlieb and coworkers [48] observed that 6 of 17 patients randomized to a 6-month aerobic training program did not tolerate exercise training; in the remaining 11 patients, both peak VO_2 and 6-minute walk distance increased significantly, but neither daily energy expenditure nor perceived quality of life improved. In 22 patients aged 75 to 90 years old who had HF, a 12-week program of once weekly exercise sessions resulted in an 11% increase in 6-minute walk distance, but no significant improvement was found in quality of life as assessed by the Living with Heart Failure Questionnaire [49].

McKelvie and coworkers [50] randomized 181 NYHA class 2 to 3 HF patients of mean age 65 years (19% women) with LV ejection fraction less than 40% to 3 months of supervised aerobic and resistance training followed by

Table 2
Randomized controlled trials of exercise training in older patients who have heart failure

Authors	n	Mean age	Women (%)	Duration	Mode	Benefits
Austin, et al [51]	200	72	34	24 weeks	Aerobic resistance	↑6-min walk — 16% ↓NYHA Class — 16% ↑QOL
Cider, et al [59]	24	63	33	5 month	resistance	No Δ Peak VO$_2$ No Δ HRV No Δ QOL
Coats, et al [41]	17	62	None	8 weeks	Row cycle	↑Peak VO$_2$ — 18% ↑HRV
Gottlieb, et al [48]	33	65	12	6 months	Cycle treadmill	↑Peak VO$_2$ – 13% ↑6-min walk – 11% No Δ – QOL
McKelvie, et al [50]	181	65	19	12 months	Cycle resistance	No Δ – 6-min walk ↑Peak VO$_2$ – 14% No Δ – QOL
Owen, et al [49]	22	81	25	12 weeks	Aerobic resistance	↑6-min walk – 11% No Δ – QOL
Pu, et al [63]	16	77	100	10 weeks	Resistance	↑Strength – 43% ↑6 min walk – 13% No Δ - Peak VO$_2$
Selig, et al [62]	39	65	15	3 months	Resistance	↑Peak VO$_2$ – 11% ↑FBF 20% ↑HRV
Tyni–Lenne, et al [61]	24	63	46	8 weeks	Resistance	↑Peak VO$_2$ — 8% ↑6-min walk—11% ↑QOL
Wielenga, et al [47]	67	64	None	12 weeks	Walk cycle	No Δ - Peak VO$_2$
Willenheimer, et al [46]	54	64	28	16 weeks	Cycle	↑QOL No Δ - Peak VO$_2$

Abbreviations: FBF, forearm blood flow; HRV, heart rate variability; QOL, quality of life; Δ, change.

9 months of home training or to a control group. Most patients received diuretics, converting enzyme inhibitors, and digitalis, and approximately 20% received beta blockers. Peak VO$_2$ in the training group increased 10% after 3 months and 14% after 12 months, whereas minimal changes occurred in controls. Modest increases in 6-minute walk distance were observed at 3 and 12 months in both groups, without significant intergroup differences. No significant changes from baseline in radionuclide cardiac function or quality of life occurred in either group.

The largest published exercise training trial of older patients with HF is that of Austin and colleagues [51], who randomized 200 60- to 89-year old outpatients (mean 72 years, 34% women) who had NYHA class 2 to 3 HF and LVEF less than 40% to 24 weeks of exercise training or standard care. Training consisted of an 8-week twice weekly hospital-based cardiac rehabilitation program followed by 16 weeks of supervised community-based exercise sessions for 1 hour per week. Throughout the 24-week program, patients performed aerobic training and low resistance/high repetition strength training and were encouraged to exercise an additional three times per week at home. Significant improvement occurred in health-related quality of life, NYHA class (from 2.4 to 2.0) and 6-minute walk distance (from 276 to 320 m) in exercisers, whereas no changes occurred in controls. In addition, fewer exercise patients (11%) than standard care patients (20%) were hospitalized by week 24, although mortality was similarly low in both groups. Peak VO_2 was not measured in this study. The low dropout rate (12%) indicates that such a training program is feasible in most older patients who have HF.

Resistance training studies in older patients who have heart failure

Although the focus of most exercise training trials to data in patients who have HF has been on enhancing the reduced aerobic capacity, another prominent characteristic of the HF syndrome is skeletal muscle atrophy [52–54]. Muscle atrophy is most pronounced in highly oxidative, fatigue-resistant Type I fibers, causing a shift toward glycolytic, more fatigue-prone Type II fibers [53]. Normative aging also is accompanied by significant loss of muscle mass [55,56], which accelerates after the sixth decade and is a major contributor to disability in the elderly. Older patients who have HF are therefore at especially high risk for skeletal muscle wasting.

Frail elderly nursing home residents in their 80s and 90s who do not have overt HF have experienced dramatic increases in strength and sizeable increases in muscle mass from high-intensity resistance training [57,58]. These improvements were accompanied by increases in gait speed; in some patients the need for walkers or canes was eliminated. Since these landmark studies, a growing literature has documented beneficial effects of resistance training in patients who have HF.

In 24 NYHA class 2 to 3 HF patients of mean age 63 years, Cider and colleagues [59] observed that those randomized to 5 months of circuit weight training twice per week increased their anaerobic threshold but experienced no improvement in peak VO_2, muscle strength, or quality of life. In an uncontrolled observational study of nine men aged 63 ± 11 years with HF, Hare and coworkers [60] documented significant enhancement of muscle strength and endurance and reduction in VO_2 at submaximal workloads, indicating enhanced walking efficiency, after 11 weeks of resistance training. In a study of 24 patients aged 63 ± 9 years who had HF, Tyni-Lenne and colleagues [61] documented increases in peak VO_2, 6-minute walk distance,

and quality of life, and reduced resting and submaximal plasma norepinephrine in those randomized to 8 weeks of resistance exercises. After 3 months
of resistance training, Selig and coworkers [62] observed an increase in peak
VO_2, skeletal muscle strength, forearm blood flow, and heart rate variability
in a randomized trial of resistance training in 39 Class 2 to 3 patients aged
65 ± 11 years (6 women) who had HF.

The relative "youth" and minimal numbers of women in the above studies of resistance training in HF patients were addressed by Pu and colleagues
[63] in a study of 16 women with HF of mean age 77 years randomized to
progressive resistance training for 10 weeks. At baseline these women had
approximately 40% lower muscle strength than those of similar age who
had other chronic diseases. Training was well tolerated and resulted in
a 43% increase in strength and 13% increase in 6-minute walk distance
but no increase in peak VO_2. Increases in type I muscle fiber area (mean
10%) and citrate synthase activity (35%) were strong predictors of improved 6-minute walk distance. Older patients who have HF thus seem to
derive significant increases in muscle strength and endurance from resistance
training. Additional studies that have combined aerobic and resistance
training in older HF patients [49,50,64,65] have demonstrated similar
benefits.

Limitations of existing training studies in older patients who have heart failure

Despite the accumulating evidence that exercise training is beneficial in
older patients with HF, several important limitations of existing studies
must be recognized. As mentioned above, few of the studies to date have enrolled a sizeable number of patients older than 75 years, representative of HF
patients in the general community [66]. Similarly, older women are severely
underrepresented in existing HF training trials. These deficiencies in recruitment of elderly patients, especially women, also are encountered in standard
cardiac rehabilitation programs, representing both a failure of clinicians to
refer such patients and logistic difficulties encountered by elderly patients in
attending these programs [27]. The latter issue can be addressed successfully
by home-based training, which elicits improvements in exercise capacity parallel to those seen in supervised programs.

Another important deficiency of existing exercise training trials in HF is
their exclusion of individuals who have preserved LV systolic function, who
represent 30% to 50% of the overall HF population [66–69]. A consistent
finding of community-based studies is that at least half of all elderly patients
who have HF fall into this category, with larger proportions of women than
men [66–69]. None of the clinical trials discussed in this review have included
patients from this large subset of the HF population. The generally normal
heart size in such patients makes it attractive to speculate that they would
derive training-induced increases in LVEDV and SV similar to those

experienced by normal people. A further limitation of existing studies is the severe under-representation of patients who have atrial fibrillation, which is seen in approximately one quarter of patients who have HF in the community [66].

Challenges and unanswered questions

Given the huge burden imposed by HF on the health, functional status, and quality of life in the elderly, exercise training in this population represents an underused therapeutic modality with enormous potential. To realize this potential, however, several obstacles must be surmounted.

The multiple comorbidities in elderly patients who have HF, including arthritis, obstructive lung disease, peripheral arterial disease, and neuromuscular disorders, provide a challenge to exercise training. Ingenuity, great care, and patience are prerequisites to successful implementation of training programs in the elderly.

Elderly patients, especially older women, often believe that they are too old to benefit from exercise training, despite the large body of data demonstrating relative improvements similar to those of younger individuals. In fact, debilitated elderly patients have the greatest potential for improvement in functional status and quality of life from such training.

Logistic factors, such as the need to care for a dependent spouse or lack of transportation, may prevent an otherwise willing elderly patient who has HF from attending a supervised rehabilitation program. Greater availability of home or community-based exercise programs may overcome such obstacles and may be more cost effective than traditional hospital-based training.

The greatest barrier to recruiting more elderly patients with HF into exercise training programs may lie within the medical community itself. Physicians and other health care providers must be educated in the benefits of exercise training in this age group so that they refer such patients to these programs.

Critical questions regarding the benefit of exercise training in the elderly remain to be answered. Perhaps the most important of these is whether such training prolongs survival or reduces morbidity in older patients who have HF. Although a few prior studies have suggested such benefits, none of these has been large enough to definitely answer this question. The ongoing Heart Failure and A Controlled Trial Investigating Outcomes of Exercise TraiNing (HF-ACTION) should fill this void [70]. This NIH-sponsored trial, which began in 2002, is randomizing 3000 patients who have NYHA class 2 to 4 systolic HF (LVEF <35%) to a program of aerobic training versus usual care. The training program consists of 36 supervised sessions in a traditional hospital-based program followed by a minimum of 12 months of home training. The primary endpoint is a combination of all-cause mortality and hospitalization. Secondary outcome measures include the change in peak VO_2 and 6-minute walk distance. To date, approximately 2000 patients have been recruited, including 30% women and 25% aged 68 years or older. In addition, the inclusion of approximately 34% African Americans will provide important data in this large subset of the HF population. Inclusion of sizeable proportions of patients who have atrial fibrillation, internal cardioverter-defibrillators, and biventricular pacemakers will allow insights regarding the usefulness of training in these subgroups. The trial is slated for completion in 2008. A substudy is addressing the role of such training on healthcare costs and quality of life. If this trial is positive, it is anticipated that Medicare will extend its coverage of cardiac rehabilitation programs to include patients who have HF, at least those with systolic dysfunction.

Future large-scale randomized trials are a necessary next step to investigate whether patients with HF and preserved LV systolic function, who are excluded from HF-ACTION, benefit from exercise training. Another important issue, especially if HF-ACTION is positive, will be to determine whether a combination of resistance and aerobic training provides greater benefit than aerobic training alone on CV endpoints, functional measures, and quality of life.

Summary

Both the aging process and HF syndrome are characterized by a striking loss of aerobic capacity caused by a combination of cardiac and peripheral factors. A significant reduction in muscle mass and strength is also common to both conditions. Although a growing literature has documented that aerobic exercise training results in improvement in peak VO_2, submaximal exercise measures, and quality of life in younger patients who have HF, few HF training studies have included meaningful numbers of elderly individuals, especially elderly women. Nevertheless, the modest data available suggest similar benefits in older as in younger patients who have HF. Resistance training may provide additional benefit in patients with HF regardless of age. Whether exercise training can reduce mortality, hospitalizations, and overall health care costs must await the outcome of the ongoing HF-ACTION trial.

References

[1] Buskirk ER, Hodgson JL. Age and aerobic power: the rate of change in men and women. Fed Proc 1987;46:1824–9.
[2] Jackson AS, Beard EF, Wier LT, et al. Changes in aerobic power of men ages 25–70 years. Med Sci Sports Exerc 1995;27:113–20.
[3] Fleg JL, Lakatta EF. Role of muscle loss in the age-associated reduction in VO_2 max. J Appl Physiol 1988;65:1147–51.

[4] Ogawa T, Spina R, Martin WH III, et al. Effects of aging, sex, and physical training on cardiovascular response to dynamic upright exercise. Circulation 1992;86:404–503.

[5] Fleg JL, Morrell CH, Bos AG, et al. Accelerated longitudinal decline of aerobic capacity in healthy older adults. Circulation 2005;112:674–82.

[6] Fleg JL, O'Connor FC, Becker LC, et al. Cardiac versus peripheral contributions to the age–associated decline in aerobic capacity. J Am Coll Cardiol 1997;29:269A.

[7] Fleg JL, O'Connor F, Gerstenblith G, et al. Impact of age on the cardiovascular response to dynamic upright exercise in healthy men and women. J Appl Physiol 1995; 78:890–900.

[8] Fleg JL, Tzankoff SP, Lakatta EG. Age–related augmentation of plasma catecholamines during dynamic exercise in healthy men. J Appl Physiol 1985;59:1033–9.

[9] Fleg JL, Schulman S, O'Connor F, et al. Effects of acute β-adrenergic receptor blockade on age-associated changes in cardiovascular performance during dynamic exercise. Circulation 1994;90:2333–41.

[10] Stelken AM, Younis LT, Jennison SH, et al. Prognostic value of cardiopulmonary exercise testing using percent achieved of predicted peak oxygen uptake for patients with ischemic and dilated cardiomyopathy. J Am Coll Cardiol 1996;27:345–52.

[11] Francis DP, Shamin W, Davies LC, et al. Cardiopulmonary exercise testing for prognosis in chronic heart failure:continuous and independent prognostic value from VE/VCO_2 slope and peak VO_2. Eur Heart J 2000;21:154–61.

[12] Mancini DM, Eisen H, Kussmaul W, et al. Value of peak exercise oxygen consumption for optimal timing of cardiac transplantation in ambulatory patients with heart failure. Circulation 1991;83:778–86.

[13] Higginbotham MB, Morris KG, Conn EH, et al. Determinants of variable exercise performance among patients with severe left ventricular dysfunction. Am J Cardiol 1983; 51:52–60.

[14] Colucci WS, Ribeiro JP, Rocco MB, et al. Impaired chronotropic response to exercise in patients with congestive heart failure. Role of post–synaptic beta-adrenergic desensitization. Circulation 1989;80:314–23.

[15] Sullivan MJ, Hawthorne MH. Exercise intolerance in patients with chronic heart failure. Prog Cardiovasc Dis 1995;38:1–22.

[16] Pina IL, Apstein CS, Balady GJ, et al. Exercise and heart failure: A statement from the American Heart Association Committee on Exercise, Rehabilitation and Prevention. Circulation 2003;107:1210–25.

[17] Fleg JL. Can exercise conditioning be effective in older heart failure patients? Heart Fail Rev 2002;7:99–103.

[18] Kitzman DW, Little WC, Brubaker PH, et al. Pathophysiologic characterization of isolated diastolic heart failure in comparison to systolic heart failure. JAMA 2002;288: 2144–50.

[19] Kitzman DW, Higginbotham MB, Cobb FR, et al. Exercise in tolerance in patients with heart failure and pressured left ventricular systolic function: failure of the Frank–Starling mechanism. J Am Coll Cardiol 1991;17:1065–72.

[20] Badenhop DJ, Cleary PA, Schoal SF, et al. Physiological adjustments to higher- and lower-intensity exercise in elders. Med Sci Sports Exerc 1983;15:496–502.

[21] Seals DR, Hagberg JM, Hurley BF, et al. Endurance training in older men and women. I. Cardiovascular response to exercise. J Appl Physiol 1984;57:1024–9.

[22] Hagberg JM, Graves JF, Limacher M, et al. Cardiovascular response of 70- to 79-year old men to exercise training. J Appl Physiol 1989;66:2589–94.

[23] Schulman SP, Fleg JL, Goldberg AP, et al. Continuum of cardiovascular performance across a broad range of fitness levels in healthy older men. Circulation 1996;94:359–67.

[24] Williams MA, Maresh CM, Esterbrooks DJ, et al. Early exercise training in patients older than 65 years compared with that in younger patients after acute myocardial infarction or coronary artery bypass grafting. Am J Cardiol 1985;55:263–6.

[25] Lavie CJ, Milani RV, Littman AB. Benefits of cardiac rehabilitation and exercise training in secondary coronary prevention in the elderly. J Am Coll Cardiol 1993;22: 678–83.

[26] Ades PA, Waldmann ML, Meyer WL, et al. Skeletal muscle and cardiovascular adaptations to exercise conditioning in older coronary patients. Circulation 1996;94:323–30.

[27] Ades PA. Cardiac rehabilitation in older coronary patients. J Am Geriatr Soc 1999;47: 98–105.

[28] Afzal A, Brawner CA, Keteyian SJ. Exercise training in heart failure. Prog Cardiovasc Dis 1998;41:175–90.

[29] Piepoli MT, Flather M, Coats AJS. Overview of studies of exercise training in chronic heart failure: the need for a prospective randomized multicentre European trial. Eur Heart J 1998; 19:830–41.

[30] Currier D, Galinier M, Pathak A, et al. Rehabilitation of patients with congestive heart failure with or without β-blockade therapy. J Card Fail 2001;7:241–8.

[31] Hambrecht R, Gielen S, Linke A, et al. Effects of exercise training on left ventricular function and peripheral resistance in patients with chronic heart failure. JAMA 2000; 283:3095–101.

[32] Jugdutt BI, Michorowski BL, Kappagoda CT. Exercise training after anterior Q wave myocardial infraction: importance of regional left ventricular function and topography. J Am Coll Cardiol 1988;12:362–72.

[33] Sullivan MJ, Higginbotham MB, Cobb FR. Exercise training in patients with severe left ventricular dysfunction: hemodynamic and metabolic effects. Circulation 1988;78: 506–15.

[34] Hambrecht R, Fiehn E, Weigl C, et al. Regular physical exercise corrects endothelial dysfunction and improves exercise capacity in patients with chronic heart failure. Circulation 1998;98:2709–15.

[35] Katz SD, Yuen J, Bijou R. Training improves endothelium–dependent vasodilation in resistance vessels of patients with heart failure. J Appl Physiol 1997;82:1488–92.

[36] Minotti, JR, Johnson EC, Hudson TC, et al. Skeletal muscle response to exercise training in congestive heart failure. J Clin Invest 1990;86:751–8.

[37] Adamopoulos S, Coats AJ, Brunotte F. Physical training improves skeletal muscle metabolism in patients with heart failure. J Am Coll Cardiol 1993;21:1101–6.

[38] Stratton JR, Dunn SF, Adamopoulos S, et al. Training partially reverses skeletal muscle metabolic abnormalities during exercise in heart failure. J Appl Physiol 1994;76:1575–82.

[39] Hambrecht R, Niebauer J, Fiehn E, et al. Physical training in patients with stable chronic heart failure. Effects on cardiorespiratory fitness and ultrastructural abnormalities of leg muscles. J Am Coll Cardiol 1995;25:1239–45.

[40] Braith RW, Welsch MA, Feigenbaum MS, et al. Neuroendocrine activation in heart failure is modified by endurance exercise. J Am Coll Cardiol 1999;34:1170–5.

[41] Coats AJS, Adamopoulos S, Radaelli A. Controlled trial of physical training in chronic heart failure. Exercise performance, hemodynamics, ventilation, and autonomic function. Circulation 1992;85:2119–31.

[42] Belardinelli R, Georgiou D, Cianci G, et al. Randomized, controlled trial of long-term moderate exercise training in chronic heart failure: effects on functional capacity, quality of life, and clinical outcome. Circulation 1999;99:1173–82.

[43] Heiat A, Gross CP, Krumholz HM. Representation of the elderly, women, and minorities in heart failure clinical trials. Arch Intern Med 2002;162:1682–8.

[44] European Heart Failure Group. Experience from controlled trials of physical training in chronic heart failure. Eur Heart J 1998;19:466–75.

[45] Rees K, Taylor RS, Singh S, et al. Exercise based rehabilitation for heart failure. The Cochrane Database Syst Rev 2004;3:CD003331.

[46] Willenheimer R, Erhardt L, Cline C, et al. Exercise training in heart failure improves quality of life and exercise capacity. Eur Heart J 1998;19:774–81.

[47] Wielenga RP, Huisveld IA, Bol E, et al. Exercise training in elderly patients with chronic heart failure. Coron Artery Dis 1998;9:765–70.
[48] Gottlieb SS, Fisher ML, Freudenberger R, et al. Effect of exercise training on peak performance and quality of life in congestive heart failure patients. J Card Fail 1999;3:188–94.
[49] Owen A, Croucher L. Effect of an exercise programme for elderly patients with heart failure. Eur J Heart Fail 2000;2:65–70.
[50] McKelvie RS, Teo KK, Roberts R, et al. Effects of exercise training in patients with heart failure: The Exercise Rehabilitation Trial (EXERT). Am Heart J 2002;144:23–30.
[51] Austin J, Williams R, Ross L, et al. Randomised controlled trial of cardiac rehabilitation in elderly patients with heart failure. Eur J Heart Fail 2005;7:411–7.
[52] Mancini DM, Walter G, Reichek N, et al. Contribution of skeletal muscle atrophy to exercise intolerance and altered muscle metabolism in heart failure. Circulation 1992;85:1364–73.
[53] Drexler H, Reide V, Munzel T, et al. Alteration of skeletal muscle in chronic heart failure. Circulation 1992;85:1751–9.
[54] Toth MJ, Gottlieb SS, Fisher ML, et al. Skeletal muscle atrophy and peak oxygen consumption in heart failure. Am J Cardiol 1997;79:1267–9.
[55] Kallman DA, Plato CC, Tobin JD. The role of muscle loss in the age-related decline of grip strength:cross-sectional and longitudinal perspectives. J Gerontol 1990;45:M82–8.
[56] Faulkner JA, Brooks SV, Zerba E. Muscle atrophy and weakness with aging: contraction-induced injury as an underlying mechanism. J Gerontol 1995;50A:124–9.
[57] Fiataroni MA, Marks EC, Ryan ND, et al. High intensity strength training in nonagenarians: effects on skeletal muscle. JAMA 1990;263:3029–34.
[58] Fiataroni MA, O'Neill EF, Ryan ND, et al. Exercise training and nutritional supplementation for physical frailty in very elderly people. N Engl J Med 1994;330:1769–75.
[59] Cider A, Tygessen H, Hedberg M, et al. Peripheral muscle training in patients with clinical signs of heart failure. Scand J Rehabil Med 1997;2:121–7.
[60] Hare DL, Ryan T, Selig SE, et al. Resistance exercise training increases muscle strength, endurance, and blood flow in patients with chronic heart failure. Am J Cardiol 1999;83:1674–7.
[61] Tyni-Lenne R, Dencker K, Gordon A, et al. Comprehensive local muscle training increases aerobic working capacity and quality of life and decreases neurohormonal activation in patients with chronic heart failure. Eur J Heart Fail 2001;3:47–52.
[62] Selig SE, Carey MF, Menzies DG, et al. Moderate-intensity resistance training in patients with chronic heart failure improves strength, endurance, heart rate variability, and forearm blood flow. J Card Fail 2004;10:21–30.
[63] Pu CT, Johnson MT, Foreman DE, et al. Randomized trial of progressive resistance training to counteract the myopathy of chronic heart failure. J Appl Physiol 2001;90:2341–50.
[64] Maiorani A, O'Driscoll G, Cheetham C, et al. Combined aerobic and resistance exercise training improves functional capacity and strength in CHF. J Appl Physiol 2000;88:1565–70.
[65] Senden PJ, Sabelis LW, Zonderland ML, et al. The effect of physical training on workload, upper leg muscle function and muscle areas in patients with chronic heart failure. Int J Cardiol 2005;100:293–300.
[66] Senni M, Tribouilloy CM, Rodeheffer RJ, et al. Congestive heart failure in the community. A study of all incident cases in Olmstead County, Minnesota, in 1991. Circulation 1998;98:2282–9.
[67] Vasan RS, Larson MG, Benjamin EJ, et al. Congestive heart failure in subjects with normal versus reduced left ventricular ejection fraction: prevalence, and mortality in a population-based cohort. J Am Coll Cardiol 1999;33:1948–55.
[68] Devereux RB, Roman MJ, Liu JE, et al. Congestive heart failure despite normal left ventricular systolic function in a population-based sample: the Strong Heart Study. Am J Cardiol 2000;86:1090–6.

[69] Kitzman DW, Gardin JM, Gottdiener JS, et al, for the Cardiovascular Health Study Research Group. Importance of heart failure with preserved systolic function in patients > or = 65 years of age. Am J Cardiol 2001;87:413–9.
[70] Whellan DJ, Lee KL, Ellis S, et al. Heart failure and a controlled trial investigating outcomes of exercise training (HF-ACTION): Design and rationale. J Card Fail 2003;9: S57.

ELSEVIER
SAUNDERS

CLINICS IN
GERIATRIC
MEDICINE

Clin Geriatr Med 23 (2007) 235–248

End-of-Life Care in the Treatment of Heart Failure in the Elderly

John Arthur McClung, MD[a,b,*]

[a]*Division of Cardiology, Westchester Medical Center/New York Medical College, Valhalla, NY 10595, USA*
[b]*Bioethics Institute, New York Medical College, Valhalla, NY 10595, USA*

The American Geriatrics Society position statement on the care of dying patients opens by stating that, "providing excellent, humane care to patients near the end of life, when curative means are either no longer possible or no longer desired by the patient, is an essential part of medicine" [1]. Although the essential nature of this discipline certainly cannot be denied, much of the literature dedicated to this topic has revolved around terminal care provided to patients who have neoplastic diagnoses. Heart failure (HF) presents its own unique challenges to the clinician who desires to make the recommendations of the American Geriatrics Society a tangible reality. This article focuses on both specific clinical recommendations and an analysis of some of the ethical issues involved in the provision of care to elderly patients in the terminal stages of HF.

How do we know we have arrived?

The ability of physicians to predict mortality accurately has been demonstrated recently to be questionable, even in cases of advanced malignancy [2,3]. Attempts to ascertain variables predictive of mortality in patients who have HF have proven to be significantly more difficult. An exhaustive review of the literature conducted during the last decade found very few consistently predictive variables. Factors accounting for this included small sample size, differing patient populations, selective acquisition of variables, interrelationship of variables, differing measurement technologies, duration of follow-up, poor reproducibility, and problems with data handling [4].

This work was supported in part by a grant from the Dr. I Fund Foundation.
* Division of Cardiology, Westchester Medical Center, Valhalla, New York 10595.
E-mail address: john.mcclung@jhu.edu

doi:10.1016/j.cger.2006.08.009
geriatric.theclinics.com

Measures that appear to have consistent independent prognostic value include New York Heart Association symptom class, echocardiographic left ventricular dimensions, radionuclide ejection fraction, and ischemic cause. Hyponatremia previously has been documented to be associated with an extremely negative prognosis; however, it is unclear whether or not this remains as robust an indicator in patients treated with angiotensin-converting enzyme (ACE) inhibitors [4,5].

Patients who have HF present with the additional challenge of sudden death, which makes the generation of prediction models even more difficult. As many as 60% of patients who have HF die suddenly; however, prediction of who is most likely to suffer sudden death remains controversial [6,7]. Recent attempts to determine who is expected to die suddenly include studies of the prognostic efficacy of B-type natriuretic peptide (BNP) and a risk factor assessment that includes ejection fraction, LV end-diastolic diameter, BNP level, presence of nonsustained ventricular tachycardia, and diabetes mellitus [8,9]. Accurate assessment of sudden death incidence is rendered all the more difficult by the increased prevalence of automatic internal cardioverter-defibrillator insertion in patients who have reduced ejection fraction, which concurrently enhances data collection about the incidence of dysrhythmia in patients who have HF and decreases the overall mortality attributable to dysrhythmia [10,11].

The estimation of overall prognosis in cardiac failure has been equally elusive. A recent study of patients in Europe with a mean age of 69.7 years previously diagnosed with HF generated a clinical model that scored age, sex, history of diabetes, history of renal insufficiency, ankle edema, weight, low blood pressure, and the absence of beta-blocker therapy by a regression coefficient. Using this model, patients who scored very high had a mortality as high as 78% over the 18-month observation period [12]. Patients who had lower scores had significantly greater variability in mortality. This observation also needs to be placed in the context of the increasingly frequent use of resynchronization therapy, which, in combination with an internal cardioverter-defibrillator, has been demonstrated to reduce overall mortality by 36% [13].

The persistence of this prognostic uncertainty renders a discussion of patient preference difficult at best. Prior work done in patients who have cancer diagnoses suggests that even a 10% probability of not surviving the next 6 months leads patients to consider different treatment options [14]. In part because of prognostic uncertainty, patients dying of HF have been documented to have both a poorer understanding of their condition and less involvement in the decision-making process regarding their care [15]. A study of 274 dying patients, 26% of whom had cardiovascular disease, found that some treatment was withheld or withdrawn in 84% of patients; however, only 35% of these patients were able to participate in the decision-making process [16].

Patients dying of HF who do not die suddenly, deteriorate gradually; however, this gradual process is interrupted by acute episodes that frequently require hospitalization (Fig. 1) [15,17]. The clinical hallmark of patients not presenting with sudden death is a combination of dyspnea and low output symptoms. Other commonly reported symptoms include pain in 78% of patients, depressed mood in 59%, insomnia in 45%, anxiety in 30%, anorexia in 43%, constipation in 37%, and nausea and vomiting in 32% [18].

Patients dying of HF either do so suddenly, suffer a chronic, slow deterioration punctuated by acute episodes, or both. In either case, there is little to no time for the physician to explore patient preferences in this population unless this is addressed early in course of the disease.

Improving communication

Interviews conducted in Great Britain with patients dying of HF and their caregivers identified several problems unique to the treatment of this patient population [14]. Patients tended not to recall receiving any written

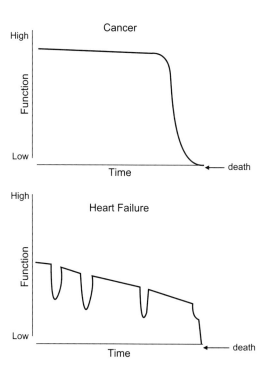

Fig. 1. Typical trajectory of disease for patients who have cancer and heart failure. Top: Patients who have cancer have a long period of preserved function followed by a precipitous drop that starts within a few months before death. Bottom: Patients who have heart failure have an overall gradual decline in function punctuated by periods of exacerbations with acute drops in function followed by a return to near their previous level. (*From* Goldstein NE, Lynn J. Trajectory of end-stage heart failure: the influence of technology and implications for policy change. Perspect Biol Med 2006;49(1):10–9, Fig. 1; with permission. © The Johns Hopkins University Press. Reproduced with permission of the Johns Hopkins University Press.)

information about their condition and often did not see an association between symptoms, such as dyspnea and edema, and their cardiac status. Similarly, patients and caregivers did not feel particularly involved in the decision-making process regarding the illness. Medication regimens were seen as difficult and burdensome despite their frequent effectiveness. The concurrent presence of comorbidity in this generally elderly population added to the burden of the primary condition. Care often was seen as fragmented, with an absence of the kinds of resources frequently available to cancer patients.

Although identification of these problems is helpful, solutions are not necessarily obvious. Initially published a decade ago, the SUPPORT study of the care of patients who have life-threatening diagnoses documented that only 47% of physicians were aware of their patients' wishes regarding cardiopulmonary resuscitation, that 50% of patients reported severe pain at least half the time, and that 38% of patients spent 10 or more days in intensive care [19]. A subsequent intervention that provided written prognostic reports and written synopses of patient preferences regarding resuscitation and pain control for the physicians and a skilled nurse practitioner who monitored the patients' progress resulted in no measurable difference in any of the indices related to communication or outcome [20]. A post-hoc analysis of 236 patients dying of HF in the databases of the SUPPORT trial and the Hospitalized Elderly Longitudinal Project (HELP) databases documented breathlessness in 65% of patients and severe pain in 42% during the last 3 days of life, whereas 40% received a major therapeutic intervention during the same time period [21].

These data clearly speak to the necessity for more robust interpersonal communication and more creative ways of providing services to this patient population. In an intervention conducted at six centers in the United States, 988 terminally ill patients (of whom 21% had heart disease) and 893 caregivers were offered a structured interview [22]. Areas surveyed included questions about symptoms, communication with health care providers, spiritual and personal meaning of dying, care needs, end-of-life plans, economic burdens, preferences regarding end-of-life care, and opinions about euthanasia and physician-assisted suicide, among others. Each respondent also was asked how stressful and how helpful the interview had been. Of the patients responding, 88.7% reported little or no stress associated with the interview, whereas 46.5% thought the interview was somewhat or very helpful. Of the caregivers responding, 89.7% reported little or no stress associated with the interview, whereas 53.4% thought it was somewhat or very helpful. This finding would suggest that the SUPPORT investigators did not go far enough in designing the intervention that was ultimately studied. The use of a more structured interview format with patients and family members might serve to improve communication initially between these individuals and their caregivers and to set the stage for more focused and interactive palliative care.

Palliative care in heart failure

The previously described uncertainty regarding the trajectory of terminal HF can induce what has been termed a "prognostic paralysis" regarding the initiation of discussion about palliative care and its actual implementation [23]. One commentator has suggested that patients who have HF should be considered candidates for palliative care if a clinician answers "no" to the question, "Would I be surprised if my patient were to die in the next 12 months?" [24]. Another suggested algorithm would initiate palliative intervention during or shortly after recovery from an acute exacerbation of HF [25]. What seems clear from the experience of many is that palliative care needs to be considered much earlier in the course of the disease process than is currently the case.

The hallmark of congestive failure is dyspnea. The initial management of dyspnea in this patient population includes standard management with diuretics, vasodilators, and positive inotropes as necessary. Refractory pleural effusions can be addressed by thoracentesis. Severe dyspnea that remains refractory to these interventions often can be palliated in the opioid-naïve patient with doses of intravenous morphine of between 2 and 5 mg administered intravenously every 5 to 10 minutes as necessary for relief. Low doses of diamorphine (1 to 2 mg) administered as an intravenous bolus have been documented to improve cardiopulmonary exercise test results even in patients who have stable HF [26]. The use of supplemental oxygen and appropriate room ventilation are also helpful.

As noted above, pain is reported in nearly 80% of patients dying of HF, whereas 41% of patients dying of HF in the SUPPORT database had moderate to severe pain during the last 3 days of life [27]. One half of these patients reported moderate to severe pain during the last 6 months of life. Treatment of pain with nonsteroidal anti-inflammatory agents in the setting of HF is relatively contraindicated because of their propensity to retain sodium and to antagonize the effect of ACE inhibitors and decrease renal function [28]. Doses of opioids similar to those effective for dyspnea are often effective for pain control in this population.

Fatigue is often a result of low output and responds to therapy with positive inotropic agents except in the very end stage of HF. Fatigue also may be related to coexistent depression, which usually is best treated pharmacologically with selective serotonin reuptake inhibitors; however, use of these agents in the absence of appropriate psychological, spiritual, and social support is often compromised by noncompliance.

Treatment of comorbidities also may be helpful. The use of continuous positive airway pressure in patients who have sleep apnea secondary to HF has been demonstrated to have no effect on survival; however, reductions in apnea and norepinephrine levels have been documented along with increases in nocturnal oxygen saturation, ejection fraction, and distance walked in 6 minutes [29]. Similarly, treatment of anemia in patients who have New York Heart Association class II to IV HF with darbepoetin alfa has been demonstrated to improve walking distance and quality of life indicators [30]. Additional comorbidities frequently documented in this patient population that require intervention include chronic obstructive pulmonary disease, arthropathies, and diabetes mellitus [31].

Patients who have HF may benefit from group visits in which palliative care issues can be addressed. A randomized study of 321 elderly patients, 33% of whom had heart disease, demonstrated that patients who received monthly group visits with their primary physician and a nurse that included health education, prevention strategies, opportunities for socialization, and mutual support had fewer emergency department visits, fewer visits to subspecialists, and fewer repeat hospital admissions compared with a control population [32]. The Heart Failure Society of America provides monographs on several related topics, including advance care planning and feelings about HF, that can serve as discussion aids [33,34].

Patients who have end-stage HF suffer from a wide variety of other problems, including the distress of living with a chronic, fatal condition; the disruption of social life, personal goals, income, faith, and daily function; and an increasing dependence on others with a reciprocal loss of self esteem [35]. As many as 60% of patients in one observational review felt that one or more of their problems were inadequately addressed [31]. Identification of these issues was easily facilitated by asking the simple question, "What are your three most troublesome problems?"

People dying of HF also have been documented to have spiritual needs that are characterized by feelings of hopelessness, isolation, and altered self image [36]. Among their concerns are the meaning of life, physical needs and practical problems of living both at home and in social settings, feelings of abandonment by the health care system, loss of dignity, changes in relationships, increasing dependence, and wishes for death. Responses to problems such as these include discussion of life goals and life closure issues, discussion of the meaning of the illness and its attendant suffering, discussion of coping ability, and the involvement of pastoral care services [35].

In many instances support services may be facilitated best by a dedicated palliative care team that has significant experience with dying patients [37]. It is now common for hospice services to accept patients who have HF for the provision of integrated services in both inpatient and outpatient settings [38].

Device therapy

The increasingly common use of device therapy has significantly reduced the morbidity and mortality associated with HF. Notwithstanding, these devices pose significant problems for the end-stage patient who may wish to minimize or reduce the intensity of his or her care. The right of a patient who has intact decision-making capacity to refuse any and all medical interventions has a long and established history in bioethics and common law [39,40]. This right applies equally to the withholding and withdrawing of therapy and clearly extends to deactivation of pacemakers and defibrillators, each of which constitutes a highly technical medical intervention. In recognition of this, discussion of device inactivation for patients who have HF at the end of life has recently been codified as a Class 1 recommendation in the 2005 update of the American College of Cardiology/American Heart Association guidelines for the management of chronic HF [41]. For patients who lack capacity, all jurisdictions have procedures for identification of an appropriate surrogate decision-maker or documentation of previously expressed health care wishes [42]. Hospitalized patients in the United States are required by law to have information recorded regarding the presence or absence of an advance directive at the time of admission and hospitals are also required to offer the opportunity for the patient to create an advance directive [43]. Notwithstanding this requirement, a recent survey of the next of kin of 100 patients dying with indwelling cardioverter defibrillators revealed that possible deactivation of the devices had been discussed antemortem in only 27 cases, whereas 8 patients were defibrillated by their device only minutes before death [44]. This situation is unfortunate given that deactivation of an implanted defibrillator has been equated to the withdrawal of other technically complex medical interventions, such as hemodialysis, a situation in which consensus has emerged that discontinuation at the request of a patient or recognized surrogate is the appropriate moral response [45].

Unlike cardioverter defibrillators, cardiac pacing, even with biventricular resynchronization, has not been shown clearly to prolong life [46]. One recent randomized, intention-to-treat trial has documented a significant reduction in all-cause mortality associated with cardiac resynchronization compared with medical therapy alone [47]. Another randomized comparison of medical therapy with both resynchronization and resynchronization with an indwelling defibrillator has demonstrated a modest reduction in death because of pump failure with cardiac resynchronization alone; however, the overall effect was negligible because of the increased prevalence of sudden death in the absence of coexistent ICD therapy [48].

Regardless of its effect on life expectancy, there is no question that a primary benefit of cardiac pacing in the patient who has HF is symptom relief. As a result, it is to be expected that informed requests for deactivation of cardiac pacing will be less frequent than those for deactivation of a defibrillator. Patients and surrogates who request deactivation need to be counseled appropriately regarding the potential negative effect this decision may have on the quality of the patient's remaining life. Additional adjustments in timing to optimize AV and VV delay using echocardiography are also helpful for relieving the symptoms of end-stage HF [49]. Should a patient or surrogate still prefer that the device be inactivated, it is important to emphasize that it can be reactivated should the extent of symptomatic deterioration be unacceptable. Notwithstanding these concerns, pacemaker therapy, including resynchronization, has been withdrawn in patients who were clearly end stage who had no obvious exacerbation of already existent severe symptoms [50]. The informed wishes of patients and surrogates who wish that device therapy be terminated need to be taken seriously and honored. Physicians who find this at odds with their own moral reasoning are not obligated to deactivate a device personally, but are obliged to inform the patient or surrogate of their objection and facilitate a transfer of care to a physician willing to accede to this request [50].

Cardiopulmonary resuscitation

Cardiopulmonary arrest, as an isolated episode, is not uncommon in patients who have HF and does not, in and of itself, portend end-stage disease [6,51]. This may account for the observation that only 23% of patients who had HF in the SUPPORT database initially preferred not to be resuscitated in the event of an arrest [52]. It probably also underpins the relatively high percentage of patients (14%) who changed their preference in favor of resuscitation during the course of their hospitalization. Those who did not want to be resuscitated were older, in higher income brackets, had lower activity status in the 2 weeks before admission, and perceived their prognosis to be worse than those who opted in favor of resuscitation. Although the numbers are too small for accurate comparison, a preference not to be resuscitated seems to have some degree of prognostic significance in and of itself. Of 19 patients subjected to cardiopulmonary resuscitation (CPR) who had expressed a preference for it, 10 were discharged alive. Of 6 patients subjected to CPR who had expressed a preference against it, only 1 survived to discharge [52]. One of the reasons that the numbers are not more robust is that the event rate in hospital in this patient population was only 4%, with most sudden death in patients who had HF occurring out of the hospital [51].

All of this simply confirms that the prognosis of patients who have HF remains variable and rapidly changeable such that decisions regarding resuscitation status, just as all medical decisions for these patients, need to be revisited frequently as clinical status changes.

For those patients who have not expressed a prior objection, recent data have suggested that family members prefer to be present during a resuscitative effort if possible, and that the presence of family members in this context is not usually disruptive [53,54]. As a result, recommendations that family members be offered the opportunity to be present during a resuscitative effort are now included in both the current American College of Physicians Ethics Manual and the American Heart Association Guidelines for Cardiopulmonary Resuscitation and Emergency Cardiovascular Care [40,54].

Palliative sedation

Patients at the very end stages of pump failure not uncommonly present with hallucinations, delirium, myoclonic jerks, and sometimes seizures that frequently exceed the capability of nonpharmacologic measures for control. Hallucinations and delirium can be pharmacologically managed in many situations with small doses of haloperidol, olanzapine, or risperidone [55]. For those patients in whom delirium is not controlled and for those who present with myoclonus and frank seizures, sedative therapy may be necessary. Commonly used medications for this purpose include midazolam, lorazepam, and propofol [55,56]. Use of these agents in this context has been termed palliative sedation.

The use of palliative sedation has given rise to a large volume of medical literature as a result of its threefold consequences of relief of suffering, removal of consciousness, and potential to shorten life, particularly in patients who have HF who commonly suffer from a combination of hypotension and reduced cardiac output. The appropriate use of palliative sedation has been justified by two commonly used ethical principles: double effect and proportionality. Double effect recognizes that a single action can have both positive and foreseen negative effects. It requires that the agent intend the positive effect, that the action itself not be morally wrong independent of its consequences, that the positive effect cannot be accomplished solely by means of the negative effect, and finally that there be proportionality between the intended and unintended effects [56].

In the case of palliative sedation, the intention is understood to be the relief of symptoms rather than a hastening of mortality. Sedation itself is not considered immoral independent of its consequences and the positive effect of symptom relief is not achieved in and of itself by the foreseen negative effect of a potentially shortened lifespan. Finally, the positive benefit of symptom relief is considered to outweigh the potentially negative effects of additional hypotension and further fall in cardiac output.

It has been argued that this kind of reasoning depends overmuch on the intention of the agent, a factor that is difficult to observe, let alone measure [57]. The difficulty of assessing adherence to the rule of double effect is suggested by a survey of physicians and nurses caring for 44 terminally ill patients in two hospitals in whom life support was being withdrawn [58]. Fully one third of physicians responding identified both the relief of pain and hastening of death as their primary intentions in prescribing palliative sedation. Proponents of the rule argue in response that the simple fact that people can have more than one intention does not invalidate the rule. It is also possible that the physicians in question who intend to hasten death do not consider this intention wrong. Under these circumstances, they do not need to appeal to the rule for justification of their actions because their decision is based on the assumption that the hastening of death is not fundamentally wrong [59,60].

Opponents of the use of the rule of double effect also argue that physicians are and should be held accountable for all foreseeable consequences of their actions rather than simply for those that they intend [61]. As such, some authors argue that the principle of proportionality alone may be a more appropriate justification for the use of palliative sedation [56].

Rendering the ethical landscape more murky still is the principle of collaboration that holds that cooperation in wrongdoing is itself immoral. This cooperation is understood to include advising, assisting, or tempting others to engage in wrongful acts [62]. This creates a morally ambiguous environment for the physician counseling patients or surrogates about potential treatment options when the intent of either the patient or the surrogate is primarily to shorten life, but the physician is morally opposed to euthanasia.

Several caveats are necessary when considering the use of palliative sedation. It is important that all other means of symptom control have been exhausted before its institution and that appropriate consultation with palliative care and pain management specialists have been obtained. Second, it is important that the patient or responsible surrogate is fully informed as to the rationale for palliative sedation and concurs with its use. Third, it is critical that other caregivers on the unit be instructed clearly as to how to proceed with appropriate protocols in place [56].

Pitfalls of palliative care

One perhaps unexpected concern in response to the gradual growth of palliative care initiatives has been the concept of "palliative care triumphalism" [63]. The carefully managed palliative efforts of dedicated professionals, including the use of palliative sedation, run the risk of ignoring the fact that death represents a chaotic disintegration of life that is fundamentally not controllable. To attempt to control it may represent an outright denial of an existential fact of the end of life. One palliative care practitioner has said that, "despite all we might say and all we might do, the process of dying includes suffering and painful separations and unfinished business. Death cannot be tamed. Death is unknown. Death is other. Death is death." [64].

This observation dovetails into previously identified components of a "good death" as perceived by multiple observers, including physicians, nurses, social workers, chaplains, hospice volunteers, patients, and recently bereaved family members [65]. Only one of the components was pain and symptom management. The other five were clear decision making, preparation for death, completion, contributing to others, and affirmation of the whole person. Implicit in these six components must be the understanding that some of them will come into conflict with others and that this, in and of itself, is not necessarily to be avoided or otherwise palliated.

This understanding was summarized a decade ago in the following fashion: "Often the most effective intervention that we can offer is time spent with patients and family, listening to concerns and acknowledging their value and touching—a physician's role that is hard to teach and harder to learn in medical education dominated by subspecialist- and procedure-oriented medical centers. We can, at a minimum, heed the powerful lessons taught by experiences with illness and death in our colleagues and loved ones." [66].

Summary

The terminal stages of HF present challenges to both the patient and the clinician that are the equal of terminal cancer, but with facets that are unique to cardiovascular disease. Among these unique characteristics are prognostic uncertainty, episodes of acute decompensation followed by relatively rapid improvement, and the relative frequency of device therapy. It is clear from the published literature that communication between patients, their family members, and caregivers remains suboptimal and needs to be enhanced through more creative endeavors than have been reported to date. This enhancement includes a more in-depth discussion of the clinical course of HF at an early stage of the illness. Palliative intervention for patients who have HF, including hospice, is clinically indicated for patients presenting with progressively increasing pump failure. Deactivation of device therapy in end-stage patients is often appropriate and needs to be discussed with both patients and appropriate surrogates. Similarly, resuscitation status needs to be reviewed on a regular basis given that preferences regarding resuscitation tend to change frequently in patients who have HF. Palliative sedation is an option for patients who have otherwise uncontrollable symptoms in the throes of end-stage disease; however, careful scrutiny is required to avoid its use in inappropriate situations.

A recent consensus conference identified five questions regarding end-of-life care for patients who have HF that are in need of further research data [67]. How can the physical and psychosocial burdens of advanced HF on patients and families best be decreased? Which patients will benefit from which interventions and how can they be counseled best? Which interventions improve quality of life and best achieve the outcomes desired by patients and family? How can care be coordinated between sites of care and barriers to evidence-based practice reduced? How can prognosis and treatment options be communicated better? These five questions effectively summarize some of the gaps that are currently present in the care of patients who have end-stage HF.

Above all, both the profession and society at large need to reacquaint themselves with the existential reality of death. Confronting this reality for what it is in ourselves, our loved ones, and our patients and their families will help to ensure that our patients are served to the best of our ability, both in their living and in their dying.

Acknowledgments

The author thanks Daniel P. Sulmasy MD, PhD, OFM and Jane G. McClung PhD for their assistance in the review of this manuscript.

References

[1] AGS Ethics Committee. American Geriatrics Society Position Statement: The care of dying patients. J Am Geriatr Soc 1995;43:577–8.

[2] Lamont EB, Christakis NA. Prognostic disclosure to patients with cancer near the end of life. Ann Intern Med 2001;134:1096–105.

[3] Lamont EB, Christakis NA. Complexities in prognostication in advanced cancer. JAMA 2003;290:98–104.

[4] Cowburn PJ, Cleland JGF, Coats AJS, et al. Risk stratification in chronic heart failure. Eur Heart J 1998;19:696–710.

[5] Lee WH, Packer M. Prognostic importance of serum sodium concentration and its modification by converting enzyme inhibition in patients with severe chronic heart failure. Circulation 1986;73:257–67.

[6] Cohn JN, Johnson G, Ziesche S, et al. A comparison of enalapril with hydralazine-isosorbide dinitrate in the treatment of chronic congestive heart failure. N Engl J Med 1991;325:303–10.

[7] Maisel A. B-type natriuretic peptide levels: diagnostic and prognostic in congestive heart failure. Circulation 2002;105:2328–31.

[8] Berger R, Huelsman M, Strecker K, et al. B-type natriuretic peptide predicts sudden death in patients with chronic heart failure. Circulation 2002;105:2392–7.

[9] Watanabe J, Shinozaki T, Shiba N, et al. Accumulation of risk markers predicts the incidence of sudden death in patients with chronic heart failure. Eur J Heart Fail 2006;8:237–42.

[10] Bardy GH, Lee KL, Mark DB, et al. Amiodarone or an implantable cardioverter-defibrillator for congestive heart failure. N Engl J Med 2005;352:225–37.

[11] Daubert JP, Zareba W, Hall WJ, et al. Predictive value of ventricular arrhythmia inducibility for subsequent ventricular tachycardia or ventricular fibrillation in multicenter automatic defibrillator implantation trial (MADIT) II patients. J Am Coll Cardiol 2006;47:98–107.

[12] Bouvy ML, Heerdink ER, Leufkens HGM, et al. Predicting mortality in patients with heart failure: a pragmatic approach. Heart 2003;89:605–9.

[13] Bristow MR, Saxon LA, Boehmer J, et al. Cardiac resynchronization therapy with or without an implantable defibrillator in advanced chronic heart failure. N Engl J Med 2004;350:2140–50.

[14] Weeks JC, Cook EF, O'Day SJ, et al. Relationship between cancer patients' predictions of prognosis and their treatment preferences. JAMA 1998;279:1709–14.

[15] Murray SA, Boyd K, Kendall M, et al. Dying of lung cancer or cardiac failure: prospective qualitative interview study of patients and their carers in the community. BMJ 2002;325:929–33.

[16] Faber-Langendoen K. A multi-institutional study of care given to patients dying in hospitals: ethical and practice implications. Arc Intern Med 1996;156:2130–6.

[17] Goldstein NE, Lynn J. Trajectory of end-stage heart failure: the influence of technology and implications for policy change. Perspect Biol Med 2006;49(1):10–9.

[18] McCarthy M, Lay M, Addington-Hall J. Dying from heart disease. J R Coll Phys London 1996;30:325–8.

[19] Covinsky K, Goldman L, Cook E, et al. The impact of serious illness on patients' families. JAMA 1994;272:1839–44.

[20] The SUPPORT Principal Investigators. A controlled trial to improve care for seriously ill hospitalized patients: the study to understand prognoses and preferences for outcomes and risks of treatments (SUPPORT). JAMA 1995;274:1591–8.

[21] Lynn J, Teno JM, Phillips RS, et al. Perceptions of family members of the dying experience of older and seriously ill patients. Ann Intern Med 1997;126:97–106.

[22] Emanuel EJ, Fairclough DL, Wolfe P, et al. Talking with terminally ill patients and their caregivers about death, dying, and bereavement: Is it stressful? Is it helpful? Arch Intern Med 2004;164:1999–2004.

[23] Stewart S, McMurray JJV. Palliative care for heart failure: time to move beyond treating and curing to improving the end of life. BMJ 2002;325:915–6.

[24] Murray SA, Boyd K, Sheikh A. Palliative care in chronic illness: we need to move from prognostic paralysis to active total care. BMJ 2005;330:611–2.

[25] Hauptman PJ, Havranek EP. Integrating palliative care into heart failure care. Arch Intern Med 2005;165:374–8.

[26] Williams SG, Wright DJ, Marshall P, et al. Safety and potential benefits of low dose diamorphine during exercise in patients with chronic heart failure. Heart 2003;89:1085–6.

[27] Levenson JW, McCarthy EP, Lynn J, et al. The last six months of life for patients with congestive heart failure. J Am Geriatr Soc 2000;48(5 Suppl):S101–9.

[28] Bleumink GS, Feenstra J, Sturkenboom MC, et al. Nonsteroidal anti-inflammatory drugs and heart failure. Drugs 2003;63:525–34.

[29] Bradley TD, Logan AG, Kimoff J, et al. Continuous positive airway pressure for central sleep apnea and heart failure. N Engl J Med 2005;353:2025–33.

[30] VanVeldhuisen DJ, Dickstein K, Cohen-Solal A, et al. Randomized, double-blind, placebo-controlled study to evaluate the effect of two dosing regimens of darbepoetin alfa on hemoglobin response and symptoms in patients with heart failure and anemia. J Am Coll Cardiol 2006;47(Suppl A):61A.

[31] Ward C. The need for palliative care in the management of heart failure. Heart 2002;87:294–8.

[32] Beck A, Scott J, Williams P, et al. A randomized trial of group outpatient visits for chronically ill older HMO members: The cooperative health care clinic. J Am Geriatr Soc 1997;45:543–9.

[33] Heart Failure Society of America. Advance care planning (Module 9). St. Paul: Heart Failure Society of America; 2005.

[34] Heart Failure Society of America. Managing feelings about heart failure (Module 6). St. Paul: Heart Failure Society of America; 2005.

[35] Albert NM, Davis M, Young J. Improving the care of patients dying of heart failure. Cleve Clin J Med 2002;69:321–8.

[36] Murray SA, Kendall M, Boyd K, et al. Exploring the spiritual needs of people dying of lung cancer or heart failure: a prospective qualitative interview study of patients and their carers. Palliat Med 2004;18:39–45.

[37] Bailey FA, Burgio KL, Woodby LL, et al. Improving processes of hospital care during the last hours of life. Arch Intern Med 2005;165:1722–7.

[38] Gibbs JSR, McCoy ASM, Gibbs LME, et al. Living with and dying from heart failure: the role of palliative care. Heart 2002;88(Suppl II):II36–9.

[39] Gostin LO. Deciding life and death in the courtroom: from *Quinlan* to *Cruzan, Glucksberg*, and *Vacco*—a brief history and analysis of constitutional protection of the "right to die." JAMA 1997;278:1523–8.

[40] Snyder L, Leffler C. Ethics manual: fifth edition. Ann Intern Med 2005;142:560–82.

[41] Hunt SA, Abraham WT, Chin MH, et al. ACC/AHA 2005 guideline update for the diagnosis and management of chronic heart failure in the adult—summary article. Circulation 2005;112:1825–52.

[42] Gillick MR. Advance care planning. N Engl J Med 2004;350:7–8.

[43] Greco PJ, Schulman KA, Lavizzo-Mourey R, et al. The Patient Self-Determination Act and the future of advance directives. Ann Intern Med 1991;115:639–43.

[44] Goldstein NE, Lampert R, Bradley E, et al. Management of implantable cardioverter defibrillators in end-of-life care. Ann Intern Med 2004;141:835–8.

[45] Berger JT. The ethics of deactivating implanted cardioverter defibrillators. Ann Intern Med 2005;142:631–4.

[46] Braun TC, Hagen NA, Hatfield RE, et al. Cardiac pacemakers and implantable defibrillators in terminal care. J Pain Symptom Manage 1999;18:126–31.

[47] Cleland J, Daubert JC, Erdmann E, et al. The effect of cardiac resynchronization on morbidity and mortality in heart failure. N Engl J Med 2005;352:1539–49.

[48] Carson P, Anand I, O'Connor C, et al. Mode of death in advanced heart failure: the comparison of medical, pacing, and defibrillation therapies in heart failure (COMPANION) trial. J Am Coll Cardiol 2005;46:2329–34.

[49] Bax JJ, Abraham T, Barold S, et al. Cardiac resynchronization therapy: Part 2—Issues during and after device implantation and unresolved questions. J Am Coll Cardiol 2005;46: 2168–82.

[50] Mueller PS, Hook CC, Hayes DL. Ethical analysis of withdrawal of pacemaker or implantable cardioverter-defibrillator support at the end of life. Mayo Clin Proc 2003;78:959–63.

[51] Stevenson LW. Rites and responsibility for resuscitation in heart failure: Tread gently on the thin places. Circulation 1998;98:619–22.

[52] Krumholz HM, Phillips RS, Hamel MB, et al. Resuscitation preferences among patients with severe congestive heart failure: results from the SUPPORT project. Circulation 1998; 98:648–55.

[53] Tsai E. Should family members be present during cardiopulmonary resuscitation? N Engl J Med 2002;346:1019–21.

[54] 2005 American Heart Association guidelines for cardiopulmonary resuscitation and emergency cardiovascular care—Part 2: Ethical issues. Circulation 2005;112(Suppl IV):IV6–11.

[55] Casarett D, Inouye S. Diagnosis and management of delirium near the end of life. Ann Intern Med 2001;135:32–40.

[56] Lo B, Rubenfeld G. Palliative sedation in dying patients: "We turn to it when everything else hasn't worked." JAMA 2005;294:1810–6.

[57] Quill TE, Dresser R, Brock DW. The rule of double effect – a critique of its role in end-of-life decision making. N Engl J Med 1997;337:1768–71.

[58] Wilson WC, Smedira NG, Fink C, et al. Ordering and administration of sedatives and analgesics during the withholding and withdrawal of life support from critically ill patients. JAMA 1992;267:949–53.

[59] Sulmasy DP, Pellegrino ED. The rule of double effect: clearing up the double talk. Arch Intern Med 1999;159:545–50.

[60] Sulmasy DP. Double effect: Intention is the solution, not the problem. J Law Med Ethics 2000;28(1):26–9.

[61] Brody H. Causing, intending, and assisting death. J Clin Ethics 1993;4:112–8.

[62] Jansen LA, Sulmasy DP. Sedation, alimentation, hydration, and equivocation: Careful conversation about care at the end of life. Ann Intern Med 2002;136:845–9.

[63] Barnard D. The skull at the banquet. In: Jansen L, editor. Death in the clinic. Lanham, MD: Rowman & Littlefield; 2006. p. 66–80.

[64] Kearney M. Mortally wounded: stories of soul pain, death, and healing. New York: Scribner; 1996. 131.

[65] Steinhauser KE, Clipp EC, McNeilly M, et al. In search of a good death: observations of patients, families, and providers. Ann Intern Med 2000;132:825–32.

[66] McCue JD. The naturalness of dying. JAMA 1995;273:1039–42.

[67] Goodlin SJ, Hauptman PJ, Arnold R, et al. Consensus statement: Palliative and supportive care in advanced heart failure. J Card Fail 2004;10:200–9.

**ELSEVIER
SAUNDERS**

Clin Geriatr Med 23 (2007) 249–253

**CLINICS IN
GERIATRIC
MEDICINE**

Index

Note: Page numbers of article titles are in **boldface** type.

0749-0690/07/$ - see front matter © 2006 Elsevier Inc. All rights reserved.
doi:10.1016/S0749-0690(06)00096-6   *geriatric.theclinics.com*